Gastrointestinal Diseases & Disorders
Sourcebook
Genetic Disorders Sourcebook,
1st Edition
Genetic Disorders Sourcebook,
2nd Edition
Head Trauma Sourcebook
Headache Sourcebook
Health Insurance Sourcebook
Health Reference Series Cumulative
Index 1999
Healthy Aging Sourcebook
Healthy Children Sourcebook
Healthy Heart Sourcebook for Women
Heart Diseases & Disorders
Sourcebook, 2nd Edition
Household Safety Sourcebook
Immune System Disorders Sourcebook
Infant & Toddler Health Sourcebook
Injury & Trauma Sourcebook
Kidney & Urinary Tract Diseases &
Disorders Sourcebook
Learning Disabilities Sourcebook,
1st Edition
Learning Disabilities Sourcebook,
2nd Edition
Liver Disorders Sourcebook
Lung Disorders Sourcebook
Medical Tests Sourcebook
Men's Health Concerns Sourcebook
Mental Health Disorders Sourcebook,
1st Edition
Mental Health Disorders Sourcebook,
2nd Edition
Mental Retardation Sourcebook
Movement Disorders Sourcebook
Obesity Sourcebook
Ophthalmic Disorders Sourcebook,
1st Edition
Oral Health Sourcebook
Osteoporosis Sourcebook
Pain Sourcebook, 1st Edition
Pain Sourcebook, 2nd Edition

Pediatric Cancer Sourcebook
Physical & Mental Issues in Aging
Sourcebook
Podiatry Sourcebook
Pregnancy & Birth Sourcebook
Prostate Cancer
Public Health Sourcebook
Reconstructive & Cosmetic Surgery
Sourcebook
Rehabilitation Sourcebook
Respiratory Diseases & Disorders
Sourcebook
Sexually Transmitted Diseases
Sourcebook, 1st Edition
Sexually Transmitted Diseases
Sourcebook, 2nd Edition
Skin Disorders Sourcebook
Sleep Disorders Sourcebook
Sports Injuries Sourcebook, 1st Edition
Sports Injuries Sourcebook, 2nd Edition
Stress-Related Disorders Sourcebook
Substance Abuse Sourcebook
Surgery Sourcebook
Transplantation Sourcebook
Traveler's Health Sourcebook
Vegetarian Sourcebook
Women's Health Concerns Sourcebook
Workplace Health & Safety Sourcebook
Worldwide Health Sourcebook

Teen Health Series

Diet Information for Teens
Drug Information for Teens
Mental Health Information
for Teens
Sexual Health Information
for Teens

Movement Disorders
SOURCEBOOK

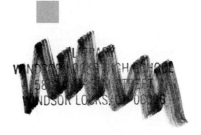

Health Reference Series

First Edition

Movement Disorders SOURCEBOOK

Basic Consumer Health Information about Neurological Movement Disorders, Including Essential Tremor, Parkinson's Disease, Dystonia, Cerebral Palsy, Huntington's Disease, Myasthenia Gravis, Multiple Sclerosis, and Other Early-Onset and Adult-Onset Movement Disorders, Their Symptoms and Causes, Diagnostic Tests, and Treatments

Along with Mobility and Assistive Technology Information, a Glossary, and a Directory of Additional Resources

Edited by
Joyce Brennfleck Shannon

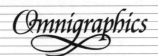

Omnigraphics

615 Griswold Street • Detroit, MI 48226

Bibliographic Note

Because this page cannot legibly accommodate all the copyright notices, the Bibliographic Note portion of the Preface constitutes an extension of the copyright notice.

Edited by Joyce Brennfleck Shannon

Health Reference Series

Karen Bellenir, *Managing Editor*
David A. Cooke, MD, *Medical Consultant*
Elizabeth Barbour, *Permissions Associate*
Dawn Matthews, *Verification Assistant*
Laura Pleva Nielsen, *Index Editor*
EdIndex, Services for Publishers, *Indexers*

* * *

Omnigraphics, Inc.

Matthew P. Barbour, *Senior Vice President*
Kay Gill, *Vice President—Directories*
Kevin Hayes, *Operations Manager*
Leif Gruenberg, *Development Manager*
David P. Bianco, *Marketing Consultant*

* * *

Peter E. Ruffner, *Publisher*

Frederick G. Ruffner, Jr., *Chairman*

Copyright © 2003 Omnigraphics, Inc.

ISBN 0-7808-628-X

Library of Congress Cataloging-in-Publication Data

Movement disorders sourcebook : basic consumer health information about neurological movement disorders, including essential tremor, Parkinson's disease, dystonia, cerebral palsy, Huntington's disease, myasthenia gravis, multiple sclerosis, and other early-onset and adult-onset movement disorders, their symptoms and causes, diagnostic tests, and treatments; along with mobility and assistive technology information, a glossary, and a directory of additional resources / edited by Joyce Brennfleck Shannon. -- 1st ed.
    p. cm. -- (Health reference series)
  Includes bibliographical references and index.
  ISBN 0-7808-0628-X
    1. Movement disorders--Popular works. I. Shannon, Joyce Brennfleck. II. Health reference series (Unnumbered)

RC376.5 .M693 2003
616.8'3--dc21

2002192486

Table of Contents

Part II: Diagnostic Tests

Part III: The Three Most Common Movement Disorders in the U.S.

Part IV: Early-Onset Neurological-Based Movement Disorders

Part V: Adult-Onset Neurological-Based Movement Disorders

Part VI: Treatments for Movement Disorders

Part VII: Quality of Life Assistance

Part VIII: Additional Help and Information

Preface

About This Book

Movement is an essential part of life. Our bodies must move to breathe, circulate blood, and digest food. Beyond these basics, movement is also an integral part of family life, work, and play. Many Americans, however, find that their ability to function is impaired by neurological movement disorders. Although cures remain elusive, treatments and mobility aids can improve quality of life, relieve pain, and allow maximum independence for affected individuals.

This *Sourcebook* provides health information about early-onset and adult-onset neurological movement disorders, including essential tremor, Parkinson's disease, dystonia, cerebral palsy, Huntington's disease, myasthenia gravis, and multiple sclerosis. Readers will learn about symptoms, causes, diagnostic tests, and treatments. Information about mobility aids and assistive technology is included, along with a glossary and directories of additional resources.

How to Use This Book

This book is divided into parts and chapters. Parts focus on broad areas of interest. Chapters are devoted to single topics within a part.

Part I: Movement Disorders Overview describes causes and symptoms of neurological movement disorders. It also identifies the health care team involved in the diagnosis and treatment of movement disorders. Muscular dystrophy—a degenerative muscular disorder—is briefly described. Readers seeking further information about muscular dystrophy may wish to consult *Muscular Dystrophy Sourcebook*, a forthcoming volume in the *Health Reference Series*.

Part II: Diagnostic Tests explains medical tests that are used in the diagnosis of movement disorders, including neurological tests, electromyography, electroencephalogram (EEG), muscle biopsy, creatine kinase test, spinal tap, and gene testing. A chapter about preparing children for test procedures is also included.

Part III: The Three Most Common Movement Disorders in the U.S. provides facts about essential tremor, Parkinson's disease, and dystonia. Information specific to the diagnosis and treatment of each disorder is presented.

Part IV: Early-Onset Neurological-Based Movement Disorders reviews the causes, diagnosis, treatment, and prognosis of movement disorders that begin in childhood, including Angelman syndrome, Louis-Bar syndrome, cerebral palsy, Rett syndrome, spina bifida, spinal muscular atrophy, and Tourette Syndrome.

Part V: Adult-Onset Neurological-Based Movement Disorders offers information about movement disorders that develop after childhood, including their causes, diagnosis, treatments, and prognosis. These include Lou Gehrig's disease, Charcot-Marie-Tooth disease, Friedreich's ataxia, Huntington's disease, Machado-Joseph disease, multiple sclerosis, Shy Drager syndrome, myasthenia gravis, post-polio syndrome, restless legs syndrome, stiff-person syndrome, Wilson's disease, and spinal cord injury.

Part VI: Treatments for Movement Disorders describes tremor control therapy, spasticity management, surgical procedures, plasmapheresis, therapeutic horseback riding, and specific treatments for dystonia and cerebral palsy.

Part VII: Quality of Life Assistance gives practical advice for living with a movement disorder, including facts about home modifications, mobility aids, service animals, and assistive technology.

Part VIII: Additional Help and Information includes a glossary of important terms and directories of on-line resources and organizations able to provide additional information.

Bibliographic Note

This volume contains documents and excerpts from publications issued by the following U.S. government agencies: Human Genome Program; National Center for Health Statistics (NCHS); National Information Center for Children and Youth with Disabilities (NICHCY); National Institute of Neurological Disorders and Stroke (NINDS); National Institutes of Health (NIH); and Warren Grant Magnuson Center.

In addition, this volume contains copyrighted documents from the following organizations and individuals: A.D.A.M., Inc.; American Association of Neurological Surgeons/Congress of Neurological Surgeons; American Hippotherapy Association; American Parkinson Disease Association, Inc.; Angelman Syndrome Foundation, Inc.; Children's Neurological Solutions; the Dystonia Medical Research Foundation; Families of Spinal Muscular Atrophy; Gale Group; Timothy C. Hain, MD; Hallervorden-Spatz Syndrome Association; Illinois Assistive Technology Project; Infinitec, Inc./United Cerebral Palsy Associations, Inc.; International Essential Tremor Foundation; International Radiosurgery Support Association; International Rett Syndrome Association; Miller-Dwan Medical Center; Moving Forward UK; Muscular Dystrophy Association; National Parkinson Foundation; National Spinal Cord Injury Association; New York University School of Medicine Department of Neurosurgery; Restless Legs Syndrome Foundation; Society for Progressive Supranuclear Palsy; Spastic Paraplegia Foundation, Inc.; Spina Bifida Association of America; Tourette Syndrome Association, Inc.; University of Alabama at Birmingham; University of California, San Francisco; University of Pittsburgh Department of Neurosurgery; Bob Vogel and *New Mobility Magazine*; Washington Assistive Technology Alliance/University of Washington Center for Technology and Disability Studies; and Wilson's Disease Association International.

Full citation information is provided on the first page of each chapter. Every effort has been made to secure all necessary rights to reprint the copyrighted material. If any omissions have been made, please contact Omnigraphics to make corrections for future editions.

Acknowledgements

Special thanks go to the many organizations, agencies, and individuals who have contributed materials for this *Sourcebook* and to the managing editor Karen Bellenir, medical consultant Dr. David

Cooke, permissions specialist Liz Barbour, verification assistant Dawn Matthews, indexer Edward J. Prucha, and document engineer Bruce Bellenir.

Note from the Editor

This book is part of Omnigraphics' *Health Reference Series*. The *Series* provides basic information about a broad range of medical concerns. It is not intended to serve as a tool for diagnosing illness, in prescribing treatments, or as a substitute for the physician/patient relationship. All persons concerned about medical symptoms or the possibility of disease are encouraged to seek professional care from an appropriate health care provider.

Our Advisory Board

The *Health Reference Series* is reviewed by an Advisory Board comprised of librarians from public, academic, and medical libraries. We would like to thank the following board members for providing guidance to the development of this series:

Dr. Lynda Baker,
Associate Professor of Library and Information Science,
Wayne State University, Detroit, MI

Nancy Bulgarelli,
William Beaumont Hospital Library, Royal Oak, MI

Karen Imarisio,
Bloomfield Township Public Library, Bloomfield Township, MI

Karen Morgan,
Mardigian Library, University of Michigan-Dearborn,
Dearborn, MI

Rosemary Orlando,
St. Clair Shores Public Library, St. Clair Shores, MI

Medical Consultant

Medical consultation services are provided to the *Health Reference Series* editors by David A. Cooke, MD. Dr. Cooke is a graduate of Brandeis University, and he received his M.D. degree from the University of Michigan. He completed residency training at the University of Wisconsin Hospital and Clinics. He is board-certified in Internal

Medicine. Dr. Cooke currently works as part of the University of Michigan Health System and practices in Brighton, MI. In his free time, he enjoys writing, science fiction, and spending time with his family.

Health Reference Series *Update Policy*

The inaugural book in the *Health Reference Series* was the first edition of *Cancer Sourcebook* published in 1989. Since then, the *Series* has been enthusiastically received by librarians and in the medical community. In order to maintain the standard of providing high-quality health information for the layperson the editorial staff at Omnigraphics felt it was necessary to implement a policy of updating volumes when warranted.

Medical researchers have been making tremendous strides, and it is the purpose of the *Health Reference Series* to stay current with the most recent advances. Each decision to update a volume will be made on an individual basis. Some of the considerations will include how much new information is available and the feedback we receive from people who use the books. If there is a topic you would like to see added to the update list, or an area of medical concern you feel has not been adequately addressed, please write to:

Editor
Health Reference Series
Omnigraphics, Inc.
615 Griswold Street
Detroit, MI 48226
E-mail: editorial@omnigraphics.com

Part One

Movement Disorders Overview

Chapter 1

Movement Disorders

Chapter Contents

Section 1.1

Definition and Description

"Movement Disorders," from *Gale Encyclopedia of Medicine,* by Richard Robinson, Gale Group. Reprinted by permission of The Gale Group. © 1999.

Definition

Movement disorders are a group of diseases and syndromes affecting the ability to produce and control movement.

Description

Though it seems simple and effortless, normal movement in fact requires an astonishingly complex system of control. Disruption of any portion of this system can cause a person to produce movements that are too weak, too forceful, too uncoordinated, or too poorly controlled for the task at hand. Unwanted movements may occur at rest. Intentional movement may become impossible. Such conditions are called movement disorders.

Abnormal movements themselves are symptoms of underlying disorders. In some cases, the abnormal movements are the only symptoms. Disorders causing abnormal movements include:

- Parkinson's disease
- Parkinsonism caused by drugs or poisons
- Parkinson-plus syndromes (progressive supranuclear palsy, multiple system atrophy, and cortical-basal ganglionic degeneration)
- Huntington's disease
- Wilson's disease
- Inherited ataxias (Friedreich's ataxia, Machado-Joseph disease, and spinocerebellar ataxias)
- Tourette syndrome and other tic disorders
- Essential tremor

4

- Restless leg syndrome
- Dystonia
- Stroke
- Cerebral palsy
- Encephalopathies
- Intoxication
- Poisoning by carbon monoxide, cyanide, methanol, or manganese.

Causes and Symptoms

Causes

Movement is produced and coordinated by several interacting brain centers, including the motor cortex, the cerebellum, and a group of structures in the inner portions of the brain called the basal ganglia. Sensory information provides critical input on the current position and velocity of body parts, and spinal nerve cells (neurons) help prevent opposing muscle groups from contracting at the same time.

To understand how movement disorders occur, it is helpful to consider a normal voluntary movement, such as reaching to touch a nearby object with the right index finger. To accomplish the desired movement, the arm must be lifted and extended. The hand must be held out to align with the forearm, and the forefinger must be extended while the other fingers remain flexed.

The Motor Cortex

Voluntary motor commands begin in the motor cortex located on the outer, wrinkled surface of the brain. Movement of the right arm is begun by the left motor cortex, which generates a large volley of signals to the involved muscles. These electrical signals pass along upper motor neurons through the midbrain to the spinal cord. Within the spinal cord, they connect to lower motor neurons, which convey the signals out of the spinal cord to the surface of the muscles involved. Electrical stimulation of the muscles causes contraction, and the force of contraction pulling on the skeleton causes movement of the arm, hand, and fingers.

Damage to or death of any of the neurons along this path causes weakness or paralysis of the affected muscles.

Antagonistic Muscle Pairs

This picture of movement is too simple; however, one important refinement to it comes from considering the role of opposing, or antagonistic, muscle pairs. Contraction of the biceps muscle, located on the top of the upper arm, pulls on the forearm to flex the elbow and bend the arm. Contraction of the triceps, located on the opposite side, extends the elbow and straightens the arm. Within the spine, these muscles are normally wired so that willed (voluntary) contraction of one is automatically accompanied by blocking of the other. In other words, the command to contract the biceps provokes another command within the spine to prevent contraction of the triceps. In this way, these antagonist muscles are kept from resisting one another. Spinal cord or brain injury can damage this control system and cause involuntary simultaneous contraction and spasticity, an increase in resistance to movement during motion.

The Cerebellum

Once the movement of the arm is initiated, sensory information is needed to guide the finger to its precise destination. In addition to sight, the most important source of information comes from the *position sense* provided by the many sensory neurons located within the limbs (proprioception). Proprioception is what allows you to touch your nose with your finger even with your eyes closed. The balance organs in the ears provide important information about posture. Both postural and proprioceptive information are processed by a structure at the rear of the brain called the cerebellum. The cerebellum sends out electrical signals to modify movements as they progress, sculpting the barrage of voluntary commands into a tightly controlled, constantly evolving pattern. Cerebellar disorders cause inability to control the force, fine positioning, and speed of movements (ataxia). Disorders of the cerebellum may also impair the ability to judge distance so that a person under- or over-reaches the target (dysmetria). Tremor during voluntary movements can also result from cerebellar damage.

The Basal Ganglia

Both the cerebellum and the motor cortex send information to a set of structures deep within the brain that help control involuntary components of movement (basal ganglia). The basal ganglia send output messages to the motor cortex, helping to initiate movements, regulate repetitive or patterned movements, and control muscle tone.

6

Circuits within the basal ganglia are complex. Within this structure, some groups of cells begin the action of other basal ganglia components and some groups of cells block the action. These complicated feedback circuits are not entirely understood. Disruptions of these circuits are known to cause several distinct movement disorders. A portion of the basal ganglia called the substantia nigra sends electrical signals that block output from another structure called the subthalamic nucleus. The subthalamic nucleus sends signals to the globus pallidus, which in turn blocks the thalamic nuclei. Finally, the thalamic nuclei send signals to the motor cortex. The substantia nigra, then, begins movement and the globus pallidus blocks it.

This complicated circuit can be disrupted at several points. For instance, loss of substantia nigra cells, as in Parkinson's disease, increases blocking of the thalamic nuclei, preventing them from sending signals to the motor cortex. The result is a loss of movement (motor activity), a characteristic of Parkinson's.

In contrast, cell loss in early Huntington's disease decreases blocking of signals from the thalamic nuclei, causing more cortex stimulation and stronger but uncontrolled movements.

Disruptions in other portions of the basal ganglia are thought to cause tics, tremors, dystonia, and a variety of other movement disorders, although the exact mechanisms are not well understood.

Some movement disorders, including Huntington's disease and inherited ataxias, are caused by inherited genetic defects. Some diseases that cause sustained muscle contraction limited to a particular muscle group (focal dystonia) are inherited, but others are caused by trauma. The cause of most cases of Parkinson's disease is unknown, although genes have been found for some familial forms.

Symptoms

Abnormal movements are broadly classified as either hyperkinetic—too much movement—and hypokinetic—too little movement. Hyperkinetic movements include:

- **Dystonia.** Sustained muscle contractions, often causing twisting or repetitive movements and abnormal postures. Dystonia may be limited to one area (focal) or may affect the whole body (general). Focal dystonias may affect the neck (cervical dystonia or torticollis), the face (one-sided or hemifacial spasm, contraction of the eyelid or blepharospasm, contraction of the mouth and jaw or oromandibular dystonia, simultaneous spasm of the

7

chin and eyelid or Meige syndrome), the vocal cords (laryngeal dystonia), or the arms and legs (writer's cramp, occupational cramps). Dystonia may be painful as well as incapacitating.

- **Tremor.** Uncontrollable (involuntary) shaking of a body part. Tremor may occur only when muscles are relaxed or it may occur only during an action or holding an active posture.
- **Tics.** Involuntary, rapid, nonrhythmic movement or sound. Tics can be controlled briefly.
- **Myoclonus.** A sudden, shock-like muscle contraction. Myoclonic jerks may occur singly or repetitively. Unlike tics, myoclonus cannot be controlled even briefly.
- **Chorea.** Rapid, nonrhythmic, usually jerky movements, most often in the arms and legs.
- **Ballism.** Like chorea, but the movements are much larger, more explosive, and involve more of the arm or leg. This condition, also called ballismus, can occur on both sides of the body or on one side only (hemiballismus).
- **Akathisia.** Restlessness and a desire to move to relieve uncomfortable sensations. Sensations may include a feeling of crawling, itching, stretching, or creeping, usually in the legs.
- **Athetosis.** Slow, writhing, continuous, uncontrollable movement of the arms and legs.

Hypokinetic movements include:

- **Bradykinesia.** Slowness of movement.
- **Freezing.** Inability to begin a movement or involuntary stopping of a movement before it is completed.
- **Rigidity.** An increase in muscle tension when an arm or leg is moved by an outside force.
- **Postural instability.** Loss of ability to maintain upright posture caused by slow or absent righting reflexes.

Diagnosis

Diagnosis of movement disorders requires a careful medical history and a thorough physical and neurological examination. Brain imaging studies are usually performed. Imaging techniques include computed tomography scan (CT scan), positron emission tomography (PET), or magnetic resonance imaging (MRI) scans. Routine blood and urine analyses are performed. A lumbar puncture (spinal tap) may be necessary. Video recording of the abnormal movement is often used to analyze movement patterns and to track progress of the disorder and its treatment. Genetic testing is available for some forms of movement disorders.

Treatment

Treatment of a movement disorder begins with determining its cause. Physical and occupational therapy may help make up for lost control and strength. Drug therapy can help compensate for some imbalances of the basal ganglionic circuit. For instance, levodopa (L-dopa) or related compounds can substitute for lost dopamine-producing cells in Parkinson's disease. Conversely, blocking normal dopamine action is a possible treatment in some hyperkinetic disorders, including tics. Oral medications can also help reduce overall muscle tone. Local injections of botulinum toxin can selectively weaken overactive muscles in dystonia and spasticity. Destruction of peripheral nerves through injection of phenol can reduce spasticity. All of these treatments may have some side effects.

Surgical destruction or inactivation of basal ganglionic circuits has proven effective for Parkinson's disease and is being tested for other movement disorders. Transplantation of fetal cells into the basal ganglia has produced mixed results in Parkinson's disease.

Alternative Treatment

There are several alternative therapies that can be useful when treating movement disorders. The progress made will depend on the individual and his/her condition. Among the therapies that may be helpful are acupuncture, homeopathy, touch therapies, postural alignment therapies, and biofeedback.

Prognosis

The prognosis for a patient with a movement disorder depends on the specific disorder.

Prevention

Prevention depends on the specific disorder.

Key Terms

Botulinum toxin. Any of a group of potent bacterial toxins or poisons produced by different strains of the bacterium. The toxins cause muscle paralysis, and thus force the relaxation of a muscle in spasm.

Cerebral palsy. A movement disorder caused by a permanent brain defect or injury present at birth or shortly after. It is frequently associated with premature birth. Cerebral palsy is not progressive.

Computed tomography (CT). An imaging technique in which cross-sectional x-rays of the body are compiled to create a three-dimensional image of the body's internal structures.

Encephalopathy. An abnormality in the structure or function of tissues of the brain.

Essential tremor. An uncontrollable (involuntary) shaking of the hands, head, and face. Also called familial tremor because it is sometimes inherited, it can begin in the teens or in middle age. The exact cause is not known.

Fetal tissue transplantation. A method of treating Parkinson's and other neurological diseases by grafting brain cells from human fetuses onto the basal ganglia. Human adults cannot grow new brain cells but developing fetuses can. Grafting fetal tissue stimulates the growth of new brain cells in affected adult brains.

Hereditary ataxia. One of a group of hereditary degenerative diseases of the spinal cord or cerebellum. These diseases cause tremor, spasm, and wasting of muscle.

Huntington's disease. A rare hereditary condition that causes progressive chorea (jerky muscle movements) and mental deterioration that ends in dementia. Huntington's symptoms usually appear in patients in their 40s. There is no effective treatment.

Levodopa (L-dopa). A substance used in the treatment of Parkinson's disease. Levodopa can cross the blood-brain barrier that protects the brain. Once in the brain, it is converted to dopamine and thus can replace the dopamine lost in Parkinson's disease.

Magnetic resonance imaging (MRI). An imaging technique that uses a large circular magnet and radio waves to generate signals from atoms in the body. These signals are used to construct images of internal structures.

Parkinson's disease. A slowly progressive disease that destroys nerve cells in the basal ganglia and thus causes loss of dopamine, a chemical that aids in transmission of nerve signals (neurotransmitter). Parkinson's is characterized by shaking in resting muscles, a stooping posture, slurred speech, muscular stiffness, and weakness.

Positron emission tomography (PET). A diagnostic technique in which computer-assisted x-rays are used to track a radioactive substance inside a patient's body. PET can be used to study the biochemical activity of the brain.

Progressive supranuclear palsy. A rare disease that gradually destroys nerve cells in the parts of the brain that control eye movements, breathing, and muscle coordination. The loss of nerve cells causes palsy, or paralysis, that slowly gets worse as the disease progresses. The palsy affects ability to move the eyes, relax the muscles, and control balance.

Restless legs syndrome. A condition that causes an annoying feeling of tiredness, uneasiness, and itching deep within the muscle of the leg. It is accompanied by twitching and sometimes pain. The only relief is in walking or moving the legs.

Tourette syndrome. An abnormal condition that causes uncontrollable facial grimaces and tics, and arm and shoulder movements. Tourette syndrome is perhaps best known for uncontrollable vocal tics that include grunts, shouts, and use of obscene language (coprolalia).

Wilson's disease. An inborn defect of copper metabolism in which free copper may be deposited in a variety of areas of the body. Deposits in the brain can cause tremor and other symptoms of Parkinson's disease.

Further Reading

Books

Martini, Frederic. *Fundamentals of Anatomy and Physiology.* Englewood Cliffs, NJ: Prentice Hall, 1989.

Watts, Ray L. and William C. Koller, eds. *Movement Disorders: Neurologic Principles and Practice*. New York: McGraw-Hill, 1997.

Periodicals

Movement Disorders. Lippincott-Raven Publishers, 12107 Insurance Way, Hagerstown, MD 21740.

Organizations

WE MOVE
204 West 84th Street
New York, NY 10024
Toll-Free: 800-437-MOV2
Fax: 212-875-8389
Website: www.wemove.org
E-mail: wemove@wemove.org

Section 1.2

A Note about Muscular Dystrophy

"NINDS Muscular Dystrophy (MD) Information Page," National Institute
of Neurological Disorders and Stroke (NINDS), reviewed 7/1/01.

What Is Muscular Dystrophy (MD)?

Muscular dystrophy (MD) refers to a group of genetic diseases characterized by progressive weakness and degeneration of the skeletal or voluntary muscles which control movement. The muscles of the heart and some other involuntary muscles are also affected in some forms of MD, and a few forms involve other organs as well. The major forms of MD include myotonic, Duchenne, Becker, limb-girdle, facioscapulohumeral, congenital, oculopharyngeal, distal, and Emery-Dreifuss. Duchenne is the most common form of MD affecting children, and myotonic MD is the most common form affecting adults. MD can affect people of all ages. Although some forms first become apparent in infancy or childhood, others may not appear until middle age or later.

Is There Any Treatment?

There is no specific treatment for any of the forms of MD. Physical therapy to prevent contractures (a condition in which shortened muscles around joints cause abnormal and sometimes painful positioning of the joints), orthoses (orthopedic appliances used for support), and corrective orthopedic surgery may be needed to improve the quality of life in some cases. The cardiac problems that occur with Emery-Dreifuss MD and myotonic MD may require a pacemaker. The myotonia (delayed relaxation of a muscle after a strong contraction) occurring in myotonic MD may be treated with medications such as phenytoin or quinine.

What Is the Prognosis?

The prognosis of MD varies according to the type of MD and the progression of the disorder. Some cases may be mild and very slowly progressive, with normal lifespan, while other cases may have more marked progression of muscle weakness, functional disability, and loss of ambulation. Life expectancy may depend on the degree of progression and late respiratory deficit. In Duchenne MD, death usually occurs in the late teens to early 20s.

What Research Is Being Done?

The NINDS supports a broad program of research on MD. The goals of these studies are to increase understanding of MD and its cause(s), develop better therapies, and, ultimately, find ways to prevent and cure the disorder.

Selected References

Dubowitz V. What's in a name? Muscular dystrophy revisited. *European Journal of Paediatric Neurology*. 1998; 2(6):279-84

Laing NG, Mastaglia FL. Inherited skeletal muscle disorders. *Annals of Human Biology*. 1999 Nov-Dec; 26(6):507-25

Moore DP, Kowalske KJ. Neuromuscular rehabilitation and electrodiagnosis 5. Myopathy. *Archives of Physical Medicine and Rehabilitation*. 2000 Mar; 81(3 Suppl 1):S32-5; quiz S36-44

Tsao CY, Mendell JR. The childhood muscular dystrophies: making order out of chaos *Seminars in Neurology*. 1999; 19(1):9-23

Urtizberea JA. Therapies in muscular dystrophy: current concepts and future prospects *European Neurology*. 2000; 43(3):127-32

Additional Information

Readers seeking further information about muscular dystrophy may wish to consult *Muscular Dystrophy Sourcebook*, a forthcoming volume in the *Health Reference Series*.

Facioscapulohumeral Dystrophy (FSHD) Society
3 Westwood Road
Lexington, MA 02420
Tel: 781-860-0501
Fax: 781-860-0599
Website: www.fshsociety.org
E-mail: info@fshsociety.org

Muscular Dystrophy Association
3300 East Sunrise Drive
Tucson, AZ 85718-3208
Toll-Free: 800-572-1717
Tel: 520-529-2000
Fax: 520-529-5300
Website: www.mdausa.org
E-mail: mda@mdausa.org

Muscular Dystrophy Family Foundation
2330 North Meridian Street
Indianapolis, IN 46208-5730
Toll-Free: 800-544-1213
Tel: 317-923-6333
Fax: 317-923-6334
Website: www.mdff.org
E-mail: mdff@mdff.org

Parent Project for Muscular Dystrophy Research
1012 North University Blvd.
Middletown, OH 45042
Toll-Free: 800-714-KIDS (5437)
Tel: 413-424-0696
Fax: 513-425-9907
Website: www.parentprojectmd.org
E-mail: ParentProject@aol.com

Chapter 2

Symptoms of Movement Disorders

Chapter Contents

Section 2.1

Stiffness, Cramps, and Twitching

"Simply Stated—Stiffness, Cramps, and Twitching," *Quest*, Volume 7, Number 3, June 2000, © Muscular Dystrophy Association. Reprinted with permission of the Muscular Dystrophy Association.

Neuromuscular diseases can cause a variety of symptoms other than muscle weakness. Some people may feel their muscles are stiff or don't respond quickly; others might complain of cramps or twitches; while still others get tired quickly during exercise.

Not all of these symptoms are painful, but some can be inconvenient or annoying. Learning the medical names and natures of these symptoms can lead to better discourse between you and your doctor, and sometimes better management of symptoms.

Cramps

A true cramp is a specific condition in which muscles undergo painful involuntary contractions (muscle shortening). The classic muscle cramp is neural in origin, meaning the contractions are caused by abnormal nerve activity rather than abnormal muscle activity. This type of contraction problem usually has a sudden onset and may be ended by stretching the muscle passively.

True cramps can occur in anyone, particularly after exercise or at night. Neuromuscular diseases in which classic cramps are common are amyotrophic lateral sclerosis (ALS) and spinal muscular atrophy (SMA).

A second kind of cramp, which doesn't involve abnormal nerve activity, occurs when a muscle is temporarily locked in a contracted state. This is technically called a contracture, but isn't to be confused with the more common use of *contracture* to indicate fixed joints. This sensation can be painful and is often described as a cramp. People with paramyotonia congenita, some forms of myotonia, rippling muscle syndrome, or metabolic myopathies due to glycolytic defects (McArdle's disease, Cori's or Forbes' disease, Tarui's disease, phosphoglycerate kinase deficiency, and lactate dehydrogenase deficiency) may experience muscle pain during exercise due to non-neural muscle cramps.

Fasciculation

Fasciculation is basically a fancy term for a twitch. Like classic cramps, fasciculations are caused by abnormal nerve activity, but they tend to involve only a small portion of the affected muscle and aren't generally painful.

While one is occurring, you may observe a small muscle "jump" under the skin. Fasciculations are common in ALS, spinal bulbar muscular atrophy, X-linked SMA, and SMA type 1 (in the tongue and mouth).

Neurologist Valerie Cwik of the University of Arizona Health Sciences Center in Tucson says that everyone gets fasciculations now and then, particularly around the eye, in the small muscle of the back of the hand between the thumb and index finger, and in the feet.

Fasciculations are made worse by stress, lack of sleep, and caffeine. They may also be seen in people with overactive thyroids, and there's a syndrome of benign (harmless) cramps and fasciculations. While some people with cramps and fasciculations develop ALS, in others the problem remains restricted to these symptoms.

Myotonia

Myotonia occurs when contracted muscles relax too slowly due to electrical problems in the muscle or nerve cells. A person with myotonia may have difficulty releasing his grip after holding an object—the sensation is sometimes described as stiffness. Myotonia can be sensitive to exercise, temperature, or diet, and occurs in paramyotonia congenita, myotonia congenita, hyperkalemic periodic paralysis, and myotonic dystrophy.

Myalgia

Myalgia, or muscle pain, can be caused by mechanical stress without muscle injury (as in classic or non-neural muscle cramps), or by injury. Muscle injury can occur in anyone who overdoes during exercise, including those with types of muscular dystrophy that render muscle cells more fragile. Muscle injury can also occur in response to problems with the immune system, as in polymyositis and dermatomyositis, or in response to a lack of energy and buildup of toxic metabolites, as in carnitine palmityl transferase deficiency.

Fatigue

Fatigue can mean a subjective feeling of tiredness or an objective measurement of a decline in muscle force with use, but is always distinguished from weakness. Fatigue is associated with myasthenia gravis, ALS, SMA, myotonic disorders, metabolic disorders (McArdle's and Tarui's diseases), and mitochondrial disease. It can be a feature of many of the muscular dystrophies as muscles weaken and greater energy is expended to move them.

Hypotonia

Hypotonia means lack of muscle tone, or absence of the normal degree of tension in the muscle at rest. The condition is seen most often in infants and children with neuromuscular problems, who may appear floppy because of the lack of muscle tone.

Hypotonia can occur in many muscle disorders, including acid maltase deficiency, mitochondrial disorders, congenital myopathies (central core disease, nemaline myopathy, and myotubular myopathy), congenital myotonic dystrophy, congenital muscular dystrophies, neonatal and infantile myasthenia gravis, SMA type 1, and "benign" congenital hypotonia.

These muscle symptoms have many different primary causes. Although not all can be treated, some respond to gentle stretching, heat, or cold, while others may respond to drug treatments. Your doctor will help you identify and possibly treat these symptoms.

Section 2.2

Spasticity: Abnormal Muscle Contraction

The information in this section is reprinted from "What Is Spasticity" with permission from Moving Forward UK, an organization committed to improving the treatment and management of spasticity. © 2002. Contact Moving Forward UK at Third Floor, 94 New Bond Street, London W1S, United Kingdom, via email at info@movingforward.org.uk, or visit their website at www.moving forward.org.uk. Excerpts from "NINDS Spasticity Information Page," National Institute of Neurological Disorders and Stroke (NINDS), reviewed 7/1/01, are also included.

What Is Spasticity?

Spasticity is not a disease in itself but a term used to describe one or more symptoms which can result from malfunctioning of the nervous system, brain, or spinal cord. Spasticity is caused by damage to the portion of the brain that serves the nerve pathways regulating muscles and controlling voluntary movement.

How Normal Movement Occurs

Despite it seeming simple, normal muscle control is actually very complex, involving several regions of the brain and spinal cord. Voluntary movement of a muscle begins when electrical signals are generated in the brain. These electrical signals pass to the spinal cord. The spinal cord then sends signals out to the surface of the muscle involved. To control physical movement we need to be able to tighten and relax the muscles controlling our joints. All joints are controlled by two opposing sets of muscles one that bends (or flexes) the joint, and another which straightens (or extends) it.

Spastic muscles are resistant to the normal stretching that occurs during use, and may remain abnormally contracted for long periods. This contraction causes stiffness or tightness of the muscles and may interfere with walking, movement, and speech.

Even when we are inactive or relaxed the body maintains muscle tone. To see this, lay your hand, palm up, on a table and let it relax. Its natural position is slightly curled up—this is the result of normal

19

muscle tone. Too little tone and limbs become floppy. But with spasticity there is too much tone. The result being fingers may become curled up or tightened. This increased tone occurs in other areas of the body too. When this increased muscle tone is left unchecked it can develop into contractures where the muscles become so tightened they can't be straightened out. This can make normal mobility impossible and can also cause painful muscular spasms.

Contractures

A contracture is an abnormal joint posture due to persistent muscle shortening. Contracture is one of the most noticeable consequences of spasticity. Once this happens it sets off a vicious cycle. When a muscle is not regularly put through its full range of motion, its tendons shorten. This makes stretching the muscle even more difficult, so even more shortening and decreased stretch occur. The muscle may also develop scar tissue, further impeding full range of movement. The outcome of untreated contracture is a fixed, often painful, abnormal posture.

Why Does Spasticity Occur?

Spasticity is a very common complication of a number of neurological conditions including cerebral palsy, brain injuries, spinal cord injuries, multiple sclerosis (MS), and stroke.

Cerebral Palsy

Cerebral Palsy (CP) is a physical impairment that affects movement. It develops as a result of a failure of part of the brain to develop either in the unborn baby or during early childhood. It can take various forms but all are characterized by movement impairment.

Multiple Sclerosis (MS)

Multiple Sclerosis is the most common neurological disorder among young adults. Its causes are unclear, although environmental, genetic, and family connections may play a role. The result is damage to a substance called myelin. Myelin is a protective sheath surrounding all the nerve fibers in the brain and spinal cord and damage to this sets off problems in the central nervous system. About three quarters of those with MS experience some form of spasticity.

Head Injuries

Head injuries occur from a variety of causes often through road traffic or other kinds of accidents. Of people who sustain severe brain damage, 30% are likely to require treatment for the spasticity that occurs.

Stroke

Strokes occur when there is an interruption of blood supply to a localized area of the brain. When the brain is deprived of blood, brain cells die or become damaged. Spasticity affects about 20% of those living with disabilities following a stroke.

What Are the Symptoms of Spasticity?

Where spasticity is present an increase of muscle tone can result in stiff limbs, restricted movement, and difficulty in undertaking normal activities such as walking, eating, and self-care. Spasticity is also often complicated by sudden violent muscle contractions (spasms) which can be very painful.

The symptoms of spasticity can range from slight muscle stiffness to deformity, permanent muscle shortening, and contracture. When spasticity pulls joints into abnormal positions or prevents normal range of movement it can be very painful as well as causing other complications (e.g. pressure sores). While spasticity can affect any muscle group, definite clinical patterns occur, creating well-recognized limb deformities.

People with spasticity usually report a feeling of tightness or stiffness in their legs or arms. Occasionally, the legs will cramp up and go into spasm, which can disrupt sleep. Spasticity often makes walking difficult, patients are often stiff-legged. Walking requires great effort and there is a general loss of grace and agility about their walk.

Symptoms include:

• Stiffness making actions less precise, particularly delicate movements (e.g. of the hands and fingers to perform certain tasks difficult).

• Muscle spasms—uncontrollable muscle contractions causing pain.

• Scissoring (involuntary crossing of the legs).

- Deformities from fixed joints.
- Fatigue caused by trying to force the limbs to do something they want to resist.

Other complications include:

- Urinary tract infections
- Chronic constipation
- Fever or other systemic illnesses
- Pressure sores

What Are the Effects of Spasticity?

Daily Living

The inability to control muscles independently can bring about difficulty in doing all kinds of every day activities from dressing, to writing, eating, and grooming. This often means relying on others to assist with these activities and a loss of independent living.

Hygiene

Stiff limbs and contractured muscles can prevent access to such areas as the palm, armpit, or groin, interfering with cleaning and skin breakdown may occur. Spasticity can also make it difficult to deal with urinary or bowel problems including inserting catheters or giving enemas.

Comfort

Spasticity can cause discomfort in sleeping and sitting. The inability to change positions to ease these activities can result in further pain, stiffness, or pressure sores.

Emotional Distress

Feelings of frustration and helplessness are common as every day tasks become difficult to manage and when there is an increasing need to rely on others for help. Lack of mobility can bring isolation. Also many people feeling conscious of the physical appearance of their spasticity want to avoid unnecessary contact with friends, family, and wider society. There may also be feelings of guilt about disrupting the lives of those closest who have to care for you.

Treatments

Treatment may include medication, injections, stretching exercises, and other physical therapy regimens to help prevent stiffness and joint contractures and reduce the severity of associated symptoms. Surgery for tendon release or for cutting the nerve-muscle pathway may be considered in some cases.

Frequently a combination of anti-spasticity treatments is far more effective than any single one. Treatment is most effective when the physician, other therapists, patient, and carers approach the problem together working towards a common goal.

In some cases, no treatment is necessary or desirable. Evaluation by a medical professional is crucial to determine the best course of treatment. For further information on treatment, please refer to Chapter 43 "Managing Spasticity."

Additional Information

March of Dimes Birth Defects Foundation
1275 Mamaroneck Avenue
White Plains, NY 10605
Toll-Free: 888-MODIMES (663-4637)
Tel: 914-428-7100
Fax: 914-428-8203
Website: www.modimes.org
E-mail: resourcecenter@modimes.org

National Multiple Sclerosis Society
733 Third Avenue, 6th Floor
New York, NY 10017-3288
Toll-Free: 800-344-4867 (FIGHTMS)
Tel: 212-986-3240
Fax: 212-986-7981
Website: www.nationalmssociety.org
E-mail: nat@nmss.org

National Organization for Rare Disorders (NORD)
55 Kenosia Avenue
P.O. Box 1968
Danbury, CT 06813-1968
Tel: 203-744-0100
Voice Mail: 800-999-NORD (6673)
Fax: 203-798-2291

National Organization for Rare Disorders (NORD) (continued)
Website: www.rarediseases.org
E-mail: orphan@rarediseases.org

United Cerebral Palsy Associations
1600 L Street, NW, Suite 700
Washington, DC 20036
Toll-Free: 800-USA-5UCP (872-5827)
Tel: 202-776-0406
Fax: 202-776-0414
Website: www.ucp.org
E-mail: webmaster@ucp.org

Section 2.3

Tremor: Rhythmic, Involuntary Muscle Contraction

"NINDS Tremor Information Page," National Institute of Neurological
Disorders and Stroke (NINDS), reviewed 7/1/01.

What Is Tremor?

Tremor is a rhythmic, involuntary muscular contraction characterized by oscillations (to-and-fro movements) of a part of the body. The most common of all involuntary movements, tremor can affect various body parts such as the hands, head, facial structures, vocal cords, trunk, and legs; most tremors, however, occur in the hands. Tremor often accompanies neurological disorders associated with aging. Although the disorder is not life-threatening, it can be responsible for functional disability and social embarrassment.

Is There Any Treatment?

There are some treatment options available for tremor; the appropriate treatment depends on accurate diagnosis of the cause. Some tremors respond to treatment of the underlying condition, for example in some cases of hysterical tremor treating the patient's underlying mental problem may cause the tremor to disappear. Also, patients with tremor due to Parkinson's disease may be treated with Levodopa drug therapy. Symptomatic drug therapy is available for several other tremors as well. For those cases of tremor in which there is no effective drug treatment, physical measures such as teaching the patient to brace the affected limb during the tremor are sometimes useful. Surgical intervention such as thalamotomy may be useful in certain cases.

What Is the Prognosis?

There are many types of tremor and several ways in which tremor is classified. The most common classification is by behavioral context or position. There are five categories of tremor within this classification: resting, postural, kinetic, task-specific, and hysterical.

Resting or static tremor occurs when the muscle is at rest, for example when the hands are lying on the lap. This type of tremor is often seen in patients with Parkinson's disease.

Postural tremor occurs when a patient attempts to maintain posture, such as holding the hands outstretched. Postural tremors include physiological tremor, essential tremor, tremor with basal ganglia disease (also seen in patients with Parkinson's disease), cerebellar postural tremor, tremor with peripheral neuropathy, post-traumatic tremor, and alcoholic tremor.

Kinetic or intention (action) tremor occurs during purposeful movement, for example during finger-to-nose testing.

Task-specific tremor appears when performing goal-oriented tasks such as handwriting, speaking, or standing. This group consists of primary writing tremor, vocal tremor, and orthostatic tremor.

Hysterical tremor (also called psychogenic tremor) occurs in both older and younger patients. The key feature of this tremor is that it dramatically lessens or disappears when the patient is distracted.

What Research Is Being Done?

NINDS investigators are currently conducting physiological studies of patients with tremors. These studies include classifying the tremor and providing appropriate therapy.

Additional Information

International Tremor Foundation
7046 West 105th Street
Overland Park, KS 66212-1803
Toll-Free: 888-387-3667
Tel: 913-341-3880
Fax: 913-341-1296
Website: www.essentialtremor.org
E-mail: staff@essentialtremor.org

Section 2.4

Myoclonus: Sudden, Involuntary Muscle Jerking

"Myoclonus Fact Sheet," National Institute of Neurological Disorders and Stroke (NINDS), reviewed 7/1/2001, and "NINDS Opsoclonus Myoclonus Information Page," National Institute of Neurological Disorders and Stroke (NINDS), reviewed 11/19/2001.

What Is Myoclonus?

Myoclonus describes a symptom and generally is not a diagnosis of a disease. It refers to sudden, involuntary jerking of a muscle or group of muscles. Myoclonic twitches or jerks usually are caused by sudden muscle contractions, called positive myoclonus, or by muscle relaxation, called negative myoclonus. Myoclonic jerks may occur alone or in sequence, in a pattern or without pattern. They may occur infrequently or many times each minute. Myoclonus sometimes occurs in response to an external event or when a person attempts to make a movement. The twitching cannot be controlled by the person experiencing it.

In its simplest form, myoclonus consists of a muscle twitch followed by relaxation. A hiccup is an example of this type of myoclonus. Other familiar examples of myoclonus are the jerks or "sleep starts" that some people experience while drifting off to sleep. These simple forms of myoclonus occur in normal, healthy persons and cause no difficulties. When more widespread, myoclonus may involve persistent, shock-like contractions in a group of muscles. In some cases, myoclonus begins in one region of the body and spreads to muscles in other areas. More severe cases of myoclonus can distort movement and severely limit a person's ability to eat, talk, or walk. These types of myoclonus may indicate an underlying disorder in the brain or nerves.

What Are the Causes of Myoclonus?

Myoclonus may develop in response to infection, head or spinal cord injury, stroke, brain tumors, kidney or liver failure, lipid storage disease, chemical or drug poisoning, or other disorders. Prolonged oxygen deprivation to the brain, called hypoxia, may result in posthypoxic myoclonus. Myoclonus can occur by itself, but most often it is one of several symptoms associated with a wide variety of nervous system disorders. For example, myoclonic jerking may develop in patients with multiple sclerosis, Parkinson's disease, Alzheimer's disease, or Creutzfeldt-Jakob disease. Myoclonic jerks commonly occur in persons with epilepsy, a disorder in which the electrical activity in the brain becomes disordered leading to seizures.

What Are the Types of Myoclonus?

Classifying the many different forms of myoclonus is difficult because the causes, effects, and responses to therapy vary widely. Listed are the types most commonly described.

- **Action myoclonus** is characterized by muscular jerking triggered or intensified by voluntary movement or even the intention to move. It may be made worse by attempts at precise, coordinated movements. Action myoclonus is the most disabling form of myoclonus and can affect the arms, legs, face, and even the voice. This type of myoclonus often is caused by brain damage that results from a lack of oxygen and blood flow to the brain when breathing or heartbeat is temporarily stopped.

- **Cortical reflex myoclonus** is thought to be a type of epilepsy that originates in the cerebral cortex—the outer layer, or "gray matter," of the brain, responsible for much of the information processing that takes place in the brain. In this type of myoclonus, jerks usually involve only a few muscles in one part of the body, but jerks involving many muscles also may occur. Cortical

27

reflex myoclonus can be intensified when patients attempt to move in a certain way or perceive a particular sensation.

- **Essential myoclonus** occurs in the absence of epilepsy or other apparent abnormalities in the brain or nerves. It can occur randomly in people with no family history, but it also can appear among members of the same family, indicating that it some- times may be an inherited disorder. Essential myoclonus tends to be stable without increasing in severity over time. Some sci- entists speculate that some forms of essential myoclonus may be a type of epilepsy with no known cause.

- **Palatal myoclonus** is a regular, rhythmic contraction of one or both sides of the rear of the roof of the mouth, called the soft palate. These contractions may be accompanied by myoclonus in other muscles, including those in the face, tongue, throat, and diaphragm. The contractions are very rapid, occurring as often as 150 times a minute, and may persist during sleep. The condi- tion usually appears in adults and can last indefinitely. People with palatal myoclonus usually regard it as a minor problem, although some occasionally complain of a clicking sound in the ear, a noise made as the muscles in the soft palate contract.

- **Progressive myoclonus epilepsy** (PME) is a group of dis- eases characterized by myoclonus, epileptic seizures, and other serious symptoms such as trouble walking or speaking. These rare disorders often get worse over time and sometimes are fa- tal. Studies have identified at least three forms of PME. *Lafora body disease* is inherited as an autosomal recessive disorder, meaning that the disease occurs only when a child inherits two copies of a defective gene, one from each parent. *Lafora body disease* is characterized by myoclonus, epileptic seizures, and dementia (progressive loss of memory and other intellectual functions). A second group of PME diseases belonging to the class of *cerebral storage diseases* usually involves myoclonus, vi- sual problems, dementia, and dystonia (sustained muscle con- tractions that cause twisting movements or abnormal postures). Another group of PME disorders in the class of *system degenera- tions* often is accompanied by action myoclonus, seizures, and problems with balance and walking. Many of these PME dis- eases begin in childhood or adolescence.

- **Reticular reflex myoclonus** is thought to be a type of gener- alized epilepsy that originates in the brainstem, the part of the brain that connects to the spinal cord and controls vital functions such as breathing and heartbeat. Myoclonic jerks usually affect the whole body, with muscles on both sides of the body affected simultaneously. In some people, myoclonic jerks occur in only a part of the body, such as the legs, with all the muscles in that part being involved in each jerk. Reticular reflex myoclonus can be triggered by either a voluntary movement or an external stimulus.

- **Stimulus-sensitive myoclonus** is triggered by a variety of external events, including noise, movement, and light. Surprise may increase the sensitivity of the patient.

- **Sleep myoclonus** occurs during the initial phases of sleep, especially at the moment of dropping off to sleep. Some forms appear to be stimulus-sensitive. Some persons with sleep myoclonus are rarely troubled by, or need treatment for, the condition. However, myoclonus may be a symptom in more complex and disturbing sleep disorders, such as restless legs syndrome, and may require treatment by a doctor.

What Is Opsoclonus Myoclonus?

Opsoclonus myoclonus is a rare neurological disorder characterized by unsteady gait, intention tremor (rhythmic, involuntary motions of the limbs during voluntary movements), myoclonus (brief, shock-like muscle spasms), and opsoclonus (irregular, rapid, horizontal, and vertical eye movements). Other symptoms may include dysphasia (difficulty speaking), dysarthria (poorly articulated speech), mutism (inability to speak), hypotonia (decreased muscle tone), lethargy, irritability, or malaise (a vague feeling of bodily discomfort). Opsoclonus myoclonus may occur in association with tumors or viral infections.

Is There Any Treatment for Opsoclonus Myoclonus?

Treatment for opsoclonus myoclonus may include corticosteroids or ACTH (adrenocorticotropic hormone). In cases where there is a tumor present, treatment such as chemotherapy, surgery, or radiation may be required.

What Is the Prognosis?

The prognosis for opsoclonus myoclonus varies depending on the symptoms and the presence and treatment of tumors. With treatment of the underlying cause of the disorder, there may be an improvement of symptoms. Spontaneous remissions (unexplained lack of disease activity) may also occur. Generally the disorder is not fatal.

What Do Scientists Know about Myoclonus?

Although some cases of myoclonus are caused by an injury to the peripheral nerves (defined as the nerves outside the brain and spinal cord, or the central nervous system), most myoclonus is caused by a disturbance of the central nervous system. Studies suggest that several locations in the brain are involved in myoclonus. One such location, for example, is in the brainstem close to structures that are responsible for the startle response, an automatic reaction to an unexpected stimulus involving rapid muscle contraction.

The specific mechanisms underlying myoclonus are not yet fully understood. Scientists believe that some types of stimulus-sensitive myoclonus may involve overexcitability of the parts of the brain that control movement. These parts are interconnected in a series of feedback loops called motor pathways. These pathways facilitate and modulate communication between the brain and muscles. Key elements of this communication are chemicals known as neurotransmitters, which carry messages from one nerve cell, or neuron, to another. Neurotransmitters are released by neurons and attach themselves to receptors on parts of neighboring cells. Some neurotransmitters may make the receiving cell more sensitive, while others tend to make the receiving cell less sensitive. Laboratory studies suggest that an imbalance between these chemicals may underlie myoclonus.

Some researchers speculate that abnormalities or deficiencies in the receptors for certain neurotransmitters may contribute to some forms of myoclonus. Receptors that appear to be related to myoclonus include those for two important inhibitory neurotransmitters: serotonin, which constricts blood vessels and brings on sleep, and gamma-aminobutyric acid (GABA), which helps the brain maintain muscle control. Other receptors with links to myoclonus include those for opiates, drugs that induce sleep, and for glycine, an inhibitory neurotransmitter that is important for the control of motor and sensory functions in the spinal cord. More research is needed to determine how these receptor abnormalities cause or contribute to myoclonus.

How Is Myoclonus Treated?

Treatment of myoclonus focuses on medications that may help reduce symptoms. The drug of first choice to treat myoclonus, especially certain types of action myoclonus, is clonazepam, a type of tranquilizer. Dosages of clonazepam usually are increased gradually until the patient improves or side effects become harmful. Drowsiness and loss of coordination are common side effects. The beneficial effects of clonazepam may diminish over time if the patient develops a tolerance for the drug.

Many of the drugs used for myoclonus, such as barbiturates, phenytoin, and primidone, are also used to treat epilepsy. Barbiturates slow down the central nervous system and cause tranquilizing or antiseizure effects. Phenytoin and primidone are effective antiepileptic drugs, although phenytoin can cause liver failure or have other harmful long-term effects in patients with PME. Sodium valproate is an alternative therapy for myoclonus and can be used either alone or in combination with clonazepam. Although clonazepam and/or sodium valproate are effective in the majority of patients with myoclonus, some people have adverse reactions to these drugs.

Some studies have shown that doses of 5-hydroxytryptophan (5-HTP), a building block of serotonin, leads to improvement in patients with some types of action myoclonus and PME. However, other studies indicate that 5-HTP therapy is not effective in all people with myoclonus, and, in fact, may worsen the condition in some patients. These differences in the effect of 5-HTP on patients with myoclonus have not yet been explained, but they may offer important clues to underlying abnormalities in serotonin receptors.

The complex origins of myoclonus may require the use of multiple drugs for effective treatment. Although some drugs have a limited effect when used individually, they may have a greater effect when used with drugs that act on different pathways or mechanisms in the brain. By combining several of these drugs, scientists hope to achieve greater control of myoclonic symptoms. Some drugs currently being studied in different combinations include clonazepam, sodium valproate, piracetam, and primidone. Hormonal therapy also may improve responses to antimyoclonic drugs in some people.

What Research Is Being Done?

Scientists are seeking to understand the underlying biochemical basis of involuntary movements and to find the most effective treatment for myoclonus and other movement disorders. The National Institute of Neurological Disorders and Stroke (NINDS), a unit of the Federal Government's National Institutes of Health (NIH), is the agency with primary responsibility for research on the brain and nervous system.

Investigators at NINDS laboratories are evaluating the role of neurotransmitters and receptors in myoclonus. If abnormalities in neurotransmitters or receptors are found to play a causative role in myoclonus, future research can focus on determining the extent to which genetic alterations are responsible for these abnormalities and on identifying the nature of those alterations. Scientists also may be able to develop drug treatments that target specific changes in the receptors to reverse abnormalities, such as the loss of inhibition, and to enhance mechanisms that compensate for these abnormalities. Identifying receptor abnormalities also may help researchers develop diagnostic tests for myoclonus. NINDS-supported scientists at research institutions throughout the country are studying various aspects of PME, including the basic mechanisms and genes involved in this group of diseases.

Additional Information

Brain Resources and Information Network (BRAIN)
P.O. Box 5801
Bethesda, MD 20824
Toll-Free: 800-352-9424
TTY: 301-468-5981
Website: www.ninds.nih.gov

Moving Forward
2934 Glenmore Avenue
Kettering, OH 45409
Tel: 937-293-0409

Myoclonus Research Foundation, Inc.
200 Old Palisade Road
Fort Lee, NJ 07024
Tel: 201-585-0770
Website: www.myoclonus.com
E-mail: research@myoclonus.com

National Organization for Rare Disorders (NORD)
P.O. Box 1968
Danbury, CT 06813-1968
Toll-Free: 800-999-NORD (6673)
Tel: 203-746-6518
Fax: 203-746-6481
Website: www.rarediseases.org
E-mail: orphan@rarediseases.org

Opsoclonus Myoclonus Support Network, Inc.
c/o 420 Montezuma Way
West Covina, CA 91791
Tel: 626-339-7949
Website: www.geocities.com/HotSprings/Spa2190

Section 2.5

Chorea: Involuntary Spasmodic Movements

"NINDS Chorea Information Page," National Institute of Neurological
Disorders and Stroke (NINDS), reviewed 9/13/2001.

What Is Chorea?

Chorea is a neurological disorder characterized by involuntary
spasmodic movements of the body. Movements are jerky and arrhyth-
mic, and may involve the whole body. Other symptoms include muscle
weakness, clumsiness, and gait disturbances. Chorea may be inherited, or the consequences of an earlier infection or autoimmune disease. The disorder is most commonly associated with Huntington's
disease (or Huntington's chorea) and Sydenham's chorea (an inflammatory reaction sometimes occurring after a streptococcal infection),
although it may be associated with other conditions as well.

Is There Any Treatment?

There is no standard course of treatment for chorea. Treatment depends on the type of chorea and the associated disorder. Treatment
for Huntington's disease is supportive, while treatment for Syndenham's chorea usually involves drugs to treat the infection, followed
by prophylactic drug therapy.

What Is the Prognosis?

The prognosis for individuals with chorea varies depending on the
type of chorea and the associated disorder. Huntington's disease is a

hereditary, progressive, and fatal neurological disorder. Syndenham's chorea is treatable and curable.

Additional Information

National Organization for Rare Disorders (NORD)
P.O. Box 1968
Danbury, CT 06813-1968
Toll-Free: 800-999-6673
Tel: 203-746-6518
Fax: 203-746-6481
Website: www.rarediseases.org
E-mail: orphan@rarediseases.org

Chapter 3

Who's Who on the Health Care Team and How to Be Its Captain

Time was when you didn't have to guess who was who in a hospital. Doctors were mostly men, and they wore white suits and carried stethoscopes in their pockets. Nurses were women, and they wore starched, white uniforms and caps. Then there were volunteers, who wore candy-striped outfits or pink smocks, and a few clerks in street clothes.

Well, all that's changed. Doctors come in both genders and may or may not wear any special clothes. Nurses may wear colorful smocks, street clothes with white jackets, or scrubs once reserved for operating room staff. And there's a virtual army of other professionals and nonprofessionals who are hard to identify.

If you don't have a scorecard, it can be hard to keep track of the players, let alone to be your team's captain. The good news is that all these members of the health care team, new and old, can help you to treat and cope with a neuromuscular disease.

If you develop an understanding of the team and its members, you'll become increasingly skilled at being its captain—using the various professionals as skilled consultants and respecting their knowledge and experience, while remaining in charge of your own, or your child's, health care.

"Who's Who on the Health Care Team and How to Be Its Captain," by Margaret Wahl, *Quest,* Volume 6, Number 1, February 1999, © Muscular Dystrophy Association (MDA). Reprinted with permission of the Muscular Dystrophy Association.

Even with the best of intentions, today's health care professionals can be so overburdened with insurance regulations, heavy patient loads, and administrative duties that things can fall through the cracks. It's up to you to make sure they don't.

You'll encounter a variety of doctors in your journey through the health care system. Here are some of them.

Neurologists

Neurologists are physicians who specialize in the nervous system and the muscles. (Strictly speaking, the study of muscles is *myology*, and the study of the nervous system is *neurology*, but there's no medical specialty in myology.)

Neurologists are interested in the diagnosis and progression of neuromuscular diseases. They also prescribe drugs to treat the symptoms or, when possible, the underlying cause of a neuromuscular disorder. They may have experience with other interventions for these disorders, such as surgery, equipment, or exercise, but usually these areas aren't their specialty.

Physiatrists (Rehabilitation Doctors)

Physiatrists are doctors who specialize in what's known as *physical medicine and rehabilitation*. Their expertise is in helping people cope with the physical effects of a disorder (for example, eating, breathing, and moving), and they're generally highly skilled in the areas of exercise, assisted ventilation, and equipment use. They usually work with other professionals, such as physical and respiratory therapists.

Cardiologists

Many forms of muscular dystrophy and some other neuromuscular disorders, such as Friedreich's ataxia, have significant effects on the heart—a muscle controlled by nerves. For this reason, you may find yourself consulting with a cardiologist, a doctor who specializes in heart problems. Your neurologist will probably make the referral and should keep in touch with the cardiologist.

Pulmonologists

Muscles that move the limbs and trunk and the nerves that control these muscles are obviously affected in neuromuscular disorders; the muscles and nerves that control breathing are also usually affected, though not quite so obviously. In recent years, there's been increasing awareness of respiratory problems in neuromuscular diseases, and you're likely to be referred at some point to the pulmonary department at your medical center, at least for an evaluation. Pulmonologists are physicians who specialize in disorders of the lungs and structures associated with the lungs, such as the muscles that control breathing. These physicians are very valuable additions to the health care team of anyone with a neuromuscular disorder. They generally work closely with respiratory therapists.

Cardiac and respiratory problems are often silent and can sometimes go unrecognized until they're very far advanced. In many neuromuscular disorders, it's a good idea to have baseline evaluations of cardiac and pulmonary functioning at the time of diagnosis and to have frequent checkups thereafter.

Orthopedists

Doctors specializing in orthopedics concern themselves with the bones and joints and their associated structures, such as the muscles and tendons attached to the bones. Bones usually aren't directly affected by neuromuscular disorders, but they do show the secondary effects of prolonged muscle weakness. Joints can become contracted—fixed in a particular position—and bracing, exercise, and sometimes surgery can be helpful in avoiding or minimizing contractures. The spine can also be pulled out of its normal alignment by muscle weakness. This condition, known as scoliosis, is particularly debilitating and may need surgical correction.

Orthopedists act as consultants for these types of problems. Orthopedics is a surgical specialty, and you'll likely also hear the term *orthopedic surgeon* in reference to these physicians.

Psychiatrists

Because the problems associated with severe disability can often lead to severe psychological distress, you or your neurologist may request a referral to a psychiatrist. Psychiatrists are medical doctors and, as such, they prescribe medications (for example, antidepressants) and other treatments for mental and emotional disorders. They also talk with patients and family members and may help people put problems in a more helpful perspective. There are other kinds of mental health professionals, such as social workers, psychologists, and mental health nurse practitioners.

37

Primary Care Physicians

The term *primary care* means care by a professional who doesn't have a specialty in a particular branch of medicine. The primary care physician specializes in care of the whole person. The term is based on the idea that one goes to a primary care provider first and is then referred to other professionals.

Neuromuscular disorders are no protection against common illnesses—such as ear infections and chickenpox in children, or high blood pressure and cancer in adults—so you'll want to have a primary care doctor as well as specialists of various kinds.

As an adult, you can choose an internist or family practitioner. For a child, you may want to choose a pediatrician, family practitioner, or adolescent medicine specialist. Pediatricians and adolescent medicine specialists are particularly sensitive to a young person's general growth and development and can help a child through the difficulties of having a chronic disorder.

Additional Health Practitioners

Many of the skilled professionals who will provide crucial support for you in the modern medical center aren't medical doctors. They're various other types of highly skilled and educated health practitioners.

Physical and Occupational Therapists

Neuromuscular disorders have obvious and sometimes devastating effects on mobility and, therefore, on many activities of daily living that require mobility.

Almost every ordinary activity—eating a meal, taking a bath or shower, using the toilet, using a computer, driving a car—can be affected by weakening muscles. And almost every one of these activities can be maintained—although in a modified form—by physical and occupational therapy.

In a general way, physical therapists deal with the large muscles and with physical strength and endurance, while occupational therapists deal more with the small muscles and with the ability to perform skilled tasks. But that isn't universally true, and there's a lot of overlap in the domains of these two professions. You'll almost certainly encounter both kinds of therapists on your journey through the health care system.

Respiratory Therapists

Physical therapists may help with exercises for the respiratory muscles, but it's really the respiratory therapist in whose domain this kind of treatment lies. Respiratory therapists work closely with neurologists, pulmonologists, and other kinds of physicians.

Respiratory therapists can help you develop an approach to supplementing the functions of weakening respiratory muscles, with monitoring and testing, devices that augment the efforts to cough and clear secretions from the respiratory tract, and devices to increase ventilation (the movement of air into and out of the lungs). They're a crucial part of the team, and your doctor can refer you to them.

Speech-Language Pathologists

Some neuromuscular disorders have a direct impact on speech because they weaken the muscles involved in speaking, and many such disorders affect swallowing. Speech-language pathologists are the professionals who attend to these forms of muscle weakness (including swallowing, although it's not reflected in the profession's name). New imaging techniques have made diagnosis of mouth and throat weakness much more effective, and these professionals can perform these tests. New electronic devices can help with speaking, and various techniques, including changes in diet, can help with swallowing. Don't overlook these therapists.

Dietitians and Nutritionists

Nutritional problems can occur in neuromuscular disorders, particularly if swallowing becomes difficult. Sometimes, special diets are suggested if you're taking certain medications, have certain kinds of heart problems, or are gaining or losing weight abnormally.

The professional title for these practitioners is *dietitian*, and a registered dietitian uses the initials R.D. The term *nutritionist* is often used in various centers, but it has no specific meaning; the nutritionist may be a nurse or other professional who has a special interest in nutrition.

Nurses

Most people are familiar with nurses, but few know how many kinds there are and fewer still can pick them out of a crowd.

- The term *registered nurse (R.N.)* means the nurse has had advanced education (usually a college degree) in nursing, including the biological and social sciences as well as nursing skills, and has passed a state licensing exam.

- The terms *licensed practical nurse (LPN)* and *licensed vocational nurse (LVN)* indicate a less extensive kind of preparation. You may encounter both kinds of nurses in the clinic or if you or your child should have to stay in the hospital.

- There are also nurses who have an even greater scope of practice than the average R.N. These are known as nurse clinicians and nurse practitioners, and both have specialized, advanced education and act independently or nearly independently in the health care system. Nurse practitioners and clinicians generally have a specialty, such as neurology or respiratory care, but their focus is slightly different from that of doctors in the same specialty. The emphasis is on health maintenance and on helping people make the best use of their abilities and resources, rather than strictly on diagnosis and treatment of disorders. You may encounter nurse clinicians and nurse practitioners in various departments of the medical center.

Social Workers

You may be introduced to social workers at many points in your health care journey. You're most likely to meet medical social workers and clinical social workers. Both are highly trained professionals, usually with master's degrees in their fields.

Medical social workers found in hospitals and clinics generally focus on the practical aspects of coping with illness and disability, such as insurance reimbursement issues and other financial problems, equipment and housing needs, transportation, and home care. They're also trained in counseling techniques. Clinical social workers function more specifically as counselors, dealing, for example, with the psychosocial issues raised by disability.

There is, of course, considerable overlap in the functions of these two kinds of social workers. In the modern medical center, social workers generally cover one area such as outpatient clinics, inpatient areas, home care, and so forth.

Genetic Counselors

Many neuromuscular disorders are genetic, so another professional who may help you and your family is the genetic counselor. This relative latecomer to the health care team combines counseling skills with a thorough grounding in the medical and scientific aspects of genetics. Genetic counselors provide information and supportive counseling, coordinate genetic testing, and connect families with community resources.

Psychologists

There are many issues raised by the presence of a serious disorder in any family, and psychologists may be the right professionals to help sort them out. Psychologists aren't medical doctors, so they do not prescribe medications or other types of medical interventions. They generally have a masters or doctoral degree, and their focus is somewhat different from that of medical doctors.

Like nurses and nurse practitioners, psychologists tend to see the person and the family in the framework of maximizing strengths and minimizing weaknesses, rather than focusing on the diagnosis and treatment of mental disorders. But, as always, there is considerable variation in the practices of these professionals and overlap between their practices and those of related mental health workers.

Remember

Being the captain of your health care team doesn't mean telling the professionals what to do, but it does mean keeping track of who they are, where they are, and when to see them. It also means understanding as far as possible the physiology of your or your child's disorder and which professionals can best help maintain a good quality of life.

Part Two

Diagnostic Tests

Chapter 4

Frequently Performed Neurological Diagnostic Tests

Neurosurgeons use a variety of diagnostic tests to help identify the specific nature of your neurological injury or disorder. In turn, the results of these tests help the neurosurgeon plan an appropriate course of treatment. Following are descriptions of some of the most frequently performed diagnostic tests by neurosurgeons.

Angiography

During this test, a series of regular x-rays are taken as a radiopaque (impenetrable by x-ray) contrast material (dye) is injected directly into an artery. The resulting radiographic image is like a map of the blood vessels. An angiogram is an accurate way of looking at arteries and veins of the head, neck, and brain, and provides information that cannot be obtained with other tests. It is often used to determine the degree of narrowing of an artery in the head or neck. It can also be used to detect the location and size of aneurysms and vascular malformations. This is an invasive test, requiring a physician to insert a catheter into the major artery near the groin and direct it *upstream* to the arteries near the brain.

Computed Tomographic Scan (CT or CAT Scan)

The computed tomographic scan (also called a CT or CAT scan) uses an x-ray beam and a computer to generate 2-dimensional images of the body. The information is displayed in a cross-section or "slice" of body tissue. Neurological CT scans focus on the head or spine.

CAT scans can help detect spinal stenosis (narrowing) or a herniated disc. They can assist in locating brain damage in patients with head injury, detect a blood clot or bleeding in patients with a stroke, detect certain brain tumors, illuminate enlarged brain ventricles (cavities) in patients with hydrocephalus, assist in planning radiation therapy for cancer of the brain, or detect bleeding in a patient with a ruptured or leaking aneurysm. CT can clearly show even the smallest bones of the body as well as surrounding muscle and blood vessels. This makes it invaluable in diagnosing and treating cranial and spinal problems.

CT scanning is fast, painless, simple, and involves little radiation exposure. If contrast material is injected, patients may experience a warm, flushed sensation or experience a metallic taste in their mouth for a few minutes. The CT scanner is a large, square machine with a donut-like hole in the center. The patient lies on a table that can move up or down and slides into and out of the center of the hold. The patient's body may be supported by pillows to help hold it still and in the proper position during the scanning process. Inside the machine, an x-ray tube on a rotating gantry moves around the patient's body to produce the images, making clicking and whirring sounds as the gantry moves. A CT scan usually takes from 15 minutes to 30 minutes; a CT exam of the head and brain can take between 10 and 45 minutes.

Discography

This test is used to determine if intervertebral discs in the spinal column are a source of pain. This test involves the placement of a needle into the disc spaces while utilizing x-ray guidance and injecting contrast material (dye). The discs are soft, cushion-like pads, which separate the hard vertebral bones of the spine. A disc may cause pain in the neck, mid-back, low back, arms, chest wall, abdomen, or legs when it bulges, herniates, tears, or degenerates.

CT and MRI scans only illustrate anatomy and cannot prove a patient's source of pain. In some cases, discs may appear abnormal on MRI or CT scans but not be the source of pain. A discogram can help identify discs that cause pain and help the neurosurgeon plan the correct surgery. A negative discogram can help avoid surgery that may not be beneficial. Because of the nature of the test, discography is usually done only if the patient's pain is significant enough to consider surgery.

During the procedure, an IV is started to administer antibiotics and relaxation medication. The patient will lie on his/her back for discography of the cervical spine and on his/her side for discography of the thoracic and lumbar spine. The physician numbs the skin, then directs a small needle, using x-ray guidance, into the space of the suspect disc. The procedure may be performed at more than one disc level at the same time. After the needle is properly positioned, a small amount of contrast is injected into each disc. Immediately thereafter, the patient is taken to the CAT scan machine where additional images are taken. Following the CAT scan, patients are taken to a recovery area and monitored for 30 to 60 minutes. A prescription for pain medication often helps with managing muscle discomfort that may occur for a few days after the procedure.

Doppler Ultrasound

This is a basic imaging test to judge the health of the carotid arteries and is done as part of an assessment of a patient's risk of stroke. It is a non-invasive test that takes about 15 to 20 minutes. The patient reclines on an exam table and the physician passes an electronic hand-held device over the body area of concern, pressing the device directly across the skin. The device transmits sound waves that are reflected from the structures in the neck and reconstructed into a picture of the outsides and inside of the artery walls. The Doppler can also use changes in the reflected sound waves to determine the velocity of blood flow through the artery. Just like stepping on a garden hose, a high velocity implies a narrower vessel. The Doppler ultrasound usually can only visualize arteries in the neck.

Electromyography (EMG)

This test is used to learn more about the functioning of peripheral nerves (those in the arms and legs). It can tell if a nerve is pinched, and give an estimate of how severely, and where it is compromised. An EMG tests for the electrical impulse coming from the brain and/ or spinal cord to the affected area. If that impulse is blocked somewhere along the spinal pathway, it may be delayed or reduced enroute to its final destination (skin, muscle, finger tips, etc.) Therefore, abnormal function could mean there is nerve injury or muscle dysfunction.

Muscles receive constant electrical signals from properly functioning nerves, and in turn they broadcast their own electrical signals.

During an EMG, the electrical activity in muscles is measured. The doctor places very thin needles (like those used in acupuncture) into the muscles to record the electrical signal from the various leg or arm muscles. If a muscle doesn't receive adequate impulses from its nerve, it broadcasts signals that indicate the muscle is confused.

The results of this test are usually correlated with the results from the Nerve Conduction Study, allowing the doctor to determine which nerves are pinched and the degree of malfunction. (See Nerve Conduction Study)

Intrathecal Contrast Enhanced CAT Scan

This test is similar to a myelogram, which utilizes contrast or x-ray dye to better visualize the spinal canal and nerve roots in the spine. This test can be performed to determine problems in the cervical, thoracic, and lumbar spine. Regardless of what area is to be studied, the physician first applies a numbing medication to the skin. Then, using x-ray guidance the physician injects a very low dose of intrathecal contrast (dye) into the patient's spinal sac (where the spinal fluid is located). Regardless of what level of the spine is to be studied, the contrast is injected in the lower back and then the patient is moved into a position that enables the flow of contrast to reach the area of interest. Contrast is heavier than water. The patient then undergoes a CAT Scan of the portion of the spine under scrutiny. The CAT Scan takes approximately 45 to 60 minutes to complete.

Magnetic Resonance Imaging (MRI)/Magnetic Resonance Angiogram (MRA)

MRI and MRA are done by a machine that uses radiofrequency energy and a strong magnetic field to provide detailed images of internal organs and tissues. The image results from the different water concentration of the various tissues. No radiation exposure is involved. The conventional MRI machine consists of a closed cylindrical magnet in which the patient must lie totally still for short periods of time. MRI causes no pain, but some patients do find it uncomfortable and even claustrophobic. However, newer, more patient-friendly MRI systems are now in increasingly widespread use. Depending on the part of the body being examined, a contrast agent may be used to enhance the visibility of certain tissue or blood vessel. This is administered via a small needle connected to an intravenous line placed in vein in the arm or hand. An MRI/MRA is a non-invasive procedure and can take from 15 minutes to approximately one hour to complete, depending on the part of the body being imaged.

MRI can be used to identify and monitor tumors of the brain and spinal cord. It can also measure small metabolic changes in the active part of the brain and therefore be used to map those parts of the brain that handle critical functions such as thought, speech, movement, and sensation. It can also document changes in chronic disorders of the nervous system such as multiple sclerosis. It is also a useful diagnostic tool for identifying diseases of the blood vessels as well as stroke. It is commonly used for patients with diseases of the pituitary gland. It is also widely used to diagnose sports-related injuries and is useful in documenting brain abnormalities related to dementia or seizures. MRI can also detect tissue abnormality in patients with diseases of the eye or inner ear.

Because the MRI can give such clear pictures of soft-tissue structures in and around bones, it also is the most sensitive exam available for spinal problems. It is particularly helpful in identifying stenosis (narrowing of the spinal canal) and herniated discs. The MRI can be critical to planning surgery, radiation therapy, treatment for stroke, or other interventions to treat brain disorders. The MRA demonstrates blood vessels in the neck and brain and can help detect abnormalities.

For an MRI of the head, the patient is placed on a sliding table and a radio antenna device called a surface coil is positioned around the upper part of the head. The patient is then positioned inside the MRI gantry. The MRI exam will generally take from 15 to 45 minutes.

The functional MRI looks at how the brain is actually functioning by identify regions of increased brain activity. Increases in microscopic vessel size, chemical changes, or heat production are all signs that a particular part of the brain is processing information and giving commands to the body. For this test, the patient performs a particular task while the imaging is taking place. The metabolism in the area of the brain responsible for that task will increase, and the signal in MR image will change. By performing specific tasks that correspond to different functions, it is possible to locate the area in the brain that governs that function. This information is helpful to a surgeon so that he/she can avoid those important areas during surgery. The patient lies on a sliding table with his or her head in a brace designed to hold the head still, then is slid under or into the cylindrical magnetic unit which creates the image. As the test progresses, the patients will be asked to perform various tasks, such as tapping the thumb of one hand against each of the fingers in that hand.

Nerve Conduction Study

This is a sensitive test usually done in conjunction with an EMG. It utilizes electrical stimulation of a specific nerve or nerves and records the nerve's ability to transmit an impulse. This study can determine that a nerve is functioning normally.

During this test, electrode patches are placed along the known course of the nerve. The nerve is then stimulated with a tiny electrical current at one point. A nerve should then transmit the signal along its course so that an electrode placed further down the arm or leg captures the signal as it passes. A normally functioning nerve will transmit the signal faster and stronger than a sick nerve.

The results of this test are usually correlated with the results from the EMG test, allowing the doctor to correlate which nerves are pinched and the degree of malfunction.

Nerve Root Block: Nerve roots exit the spinal cord and form nerves that travel into the arms or legs. These nerves allow movement of the arms, chest wall, and legs. These nerve roots may become inflamed and painful because of irritation from a bony spur or herniated disc in the spine. This test provides important information about which nerve is causing pain by temporarily numbing the nerve root of concern. If the patient's pain is reduced after the injection, that nerve is most likely causing the pain. If the pain level is unchanged, that nerve is most likely not causing the patient's pain. By confirming or eliminating the exact source of pain, the test allows the physician to develop appropriate treatment, which could include further nerve blocks and/or surgery.

Nuclear Imaging—PET (Positron Emission Tomography) and SPECT (Single Photon Emission Computed Tomography) Scans

PET and SPECT are part of the family of nuclear imaging techniques that use small amounts of radioactive isotopes (radionuclides) to measure cellular and/or tissue metabolism. Radionuclides are absorbed by healthy tissue at a different rate than tissue that is diseased.

A PET image can map the biological function of an organ, detect subtle metabolic changes, and may be used to determine if a tumor is benign or malignant. The PET scan utilizes a machine called a cyclotron, which is an accelerator that propels charged particles using alternating voltage in a magnetic field to generate radioisotopes. The patient is injected with a radionuclide specific to the function or type of metabolism being tested for. The radionuclide will collect in that specific area of the body. The patient lies on a scanning table while a ring-shaped machine is positioned over the target area of the body. Detectors in the ring pick up gamma rays emitted from the body tissues. A computer analyzes the data and produces cross-sectional images on film and/or a video monitor.

A SPECT Scan is used to determine blood flow to tissue, which helps discover how well an organ may be working. It is very sensitive and useful in detecting stress fracture, spondylosis (a degenerative disease of the spinal column), infection (such as discitis), and tumor. As with a PET Scan, a radionuclide is injected intravenously into the patient and it circulates through the blood. A camera then rotates around the patient, picking up images cast by the radionuclide. The information is then transferred to a computer that converts the data into film images. The images are projected as cross-sections of the body and can be rendered into a 3-D format.

Chapter 5

Muscle Biopsy

A muscle biopsy is a surgical procedure in which one or more small pieces of muscle tissue are removed for further microscopic or biochemical examination. The procedure, often used in the diagnosis of a neuromuscular disorder, is considered minor surgery and is usually performed under local anesthetic.

A doctor is likely to call for a muscle biopsy after looking at preliminary blood tests, performing an electromyogram (EMG) and physical examination, and determining that the patient's symptoms indicate an underlying neuromuscular disorder. The muscle biopsy can help distinguish between muscular and neurological problems and can help pinpoint the exact neuromuscular disorder present.

Not everyone suspected of having a neuromuscular disease requires a muscle biopsy. In some cases, diagnosis can be made by symptoms and a DNA test based on a blood sample.

Open or Needle Biopsy

There are two types of muscle biopsy. The open biopsy involves the removal of one or more small pieces of muscle tissue with sharp scissors.

The neuromuscular specialist selects a muscle, usually the biceps, triceps, deltoid, or quadriceps muscle, that should yield the most

"Simply Stated: Muscle Biopsies," *Quest*, Volume 7, Number 4, August 2000 © Muscular Dystrophy Association (MDA). Reprinted with permission of the Muscular Dystrophy Association. The section "Muscle Biopsy Test" is from "Muscle Biopsy," © 2001 A.D.A.M., Inc., reprinted with permission.

information about the disease. Usually moderately affected muscles are chosen; the weakest muscles may already be too degraded for analysis. The procedure involves a 2-to-3-inch incision, which is then closed with stitches and may feel sore for a few days.

In a needle biopsy, used since the 1960s, a pea-sized muscle sample is collected with a large bore needle. Although this is less invasive than the open biopsy, the doctor loses the ability to examine the muscle visually first, and the specimen collected is smaller.

Analyzing the Sample

When the muscle samples are sent to a laboratory for analysis, the technicians cut them into many thin sections for examination. Using different tests on different sections, they look at the tissue's overall appearance, chemical activities in the tissue, and the presence or absence of critical proteins. The information these tests provide helps determine exactly what disease and what form of it the person has.

Histology tests (histo means tissue) employ chemical stains to see the muscle's overall appearance and the structure of the muscle cells. This analysis can yield information about muscle degeneration and regeneration, fiber type abnormalities, mitochondrial abnormalities, scar tissue, inflammation, and other clues to specific disorders.

Histochemistry uses stains to detect chemical activities in the cells, including the actions of specific enzymes and metabolic processes. A lab that performs only histology may miss important metabolic abnormalities.

Immunohistochemistry uses antibodies to detect the presence or absence of proteins. This analysis can show whether the cells are missing dystrophin (indicating Duchenne or Becker MD), sarcoglycans (limb-girdle MD), merosin (congenital MD), or other proteins whose absence causes specific muscular dystrophies. Specific antibodies can also be used to identify the nature of inflammatory cells found in the muscle.

The lab may also use electron microscopy to get very high magnification views of the cellular structure, which can confirm structural abnormalities, like the presence of nemaline rods.

Finally, a DNA analysis can be performed on a muscle sample to detect a genetic mutation. Although a blood sample is usually adequate for a DNA test, a muscle sample may be needed to test for mitochondrial DNA mutations.

Multiple Biopsies

Yadollah Harati, a neurologist and director of the Muscle and Nerve Pathology Laboratory at Baylor College of Medicine in Houston, usually takes as many as five separate muscle samples from different regions of the muscle incision. Several are analyzed and at least one is frozen for future use. Harati believes no biopsy should be done unless the amount of tissue removed is adequate for a complete study.

Having at least three muscle samples gives the lab an adequate amount of tissue to work with. In some disorders, particularly patchy disorders like the inflammatory myopathies, signs of the disease may not be present in all regions of the muscles, so more samples give a better chance of accuracy.

It's important that the tissue samples be frozen promptly and properly after the biopsy and be stored carefully. If they're not handled and stored correctly, the results may be inaccurate.

Your doctor may occasionally recommend a new biopsy even though you've had one in the past, especially if you've been given a tentative diagnosis or now suspect your diagnosis was incorrect. With many new muscle-protein antibodies now available for testing biopsy samples, as well as new understanding of mitochondrial disorders and new DNA tests, a new biopsy may be desirable.

According to Harati, tissue that was frozen promptly after removal and maintained carefully is useful for many years. In autoimmune diseases, tissue changes over time in your body may necessitate a new biopsy for the most accurate diagnosis.

Getting Results

The analysis of a muscle biopsy sample is a very tedious and labor-intensive process in which many sections of the muscle must be cut, many different types of procedures performed, and the results carefully analyzed. Harati's lab usually performs a few basic histology tests immediately after the biopsy and then, based on these results, determines what further tests should be made. His lab typically makes an initial report on the day of the biopsy and a full report in two to three weeks.

Muscle Biopsy Test

Alternative names: biopsy—muscle

Definition

A procedure involving removal and examination of a piece of muscle tissue.

How the Test Is Performed

A muscle biopsy can usually be obtained under local anesthesia. A needle biopsy may be adequate in children and adults with chronic conditions. A needle inserted into the muscle. A small "plug" of tissue remains in the needle when it is removed from the muscle; this tissue is sent to the pathologist for examination. More than one needle insertion may be needed to obtain a large enough specimen.

Open biopsy may be needed, particularly when focal (localized) and/or patchy conditions are suspected. This involves a small incision through the skin and into the muscle, so that a sample of muscle tissue can be removed from the affected area.

The muscle chosen for biopsy sampling must be appropriate for the symptoms or suspected condition. The health care provider cannot use a muscle that has recently been traumatized by an EMG needle or that is affected by pre-existing disease such as coincidental nerve compression.

How to Prepare for the Test

No fasting or other special preparation is usually necessary. The muscle chosen for biopsy must be exposed (this may require loose clothing or a hospital gown). You must sign an informed consent form.

Infants and Children

The physical and psychological preparation you can provide for this or any test or procedure depends on your child's age, interests, previous experience, and level of trust.

How the Test Will Feel

During the biopsy, there is usually minimal or no discomfort. Some pressure or tugging sensations may be noted. The anesthetic may burn or sting when injected (before the area becomes numb). After the anesthetic wears off, the area may be sore for about 1 week.

What the Risks Are

- infection (a slight risk any time the skin is broken)
- bleeding of the site
- bruising of the area
- damage to the muscle tissue or other tissues in the area (very rare)

Note: The risks are minimal.

Why the Test Is Performed

A muscle biopsy may be performed to:

- distinguish between neurogenic (nerve) and myopathic (primarily muscle) disorders
- identify specific muscular disorders such as muscular dystrophy or congenital myopathy
- identify metabolic defects of the muscle
- diagnose diseases of the connective tissue and blood vessels (such as polyarteritis nodosa)
- diagnose infections that affect the muscles (such as trichinosis or toxoplasmosis)

Normal Values

Normal muscle and related tissue anatomy. A microscopic examination with and without staining that shows no abnormalities is normal.

What Abnormal Results Mean

A muscle biopsy can reveal conditions such as:

- atrophy (loss of muscle mass)
- necrosis (tissue death) of muscle fibers
- inflammation of the muscle
- necrotizing vasculitis
- myopathic changes (destruction of the muscle)

- muscular dystrophy, indicated by antibody staining of the muscle biopsy specimen that can show deficient dystrophin

Disorders include:

- traumatic muscle damage
- Duchenne's muscular dystrophy
- polymyositis
- dermatomyositis

Additional conditions under which the test may be performed:

- Becker's muscular dystrophy
- Charcot-Marie-Tooth disease (hereditary)
- common peroneal nerve dysfunction
- eosinophilic fasciitis
- facioscapulohumeral muscular dystrophy (Landouzy-Dejerine)
- familial periodic paralysis
- Friedreich's ataxia
- necrotizing vasculitis
- polymyalgia rheumatica
- senile cardiac amyloid
- thyrotoxic periodic paralysis

Cost

The estimated cost is $313.

The information provided herein should not be used for diagnosis or treatment of any medical condition. A licensed physician should be consulted for diagnosis and treatment of any and all medical conditions.

Chapter 6

Creatine Kinase Test

Almost everyone with a neuromuscular disorder has had, or will have, a creatine kinase test. But what exactly is creatine kinase (CK), and why are its levels measured in neuromuscular diseases?

CK, also known as phosphocreatine kinase, or CPK, is a type of protein called an enzyme. It catalyzes, or encourages, a biochemical reaction to occur. The normal function of CK in our cells is to add a phosphate group to creatine, turning it into the high-energy molecule phosphocreatine. Phosphocreatine is burned as a quick source of energy by our cells.

However, the normal function of CK isn't as relevant, in this case, as what happens to CK when muscle is damaged. During the process of muscle degeneration, muscle cells break open and their contents find their way into the bloodstream. Because most of the CK in the body normally exists in muscle, a rise in the amount of CK in the blood indicates that muscle damage has occurred, or is occurring.

To measure CK levels, a blood sample is taken and separated into fractions that contain cells and a fraction that doesn't—the serum. The amount of CK in the serum is reported in units (U) of enzyme activity per liter (L) of serum. In a healthy adult, the serum CK level varies with a number of factors (gender, race, and activity), but normal range is 22 to 198 U/L (units per liter).

"Simply Stated: The Creatine Kinase Test," *Quest*, Volume 7, Number 1, February 2000 © Muscular Dystrophy Association (MDA). Reprinted with permission of the Muscular Dystrophy Association. The section "Creatinine Test" is from "Creatinine: Test" © 2001 A.D.A.M., Inc., reprinted with permission.

Higher amounts of serum CK can indicate muscle damage due to chronic disease or acute muscle injury. For this reason, if you're scheduled to have blood drawn for a CK test to diagnose a potential muscle disorder, you should limit your exercise to normal activities before the test.

CK tests are used to evaluate neuromuscular diseases in five basic ways:

1. To confirm a suspected muscle problem before other symptoms occur.

2. To determine whether symptoms of muscle weakness are caused by a muscle or a nerve problem.

3. To differentiate between some types of disorders such as dystrophies versus congenital myopathies.

4. To detect carriers of neuromuscular disorders, particularly in Duchenne muscular dystrophy. A carrier has a genetic defect, but doesn't get the full-blown disease. A carrier's child may have the full disease.

5. To follow the course of a disease that fluctuates (primarily the inflammatory myopathies), or to document episodes of acute muscle injury, as might occur in some metabolic myopathies.

Because elevated CK levels indicate muscle damage, many parents wonder why their children with Duchenne muscular dystrophy (DMD) had higher CK levels when they were younger and had more muscle function. This seeming paradox occurs because muscle degeneration is more rapid at the earlier stages and, possibly, because there's more muscle bulk available to release CK into the circulation at this time.

CK levels can be slightly elevated (500 U/L) in nerve disorders like Charcot-Marie-Tooth disease, amyotrophic lateral sclerosis, or spinal muscular atrophy, or grossly elevated (3,000 to 3,500 U/L) in DMD or inflammatory myopathies.

During episodes of acute muscle breakdown (rhabdomyolysis), CK levels can temporarily go off the scale, topping out at 50,000 to 200,000 U/L. At the same time, some neuromuscular disorders, such as the congenital myopathies (nemaline, central core disease, and others) and myasthenia gravis, may not trigger any elevation of CK levels. CK levels don't always reflect the level of functional impact on the individual.

Creatinine Test

Definition

A test that measures the amount of creatinine in the blood.

How the Test Is Performed

Adult or child: Blood is drawn from a vein (venipuncture), usually from the inside of the elbow or the back of the hand. The puncture site is cleaned with antiseptic, and a tourniquet (an elastic band) or blood pressure cuff is placed around the upper arm to apply pressure and restrict blood flow through the vein. This causes veins below the tourniquet to distend (fill with blood). A needle is inserted into the vein, and the blood is collected in an airtight vial or a syringe. During the procedure, the tourniquet is removed to restore circulation. Once the blood has been collected, the needle is removed, and the puncture site is covered to stop any bleeding.

Infant or young child: The area is cleansed with antiseptic and punctured with a sharp needle or a lancet. The blood may be collected in a pipette (small glass tube), on a slide, onto a test strip, or into a small container. Cotton or a bandage may be applied to the puncture site if there is any continued bleeding.

How to Prepare for the Test

Fast for 6 hours before the test. The health care provider may advise you to discontinue drugs that may affect the test (see special considerations).

Infants and children: The physical and psychological preparation you can provide for this or any test or procedure depends on your child's age, interests, previous experience, and level of trust.

How the Test Will Feel

When the needle is inserted to draw blood, some people feel moderate pain, while others feel only a prick or stinging sensation. Afterward, there may be some throbbing.

What the Risks Are

Risks include:

- excessive bleeding
- fainting or feeling lightheaded
- hematoma (blood accumulating under the skin)
- infection (a slight risk any time the skin is broken)
- multiple punctures to locate veins

Why Is the Test Performed

A measurement of the serum creatinine level is used to evaluate kidney function.

Creatinine is a breakdown product of creatine, which is an important constituent of muscle. Creatinine can be converted to the ATP molecule, which is a high-energy source. The daily production of creatine and subsequently creatinine, depends on muscle mass, which fluctuates very little.

Creatinine is excreted from the body entirely by the kidneys. With normal renal excretory function, the serum creatinine level should remain constant and normal.

Normal Values

The usual value is 0.8 to 1.4 mg/dl. (Note: mg/dl = milligrams per deciliter)

What Abnormal Results Mean

Greater-than-normal levels may indicate:

- acromegaly (rare)
- acute tubular necrosis (rare)
- dehydration
- diabetic nephropathy
- eclampsia
- gigantism (rare)
- glomerulonephritis
- muscular dystrophy
- pre-eclampsia
- pyelonephritis
- reduced renal blood flow (shock, congestive heart failure)

- renal failure
- rhabdomyolysis
- urinary tract obstruction

Lower-than-normal levels may indicate:

- muscular dystrophy (late stage)
- myasthenia gravis

Additional conditions under which the test may be performed:

- acute nephritic syndrome
- Alport syndrome
- atheroembolic renal disease
- chronic renal failure
- complicated UTI (pyelonephritis)
- Cushing's syndrome
- dementia due to metabolic causes
- dermatomyositis
- digitalis toxicity
- ectopic Cushing's syndrome
- end-stage renal disease
- epilepsy
- generalized tonic-clonic seizure
- Goodpasture's syndrome
- hemolytic-uremic syndrome (HUS)
- hepatorenal syndrome
- IgM mesangial proliferative glomerulonephritis
- interstitial nephritis
- lupus nephritis
- malignant hypertension (arteriolar nephrosclerosis)
- medullary cystic disease
- membranoproliferative GN I
- membranoproliferative GN II
- noninsulin-dependent diabetes mellitus (NIDDM)
- polymyositis (adult)

- prerenal azotemia
- primary amyloid
- rapidly progressive (crescentic) glomerulonephritis
- secondary systemic amyloid
- thrombotic thrombocytopenic purpura
- Wilms' tumor

Cost

The estimated cost is $21.

Special Considerations

Drugs that can increase creatinine measurements include aminoglycosides (for example, gentamicin), cimetidine, heavy metal chemotherapeutic agents (for example, Cisplatin), and nephrotoxic drugs such as cephalosporins (for example, cefoxitin).

The information provided herein should not be used for diagnosis or treatment of any medical condition. A licensed physician should be consulted for diagnosis and treatment of any and all medical conditions.

Chapter 7

Electromyography (EMG) and Nerve Conduction Velocities (NCVs)

Diagnosis of neuromuscular disease hinges on a doctor's ability to identify a specific defect of neuromuscular function. Sometimes, a doctor can infer this functional defect—and the disease associated with it—by giving a physical exam, doing a blood test, or looking at the anatomy of nerves and muscles.

But other times, the doctor may have to directly evaluate the functions of nerves and muscles and the connections between them by using two complementary techniques—nerve conduction velocity testing (NCVs) and electromyography (EMGs).

Action Potentials

Both NCV and EMG rely on the fact that the activity of nerves and muscles produces electrical signals called action potentials. A nerve is actually a bundle of axons, cables that conduct action potentials from one end of a nerve cell (or neuron) to the other.

In motor neurons (neurons that connect to muscle), these action potentials travel toward the muscle, where they cause release of a chemical called acetylcholine. Acetylcholine opens tiny pores in the muscle, and the flow of sodium and potassium ions through these

"Simply Stated: Electromyography and Nerve Conduction Velocities," *Quest*, Volume 7, Number 5, October 2000, © Muscular Dystrophy Association (MDA). Reprinted with permission of the Muscular Dystrophy Association. The section "Test Preparation and Procedure" is from "Procedures/Diagnostic Tests: Electromyography," Warren Grant Magnuson Clinical Center, 1999.

pores creates action potentials in the muscle, leading to contraction. In NCV and EMG, these tiny electrical events are amplified electronically, then visualized on a TV-like monitor called an oscilloscope and even heard using audio equipment.

NCV and Axons

NCV measures action potentials conducted by axons, so doctors use it for diagnosing diseases that primarily affect nerve function, such as different forms of Charcot-Marie-Tooth disease (CMT). It's done by placing surface electrodes (similar to those used for electrocardiograms) on the skin at various points over a nerve. One electrode delivers a mild electrical shock to the nerve, stimulating it to generate an action potential. The other electrodes record the action potential as it's conducted through the nerve.

Doctors often use NCV to determine the speed of nerve conduction (hence, its name). Conduction speed is influenced by a coating around axons, called myelin. Myelin insulates each axon and normally forces action potentials to jump quickly from one end of the axon to the other. If the myelin breaks down (as in CMT1), the action potential travels more slowly.

NCV also can measure the strength of the action potential in the nerve, which is proportional to the number of axons that contribute to it. If axons degenerate (as in amyotrophic lateral sclerosis) or become clogged with debris (as in CMT2), the action potential becomes smaller.

EMG and Muscle

An electromyogram measures the action potentials produced by muscles, and is therefore useful for diagnosing diseases that primarily affect muscle function, including the muscular dystrophies. Also, some EMG data can reveal defects in nerve function. In EMG, the doctor inserts a needlelike electrode into a muscle. The electrode records action potentials that occur when the muscle is at rest and during voluntary contractions directed by the doctor.

While a healthy muscle appears quiet at rest, spontaneous action potentials are seen in damaged muscles or muscles that have lost input from nerve cells (as in ALS or myasthenia gravis). During voluntary contraction, dystrophic (wasted) muscles show very small action potentials, and myotonic (stiff) muscles show prolonged trains of action potentials. Altered patterns of muscle action potentials can indicate defects in nerve function.

A Little Discomfort

Though NCVs and EMGs are valuable tools for doctors, they can be distressing for patients. Some people find the electric shocks of the NCV or the needle penetration of the EMG uncomfortable or even painful. Young children might struggle during the tests, making it difficult for doctors to carefully monitor nerve and muscle activity. To ease discomfort, topical anesthetic can be applied to the skin—but it won't prevent muscle pain during the EMG. Sometimes sedating medications are needed to keep a child calm.

Partly because of these factors, NCVs and EMGs are generally used when it's not possible to gather the right information from other diagnostic tests. Muscle biopsy (excising and examining muscle tissue; see Chapter 5 "Muscle Biopsy") can reveal hallmark anatomical features of some neuromuscular diseases, making EMG and NCV unnecessary. Genetic tests are now available for diagnosing some diseases, and in those cases, EMG and NCV usually can be bypassed.

Nonetheless, NCV and EMG remain the gold standards for evaluating the function of nerve and muscle. So, when a doctor suspects that a patient has a neuromuscular disease that isn't clearly associated with anatomical or genetic defects (like some types of CMT, or myasthenia gravis), NCV and EMG are among the most valuable diagnostic tools.

Test Preparation and Procedure

- There is no special preparation for electromyography.

- The examination is done by a neurologist. A technologist also does some portions of the test.

- A neurologist will do a neurological exam to locate the muscles and nerves to be studied. Once they are located, they will be studied—first by nerve conduction studies; then electromyography.

- Nerve conduction studies show how well your nerves pass electrical messages. Several nerves are studied, usually in the arm and leg. First, electrodes will be placed on your skin. Through these electrodes, the nerves will be stimulated by a weak electrical pulse. This pulse may feel like tapping, and the muscles will twitch as they respond. The electrical messages made by the nerves will be recorded by other electrodes placed on your skin, usually in the leg or arm.

67

- For electromyography, a fine, sterile needle will be inserted into the muscle. During the insertion, you will feel discomfort similar to that of taking a blood sample. Then, you will be asked to relax and do slight muscle contractions. The electrical activity from your working muscle will then be measured.

- The procedure may last up to 3 hours.

After the Procedure

The electrical procedure is completely harmless and has no lasting side effects. You may have a bruise or soreness at the needlestick site. Neurologists will interpret the results and send a detailed report to your referring doctor. Your referring doctor will discuss the results with you.

If you have questions about the procedure, ask your doctor or nurse who are ready to assist you.

Chapter 8

Spinal Tap

Alternative names: spinal tap; ventricular puncture; lumbar puncture; cisternal puncture; and collecting a spinal fluid specimen

Definition

CSF collection is a procedure to obtain a specimen of cerebrospinal fluid (CSF). CSF is the fluid that bathes, cushions, and protects the brain and spinal cord. It flows through the skull and spine in the subarachnoid space, which is the area internal to the arachnoid membrane.

How the Test Is Performed

Lumbar puncture (spinal tap) is the most common means of collecting a specimen of CSF. You are positioned on your side with your knees curled up to your abdomen and your chin tucked in to your chest. (Occasionally this procedure is performed with the person sitting bent forward).

The skin is scrubbed, and a local anesthetic is injected over the lower spine. The spinal needle is inserted, usually between the 3rd and 4th lumbar vertebrae.

Once the needle is properly positioned in the subarachnoid space, pressures can be measured and fluid can be collected for testing. After

"CSF Collection," updated 7/26/01 by Galit Kleiner-Fisman MD, FRCP(C), Department of Neurology, University of Toronto, Toronto, Ontario, Canada. © 2001 A.D.A.M., Inc. Reprinted with permission.

the sample is collected, the needle is removed, the area is cleaned, and a bandage is applied. You will be asked to remain flat, or nearly flat, for 6 to 8 hours after the test.

Lumbar puncture (with fluid collection) may also be part of other procedures, particularly a myelogram (X-ray or CT scan after dye has been inserted into the CSF).

Alternative methods of obtaining CSF are rarely used, but may be indicated if there is a problem such as lumbar deformity or infection, which would make lumbar puncture impossible or unreliable.

Cisternal puncture involves insertion of a needle below the occipital bone (back of the skull). It can be hazardous because the needle is inserted close to the brain stem.

Ventricular puncture is even more rare, but may be indicated when sampling of CSF is necessary in people with possible impending brain herniation. It is usually performed in the operating room. A hole is drilled in the skull and a needle is inserted directly into the lateral ventricle of the brain.

How to Prepare for the Test

You must sign a consent form. You must be prepared to remain in the hospital for at least the 6 to 8 hours, and you must remain flat.

Infants and children: The physical and psychological preparation you can provide for this or any test or procedure depends on your child's age, interests, previous experience, and level of trust.

How It Feels

The position may be uncomfortable, but it is imperative that you remain in the curled position to avoid moving the needle and possibly injuring the spinal cord.

The scrub will feel cold and wet. The anesthetic will sting or burn when first injected. There will be a hard pressure sensation when the needle is inserted, and there is usually some brief pain when the needle goes through the meninges. This pain should stop in a few seconds.

Overall, discomfort is minimal to moderate. The entire procedure usually takes about 30 minutes, but it may take longer. The actual pressure measurements and fluid collection only takes a few minutes.

Risks

Risks of lumbar puncture include:

- Hypersensitivity (allergic) reaction to the anesthetic.
- Discomfort during the test.
- Headache after the test.
- Bleeding into the spinal canal.
- Brain herniation (if performed on a person with increased intracranial pressure), and resulting in brain damage or death.
- Damage to the spinal cord (particularly if the person moves during the test).
- Cisternal puncture or ventricular puncture carry additional risk of damage to the brainstem or brain tissue and risk of bleeding within the brain; resulting in incapacitation or death.

Why the Test Is Performed

This test is performed to measure pressures within the cerebrospinal fluid and to collect CSF for testing. CSF collection can be a diagnostic test for many neurologic disorders, particularly infections and brain/spinal cord damage.

Normal Values

- Pressure: 50 to 180 mm H20
- Appearance: clear, colorless
- CSF total protein: 15 to 45 mg/100 ml
- Gamma globulin: 3 to 12% of the total protein
- CSF glucose: 50 to 80 mg/100 ml (or approximately 2/3 of serum glucose level)
- CSF cell count: 0 to 5 WBCs, no RBCs
- chloride: 110 to 125 mEq per liter

Note: mg/ml = milligrams per milliliter; mEq/L = milliequivalent per liter

What Abnormal Results Mean

- *Pressure, increased:* increased intracranial pressure (pressure within the skull) from trauma or infection

- *Pressure, decreased:* obstruction to the flow of CSF above the puncture site (spinal cord tumor), shock, fainting, diabetic coma

- Appearance
  - *Cloudy:* infection, white blood cells in the CSF, protein in the CSF, microorganisms
  - *Bloody or reddish colored:* bleeding within the brain or subarachnoid space, spinal cord obstruction, traumatic lumbar puncture (first specimen bloody, rest clear)
  - *Brown, orange, yellow color:* elevated protein in the CSF, old (greater than 3 days) blood in the CSF

- *Protein, increased:* blood in the CSF, diabetes, polyneuritis, tumors, trauma, any inflammatory or infectious condition

- *Protein, decreased:* rapid CSF production

- *Gamma globulin, increased:* demyelinating disease (e.g. multiple sclerosis), neurosyphilis, Guillain-Barré syndrome

- *Glucose, increased:* systemic hyperglycemia (elevated blood sugar)

- *Glucose, decreased:* systemic hypoglycemia (low blood sugar), bacterial or fungal infection (such as meningitis), tuberculosis, carcinomatous meningitis

- *WBC, increased:* active meningitis, acute infection, beginning of a chronic illness, tumor, abscess, brain infarction (stroke), demyelinating disease (such as MS)

- *RBC*: bleeding into the spinal fluid, traumatic lumbar puncture

Additional conditions under which the test may be performed:

- Chronic inflammatory polyneuropathy
- Dementia due to metabolic causes
- Encephalitis
- Epilepsy
- Febrile seizure (children)

- Generalized tonic-clonic seizure
- Hydrocephalus Inhalation anthrax
- Normal pressure hydrocephalus (NPH)
- Pituitary tumor
- Reye's syndrome

Special Considerations

This test should not be performed on people in which increased intracranial pressure is suspected.

The information provided herein should not be used for diagnosis or treatment of any medical condition. A licensed physician should be consulted for diagnosis and treatment of any and all medical conditions.

Chapter 9

Electroencephalogram (EEG)

Alternative names: electroencephalogram; brain wave test

Definition

The brain cells communicate by producing tiny electrical impulses. In the EEG, electrodes are placed on the scalp over multiple areas of the brain to detect and record the electrical impulses within the brain. Certain abnormalities can be detected by observation of the pattern of brain waves.

How the Test Is Performed

The test is performed by an EEG technician in a specially-designed room that may be in the health care provider's office or in the hospital. You will be asked to lie on your back on the table or in a reclining chair.

The technician will apply between 16 and 25 flat metal discs (electrodes) in different positions on your scalp. The discs are held in place with a sticky paste. The electrodes are connected by wires to an amplifier and the recording machine.

The recording machine converts the electrical signals into a series of wavy lines which are drawn onto a moving piece of graph paper.

"EEG," updated 7/14/01 by Galit Kleiner-Fisman, M.D., FRCP, Department of Neurology, Toronto Western Hospital and the University of Toronto, Toronto, Canada, © 2001 A.D.A.M., Inc. Reprinted with permission.

You will need to lie still with your eyes closed because movement can alter the results.

You may be asked to do certain things during the recording, such as breathe deeply and rapidly for several minutes or look at a very bright flickering light.

How to Prepare for the Test

You will need to wash your hair the night before the test. No oils, sprays, or lotion should be used on your hair. The health care provider may want you to discontinue some medications before the test. You should avoid all foods containing caffeine for 8 hours before the test.

Sometimes it is necessary to sleep during the test, so you may be asked to reduce your sleep time the night before.

Infants and children: The physical and psychological preparation you can provide for this or any test or procedure depends on your child's age, interests, previous experiences, and level of trust.

How It Feels

Nothing will be felt during the procedure.

Risks

The procedure is very safe. If you have a seizure disorder, a seizure may be triggered by the flashing lights or hyperventilation. The health care provider is trained to take care of you if this happens.

Why the Test Is Performed

The EEG is used to help diagnose the presence and type of seizure disorders, confusion, head injuries, brain tumors, infections, degenerative diseases, and metabolic disturbances that affect the brain. It is also used to evaluate sleep disorders and to investigate periods of unconsciousness. The EEG may be done to confirm brain death in a comatose patient. The procedure cannot be used to read the mind, measure intelligence, or diagnose mental illness.

Normal Values

The brain waves have a normal frequency, amplitude, and characteristics.

What Abnormal Results Mean

Abnormal findings may indicate seizure disorders (epilepsy, convulsions), any structural brain abnormality such as a brain tumor, brain abscess (infection), head injury, encephalitis (inflammation of the brain), hemorrhage (abnormal bleeding caused by a ruptured blood vessel), cerebral infarct (tissue that is dead because of a blockage of the blood supply), or a sleep disorder such as narcolepsy (sleep epilepsy). Lastly, an EEG may confirm brain death.

Additional conditions under which the test may be performed:

- Arteriovenous malformation (cerebral)
- Benign positional vertigo
- Cerebral aneurysm
- Complicated alcohol abstinence (delirium tremens)
- Creutzfeldt-Jacob disease
- Delirium
- Dementia
- Dementia due to metabolic causes
- Febrile seizure (children)
- Generalized tonic-clonic seizure
- Hepatic encephalopathy
- Hepatorenal syndrome
- Insomnias
- Labyrinthitis
- Ménière's disease
- Metastatic brain tumor
- Multiple sclerosis
- Optic glioma
- Partial (focal) seizure
- Partial complex seizure
- Petit mal seizure
- Pick's disease
- Senile dementia/Alzheimer's type
- Shy-Drager syndrome
- Syphilitic aseptic meningitis
- Temporal lobe seizure

The information provided herein should not be used for diagnosis or treatment of any medical condition. A licensed physician should be consulted for diagnosis and treatment of any and all medical conditions.

Chapter 10

Gene Testing

What Is Gene Testing? How Does It Work?

Gene tests (also called DNA-based tests), the newest and most sophisticated of the techniques used to test for genetic disorders, involve direct examination of the DNA molecule itself. Other genetic tests include biochemical tests for such gene products as enzymes and other proteins and for microscopic examination of stained or fluorescent chromosomes. Genetic tests are used for several reasons, including:

- carrier screening, which involves identifying unaffected individuals who carry one copy of a gene for a disease that requires two copies for the disease to be expressed;

- prenatal diagnostic testing;

- newborn screening;

- presymptomatic testing for predicting adult-onset disorders such as Huntington's disease;

- presymptomatic testing for estimating the risk of developing adult-onset cancers and Alzheimer's disease;

- confirmational diagnosis of a symptomatic individual; and

- forensic/identity testing.

"Gene Testing," Human Genome Project Information, U.S. Department of Energy Office of Science, Office of Biological and Environmental Research, Human Genome Program, 2001.

In gene tests, scientists scan a patient's DNA sample for mutated sequences. A DNA sample can be obtained from any tissue, including blood. For some types of gene tests, researchers design short pieces of DNA called probes, whose sequences are complementary to the mutated sequences. These probes will seek their complement among the three billion base pairs of an individual's genome. If the mutated sequence is present in the patient's genome, the probe will bind to it and flag the mutation. Another type of DNA testing involves comparing the sequence of DNA bases in a patient's gene to a normal version of the gene. Cost of testing can range from hundreds to thousands of dollars, depending on the sizes of the genes and the numbers of mutations tested.

What Are Some of the Pros and Cons of Gene Testing?

Gene testing already has dramatically improved lives. Some tests are used to clarify a diagnosis and direct a physician toward appropriate treatments, while others allow families to avoid having children with devastating diseases or identify people at high risk for conditions that may be preventable. Aggressive monitoring for and removal of colon growths in those inheriting a gene for familial adenomatous polyposis, for example, has saved many lives. On the horizon is a gene test that will provide doctors with a simple diagnostic test for a common iron-storage disease, transforming it from a usually fatal condition to a treatable one.

The recently commercialized gene tests for adult-onset disorders such as Alzheimer's disease and some cancers are the subject of most of the debate over gene testing. These tests are targeted to healthy (presymptomatic) people who are identified as being at high risk because of a strong family medical history for the disorder. The tests give only a probability for developing the disorder. One of the most serious limitations of these susceptibility tests is the difficulty in interpreting a positive result because some people who carry a disease-associated mutation never develop the disease. Scientists believe that these mutations may work together with other, unknown mutations or with environmental factors to cause disease.

A limitation of all medical testing is the possibility for laboratory errors. These might be due to sample misidentification, contamination of the chemicals used for testing, or other factors. Many in the medical establishment feel that uncertainties surrounding test interpretation, the current lack of available medical options for these diseases, the tests' potential for provoking anxiety, and risks for discrimination and social stigmatization could outweigh the benefits of testing.

For What Diseases Are Gene Tests Available?

Some gene tests available as of 1998 from clinical genetics laboratories approved by New York State follow. Test names and a description of the diseases or symptoms appear in parentheses. Susceptibility tests, noted by an asterisk, provide only an estimated risk for developing the disorder.

Some currently available DNA-based gene tests:

- Alpha-1-antitrypsin deficiency (AAT; emphysema and liver disease)

- Amyotrophic lateral sclerosis (ALS; Lou Gehrig's Disease; progressive motor function loss leading to paralysis and death)

- Alzheimer's disease* (APOE; late-onset variety of senile dementia)

- Ataxia telangiectasia (AT; progressive brain disorder resulting in loss of muscle control and cancers)

- Gaucher disease (GD; enlarged liver and spleen, bone degeneration)

- Inherited breast and ovarian cancer* (BRCA 1 and 2; early-onset tumors of breasts and ovaries)

- Hereditary nonpolyposis colon cancer* (CA; early-onset tumors of colon and sometimes other organs)

- Charcot-Marie-Tooth (CMT; loss of feeling in ends of limbs)

- Congenital adrenal hyperplasia (CAH; hormone deficiency; ambiguous genitalia and male pseudohermaphroditism)

- Cystic fibrosis (CF; disease of lung and pancreas resulting in thick mucous accumulations and chronic infections)

- Duchenne muscular dystrophy/Becker muscular dystrophy (DMD; severe to mild muscle wasting, deterioration, weakness)

- Dystonia (DYT; muscle rigidity, repetitive twisting movements)

- Fanconi anemia, group C (FA; anemia, leukemia, skeletal deformities)

- Factor V-Leiden (FVL; blood-clotting disorder)

- Fragile X syndrome (FRAX; leading cause of inherited mental retardation)

- Hemophilia A and B (HEMA and HEMB; bleeding disorders)
- Huntington's disease (HD; usually midlife onset; progressive, lethal, degenerative neurological disease)
- Myotonic dystrophy (MD; progressive muscle weakness; most common form of adult muscular dystrophy)
- Neurofibromatosis type 1 (NF1; multiple benign nervous system tumors that can be disfiguring; cancers)
- Phenylketonuria (PKU; progressive mental retardation due to missing enzyme; correctable by diet)
- Adult Polycystic Kidney Disease (APKD; kidney failure and liver disease)
- Prader Willi/Angelman syndromes (PW/A; decreased motor skills, cognitive impairment, early death)
- Sickle cell disease (SS; blood cell disorder; chronic pain and infections)
- Spinocerebellar ataxia, type 1 (SCA1; involuntary muscle movements, reflex disorders, explosive speech)
- Spinal muscular atrophy (SMA; severe, usually lethal progressive muscle-wasting disorder in children)
- Thalassemias (THAL; anemias—reduced red blood cell levels)
- Tay-Sachs Disease (TS; fatal neurological disease of early childhood; seizures, paralysis)

Chapter 11

Preparing Children for Test Procedures

Definition

Proper preparation for a test or procedure that can reduce your child's anxiety, encourage cooperation, and help develop coping skills.

Research has shown that preparatory interventions are effective in reducing some signs of distress in children such as crying or resisting the procedure; this led to other findings suggesting that with preparation children report less pain and exhibit physiologic signs showing less distress.

Before the test, know that your child probably will cry, and restraints may be used. You can try the use of play in demonstrating what will happen during the test and in discovering your child's concerns. Explaining the procedure will also be of value in reducing your child's anxiety. Make sure your child understands that the procedure is not a punishment, and focus on the pleasurable things that will happen after the test. But the most important way you can help your child through this procedure is by being there, and showing you care.

Pre-Procedure Preparation

Limit your explanations about the procedure to 10 or 15 minutes, because preschoolers have a limited attention span. Any preparation should take place directly before the test or procedure.

"Preschooler Test/Procedure Preparation," © 2001 A.D.A.M, Inc. Reprinted with permission.

Here are some general guidelines for preparing your child for a test or procedure:

- Explain the procedure in language your child understands, and use concrete terms, avoiding abstract terminology.

- Make sure your child understands the exact body part to be involved and that the procedure will be limited to that area.

- If the procedure affects part of the body that serves a noticeable function (such as speech, hearing, or urination), explain how the procedure will affect or not affect the function.

- While talking about the procedure with your child, avoid words that have more than one meaning.

- Give your child permission to yell, cry, or otherwise express any pain verbally.

- If you think your child has not understood something you are explaining, ask if he or she understands, and be certain that you define all new terms in simple language.

- To the best of your ability, describe how the test will feel.

- Allow your child to practice different positions or movements that will be required for the particular test or procedure, such as the fetal position for a lumbar puncture.

- Save topics or subjects that you think will cause your child the most stress for last.

- Be honest with your child about discomfort that may be felt, but don't dwell on the topic, since this could instill undue concern in your child.

- Stress the benefits of the procedure and anything that the child may find pleasurable afterwards, such as feeling better, or going home.

- Explain that the procedure is not a punishment.

Play Preparation

Play and third-person communication can be wonderful and revealing ways of demonstrating the procedure for your child, and identifying his or her concerns. This technique needs to be individualized for each child, and most health care facilities that are oriented toward children, such as a children's hospital, use this same technique to prepare your child. Given the age of your child, this type of interaction may not increase his or her level of understanding, but each child is unique in abilities. This type of communication can take some practice.

Children asked direct questions about their feelings often avoid answering or are elusive. Of course, some children are more than happy to share their feelings with you, but as anxiety and fear increase it is not uncommon for a child to withdraw.

Most young children have an object of importance they keep close to them. This object or toy can be a tool for a type of interaction called third-party communication. It is less threatening for your child to communicate concerns through the toy or object than to express them directly. For example, take a 4-year old girl who is clearly afraid, has a doll named Becky, and is going to have her blood drawn. You could look at the girl and tell her that Becky looks like she might feel afraid. Your child may or may not share those feelings at this point, and additional questioning along this line may be necessary.

The same object or doll can be a productive tool for explaining the procedure. Children of this age are very concrete thinkers. Concrete thinking involves taking everything literally, and an inability to make deductions or generalizations. For example, if you say you feel fine to a concrete thinker, he or she may interpret that by thinking your feeling or touch sensation is intact. For younger children who have a limited vocabulary, concrete thinking means they need visual examples, and it is helpful if they can experiment themselves.

Once you are familiar with the procedure through information obtained from your health care provider, briefly demonstrate on the toy or object what your child will experience during the procedure. For example, show positioning, bandages, stethoscopes, cleaning the skin, how incisions are made, injections are given, or IVs are inserted. Medical toys are available, or you can ask whether your health care provider can share some of the noninvasive items you need for the demonstration and play period. After your demonstration, allow your child to play with some of the noninvasive items. The way he or she plays can also give you clues regarding concerns and fears.

Regardless of the test or procedure performed, your child will probably cry. This is a normal response to the strange environment, unfamiliar people, restraints, and separation from you. Your child will cry more for these reasons than because the test or procedure is uncomfortable. Knowing this from the onset may help relieve some of your anxiety about what to expect. Having specific information about the test may further reduce your anxiety. For more information please see the appropriate test.

Why Restraints?

Your child may be restrained by hand or with physical devices. Children of this age may be unwilling or unable to follow the necessary requests of your health care provider, so restraints may be used to ensure your child's safety.

Most tests and procedures require extreme accuracy to obtain the desired outcome, whether that be correct placement of an IV, or accurate test results, and in some cases, to avoid injuring the child.

For example, if your child needs an x-ray, clear test results require there be no movement. Furthermore, in radiological and nuclear studies while the films are taken, all staff temporarily leave the room. In these situations, restraints are used for your child's safety. If a venipuncture is performed to obtain a blood sample or start an IV, restraints are important in preventing injury to your child. If your child moves while the needle is being inserted, trauma could damage the venous system, bone, tissue, or nerves.

Most tests and procedures require extreme accuracy to obtain the desired outcome, whether to place an IV correctly, ensure accurate test results, or to avoid injuring the child.

Your health care provider will use every means to ensure the safety and comfort of your baby. Besides restraints, other measures include medications, observation, and monitors.

During the Procedure

Your presence helps your child during the procedure, especially if the procedure allows you to maintain physical contact. If the procedure is performed at the hospital or your health care provider's office, you will most likely be given the opportunity to be present.

If you are not asked to be by your child's side and would like to be, ask your health care provider if this is possible. If you think you may become ill or anxious, consider keeping your distance but remaining in your child's line of vision. If you are not able to be present, leaving a familiar object with your child may be comforting.

Other considerations:

- Ask your health care provider to limit the number of strangers entering and leaving the room during the procedure, since this can raise anxiety.

- Ask that the care provider who has spent the most time with your child perform the procedure.

- Ask that anesthetics be used where appropriate to reduce the level of discomfort your child will feel.

- Ask that painful procedures not be performed in the hospital bed, so that the child does not come to associate pain with the hospital room.

- Imitate the behavior you or your health care provider need the child to do, such as opening the mouth.

The information provided herein should not be used for diagnosis or treatment of any medical condition. A licensed physician should be consulted for diagnosis and treatment of any and all medical conditions.

Part Two

The Three Most Common Movement Disorders in the U.S.

Chapter 12

Essential Tremor

Of the 20-plus different kinds of tremor, essential tremor is the most common. There are medical treatments that can help people with tremor live a fuller life, but only a small percentage of those with this condition get medical help.

There are a number of things you can do to minimize the degree to which ET interferes with life and work. Here are a few practical suggestions:

- Become informed about your condition and learn as much as you can about living with ET.

- Instead of restricting your life because of what others may think, explain your condition simply and honestly when you meet new people.

- If your child has ET, you may want to talk to teachers in person about the neurological basis for symptoms.

- Find ways to reduce stress and learn some relaxation techniques.

- Avoid things that may worsen tremor, such as caffeine and certain prescription medications.

This chapter includes "Coping with Essential Tremor: Welcome," "What Is Tremor?" "What Is Essential Tremor?" and "Frequently Asked Questions," from www.essentialtremor.org © 2000 The International Essential Tremor Foundation, reprinted with permission.

- Contact IETF for an information packet or information about joining or starting a support group for ET.

Frequently Asked Questions about Essential Tremor

What Causes Essential Tremor (ET)?

Essential tremor is due to abnormal communication between certain areas of the brain, including the cerebellum, thalamus, and brain stem.

In the majority of people with ET, the tremor seems to be inherited as an autosomal dominant trait. This means that each child of a parent with ET has approximately a 50% chance of inheriting a gene that causes ET. However, not everyone who inherits a gene develops symptoms. Some people have ET and do not have a family history of tremor, suggesting the possibility of other causes. Researchers have already located two genes that predispose to ET and are currently trying to locate others. However, at this time, there is no generic test for ET. Identifying genes may allow scientists to find a cure.

At What Age Does ET Start?

Though ET may first appear at any age between childhood and old age, onset is rare before the age of 10. Most commonly, onset is after age 40, but it can occur in younger people. Men and women are affected equally, and in the majority of cases there is a family history of ET. Life expectancy is no different for people with ET.

Does ET Worsen with Age?

No one can predict how much your tremor will worsen with time. The course of ET is variable and may be progressive over many decades.

What Does It Take to Diagnose ET?

Doctors who are trained to evaluate tremor can accurately diagnose ET on the basis of the symptoms and a neurological examination. So far, there are no specific blood, urine, or other tests for ET. Your doctor may want to investigate other causes of tremor such as thyroid disease, caffeine excess, or medication side effects. During your physical exam, your doctor will be gathering as much information as possible about your tremor. Here are some questions you may be asked:

- What body part is affected?

- How long have you had the tremor?

- Did it come on suddenly?

- What makes your tremor worse?

- What makes your tremor better?

- Do you drink a lot of caffeine-containing or alcoholic drinks?

- Do any family members have tremor?

- Have you ever had a head injury?

- Does alcohol temporarily reduce the tremor?

- Does the tremor worsen when you do certain tasks or when you're under emotional stress?

- Does the tremor disappear during sleep?

- What medications are you taking? (Certain drugs may cause tremor, so it's a good idea to bring a list of the medications you are taking or the actual pill containers themselves.

Does It Help to Look at the Brain?

A brain scan is not required to diagnose ET. Your doctor might order a magnetic resonance imaging (MRI) scan or a computerized axial tomography (CAT) scan if there is a suspicion of some other cause of tremor. ET does not have associated abnormality on routine scans.

Is All Shaking Caused by ET?

Many things cause tremor, and not all tremors are ET. There are more than 20 kinds of tremors. For instance, excessive caffeine, alcohol withdrawal, problems with thyroid or copper metabolism, or the use of certain medications may cause tremor. A major difference between ET and other tremor types is that in ET tremor is the only symptom, and muscle tone, strength, and balance are not usually affected.

What Else Causes Tremor?

Other causes of tremor include:

- Enhanced physiologic tremor

- Parkinson's disease
- Dystonic tremor
- Tremor due to medications

Because tremor is a feature of so many conditions, ET can be mistaken for something else. Some people have both ET and another disorder that causes tremor. ET is most often confused with some of the conditions listed previously, especially Parkinson's disease (PD). PD causes a tremor that occurs at rest, not action. It also causes progressive slowness, stiffness, and loss of balance. Medications for PD do not help ET symptoms. Note that many prescriptions, over-the-counter, and illicit drugs, as well as some herbal remedies, can cause or worsen tremor. Tell your doctor about all the medications you are taking.

What Medications Do Help?

If you have mild ET, you may not need treatment. There is no evidence that early treatment stops or slows the natural progression of ET symptoms. With adequate knowledge, many people learn ways to live well with ET. If possible, you should be taken off any medications that may be aggravating tremor.

If ET is interfering with your ability to work or perform daily tasks, or you find it socially disabling, you may want to consider available therapies. It is important to have realistic expectations for therapy. At present, there is no cure for ET. For the oral medications, a 50% reduction of tremor severity is considered good. The goals of treatment are to:

- Reduce tremor severity
- Improve ability to function
- Decrease social handicap

Achieving these goals can sometimes take time, so be patient. While almost two-thirds of people with ET benefit from medical therapies, your doctor may have to try two or three different medicines before finding the one that works best for you.

The main medications used to treat ET are propranolol (Inderal) and primidone (Mysoline). Both can be quite effective.

Propranolol (Inderal): Propranolol is in a class of drugs called beta-blockers. Propranolol has been used for many years, primarily for reducing high blood pressure. It is not clear exactly how it works in treating essential tremor. Other beta-blockers may also be used. Features of propranolol include the following.

- You may experience tremor reduction 1-2 hours after taking a single 10-40 mg dose of the short-acting formulation. This effect usually wears off in about 4 hours.

- Propranolol may be prescribed to be taken as needed, or on a daily basis. A once-daily long-acting preparation is available.

- 60% of people with ET are helped by propranolol. It is most effective against hand tremor and may be effective for tremor of the head, voice, and tongue.

- Individual response is variable. Complete tremor reduction is rare.

- Side effects are usually mild and are more frequent at higher doses (more than 120 mg/day of propranolol). The main side effects are decreased pulse rate and blood pressure. Less common side effects are fatigue, depression, impotence, nausea, weight gain, rash, and diarrhea. If you experience unpleasant side effects, be sure to tell your doctor. Often the dosage or drug can be changed.

- If you have heart failure, diabetes mellitus, or asthma, talk to your general medical doctor prior to taking propranolol. Do not abruptly stop this medication without first consulting with your physician.

Primidone (Mysoline): Primidone is an epilepsy medicine that was unexpectedly found to reduce tremor. It is now used widely for tremor reduction. Some features of primidone are:

- Approximately 60% of people with ET are helped by primidone. Benefit usually persists for 24 hours for each dose.

- Dizziness, fatigue, drowsiness, and flu-like symptoms—most of which subside after a couple of days. You can reduce the chance of these symptoms by starting with an extremely small dose at bedtime. If you experience more serious side effects, tell your doctor.

- One quarter of the 50 mg tablet (12.5 mg) or small amounts of the pediatric elixir may be appropriate as initial dose. Only branded Mysoline is available as a 50 mg tablet and pediatric suspension.

- Although primidone may have more initial side effects than propranolol, there are few long-term problems, and primidone may be used successfully for many years. Occasional dose adjustments may be needed.

Combination and other therapies: If your tremor is not well controlled by a beta-blocker or by primidone alone, you may experience better results when you take both medicines together. If combination therapy is not helpful, your doctor may then recommend one of the benzodiazepines such as clonazepam (Klonopin), diazepam (Valium), alprazolam (Xanax), or lorazepam (Ativan). The most common side effect is drowsiness. There is a risk of physical dependence and withdrawal. Although no scientific support is available, other drugs may be used.

Botulinum toxin injections: If medications fail, another therapy may be tried that involves injections of Botulinum toxin into muscles. Botulinum toxin injections have been useful in the treatment of some patients with head and voice tremors. The toxin must be placed into target muscles by a trained specialist, and repeat injections may be needed. Transient weakness of the injected muscles is a potential side effect. This treatment can be expensive, so check with your insurance provider regarding coverage.

What about Thalamic Stimulations and Other Surgery?

If treatment with medications is not effective and ET is very disabling or is putting your livelihood at risk, your doctor may suggest a surgical technique, such as thalamotomy or thalamic stimulation (Activa tremor control therapy). Surgical procedures are expensive but may be beneficial.

Thalamotomy: This is a surgical procedure that involves making a small hole (the size of a dried pea) in a part of the brain called the thalamus. A surgery on one side of the brain produces its effect on the opposite side of the body. The surgery destroys the faulty circuit or brain cells that modulate tremor. At the present time, thalamotomy surgery on both sides of the brain is not recommended as there is an unacceptable risk of loss of speech or other problems.

Approximately 80% of patients have experienced improvement in tremor after this procedure. When effective, medications may be reduced or even discontinued. The procedure may be especially beneficial for people with severe hand, arm, or leg tremors that do not respond to medication. Approximately 1 in 20 people suffers some complication from surgery, 1 in 100 people suffers stroke or death. You should discuss these issues with your neurologist and neurosurgeon.

Thalamic stimulation: Thalamic stimulation is an alternative to thalamotomy. It involves implanting an electrode (a fine wire) deep in the center of the brain. The electrode is connected to a stimulation device, similar to a pacemaker, which is placed under the skin below the collarbone. By sending electrical currents through the electrode, you can interrupt communication between tremor cells. Tremor reduction occurs within seconds of activation and can be dramatic. Significant or complete tremor reduction occurred in approximately 80% of people with this procedure. Tremor medications can often be reduced or even stopped.

The main advantages of this procedure are that implantation on both sides of the brain is possible, the device can be adjusted for optimal effect, and it may be removed, which allows you to keep your options open in case new therapies develop. The risks are similar to thalamotomy. While the surgery is expensive, the procedure and device are FDA-approved and are covered by most insurance providers.

What Other Treatments Are There?

Though there is no evidence that so-called alternative therapies are helpful for ET, people have tried a variety of treatments. No good scientific studies are available to encourage the use of alternative therapies. Always talk to your doctor before starting any alternative therapies. While some herbs that induce relaxation may be helpful, others, such as a Chinese herb called ma huang, can worsen tremor. Many people have tried acupuncture, hypnosis, and massage therapy. People whose tremor worsens with stress or anxiety may find biofeedback helpful. Others have found physical and occupational therapy to be helpful in terms of providing suggestions for using wrist weights, plate guards, and other adaptive devices. These devices can provide considerable benefit in activities of daily living.

What about Pregnancy and ET?

Tremor severity may fluctuate during pregnancy and after delivery. You should discuss the use of ET medications with your physician before getting pregnant, as some medications put the developing baby at risk.

How about Alcohol and ET?

Adults with ET often notice that consumption of alcohol reduces their tremors for 1-2 hours. While it is true that alcohol can temporarily reduce tremor, it may not be an appropriate form of treatment. Use of alcohol to reduce tremor should be discussed with your physician.

Additional Information

International Essential Tremor Foundation
7046 W. 105th Street
Overland Park, KS 66212-1803
Toll-Free: 888-387-3667
Tel: 913-341-3880
Fax: 913-341-1296
Website: www.essentialtremor.org
E-mail: staff@essentialtremor.org

The International Essential Tremor Foundation can be a valuable resource, whether you're seeking the latest research data, seeking medical help, checking out answers to frequently asked questions or looking for a support group of like-minded people in your area.

Chapter 13

Parkinson's Disease

Parkinson's disease may be one of the most baffling and complex of the neurological disorders. Its cause remains a mystery but research in this area is active, with new and intriguing findings constantly being reported.

Parkinson's disease was first described in 1817 by James Parkinson, a British physician who published a paper on what he called "the shaking palsy." In this paper, he set forth the major symptoms of the disease that would later bear his name. For the next century and a half, scientists pursued the causes and treatment of the disease. They defined its range of symptoms, distribution among the population, and prospects for cure.

In the early 1960s, researchers identified a fundamental brain defect that is a hallmark of the disease: the loss of brain cells that produce a chemical—dopamine—that helps direct muscle activity. This discovery pointed to the first successful treatment for Parkinson's disease and suggested ways of devising new and even more effective therapies.

Society pays an enormous price for Parkinson's disease. According to the National Parkinson Foundation, each patient spends an average

Excerpts from "Parkinson's Disease—Hope Through Research," National Institute of Neurological Disorders and Stroke (NINDS), reviewed July 1, 2001; "Difficulty Walking in Parkinson Disease," by Alireza Minagar MD and Abraham Lieberman MD, © 2000 National Parkinson Foundation, Inc., reprinted with permission; and "Researchers Find Genetic Links for Late-Onset Parkinson's Disease," by Natalie Frazin, news release, Wednesday, December 19, 2001, National Institute of Neurological Disorders and Stroke (NINDS).

of $2,500 a year for medications. After factoring in office visits, Social Security payments, nursing home expenditures, and lost income, the total cost to the Nation is estimated to exceed $5.6 billion annually.

What Is Parkinson's Disease?

Parkinson's disease belongs to a group of conditions called motor system disorders. The four primary symptoms are tremor or trembling in hands, arms, legs, jaw, and face; rigidity or stiffness of the limbs and trunk; bradykinesia or slowness of movement; and postural instability or impaired balance and coordination. As these symptoms become more pronounced, patients may have difficulty walking, talking, or completing other simple tasks.

The disease is both chronic, meaning it persists over a long period of time, and progressive, meaning its symptoms grow worse over time. It is not contagious nor is it usually inherited—that is, it does not pass directly from one family member or generation to the next.

Parkinson's disease is the most common form of parkinsonism, the name for a group of disorders with similar features. These disorders share the four primary symptoms described, and all are the result of the loss of dopamine-producing brain cells. Parkinson's disease is also called primary parkinsonism or idiopathic Parkinson's disease; idiopathic is a term describing a disorder for which no cause has yet been found. In the other forms of parkinsonism either the cause is known or suspected or the disorder occurs as a secondary effect of another, primary neurological disorder.

What Causes the Disease?

Parkinson's disease occurs when certain nerve cells, or neurons, in an area of the brain known as the substantia nigra die or become impaired. Normally, these neurons produce an important brain chemical known as dopamine. Dopamine is a chemical messenger responsible for transmitting signals between the substantia nigra and the next relay station of the brain, the corpus striatum, to produce smooth, purposeful muscle activity. Loss of dopamine causes the nerve cells of the striatum to fire out of control, leaving patients unable to direct or control their movements in a normal manner. Studies have shown that Parkinson's patients have a loss of 80 percent or more of dopamine-producing cells in the substantia nigra. The cause of this cell death or impairment is not known but significant findings by research scientists continue to yield fascinating new clues to the disease.

One theory holds that free radicals—unstable and potentially damaging molecules generated by normal chemical reactions in the body—may contribute to nerve cell death thereby leading to Parkinson's disease. Free radicals are unstable because they lack one electron; in an attempt to replace this missing electron, free radicals react with neighboring molecules (especially metals such as iron), in a process called oxidation. Oxidation is thought to cause damage to tissues, including neurons. Normally, free radical damage is kept under control by antioxidants, chemicals that protect cells from this damage. Evidence that oxidative mechanisms may cause or contribute to Parkinson's disease includes the finding that patients with the disease have increased brain levels of iron, especially in the substantia nigra, and decreased levels of ferritin, which serves as a protective mechanism by chelating or forming a ring around the iron, and isolating it.

Some scientists have suggested that Parkinson's disease may occur when either an external or an internal toxin selectively destroys dopaminergic neurons. An environmental risk factor such as exposure to pesticides or a toxin in the food supply is an example of the kind of external trigger that could hypothetically cause Parkinson's disease. The theory is based on the fact that there are a number of toxins, such as 1-methyl-4-phenyl-1,2,3,6,-tetrahydropyridine (MPTP), and neuroleptic drugs, known to induce parkinsonian symptoms in humans. So far, however, no research has provided conclusive proof that a toxin is the cause of the disease.

A relatively new theory explores the role of genetic factors in the development of Parkinson's disease. Fifteen to twenty percent of Parkinson's patients have a close relative who has experienced parkinsonian symptoms (such as a tremor). Several causative genes have been identified, usually causing young-onset parkinsonism. Mutations in the gene for the protein alpha-synuclein, located on chromosome 4 results in autosomal dominant parkinsonism. The function of this protein is not known. The most commonly occurring genetic defect affects the gene for the protein called parkin on chromosome 6. Mutations in this gene result in autosomal recessive parkinsonism that is slowly progressive with onset before the age of 40. After studies in animals showed that MPTP interferes with the function of mitochondria within nerve cells, investigators became interested in the possibility that impairment in mitochondrial DNA may be the cause of Parkinson's disease, and families with maternal inheritance of parkinsonism, suggesting mitochondrial DNA defects, are being actively investigated. Mitochondria are essential organelles found in all animal cells that convert the energy in food into fuel for the cells.

Yet another theory proposes that Parkinson's disease occurs when, for unknown reasons, the normal, age-related wearing away of dopamine-producing neurons accelerates in certain individuals. This theory is supported by the knowledge that loss of antioxidative protective mechanisms is associated with both Parkinson's disease and increasing age.

Many researchers believe that a combination of these four mechanisms—oxidative damage, environmental toxins, genetic predisposition, and accelerated aging—may ultimately be shown to cause the disease.

Researchers Find Genetic Links for Late-Onset Parkinson's Disease, by Natalie Frazin

Recent studies provide strong evidence that genetic factors influence susceptibility to the common, late-onset form of Parkinson's disease (PD). The findings improve scientists' understanding of how PD develops and may lead to new treatments or even ways of preventing the disease.

Until 1996, few people believed there was a genetic component to PD. The prevailing evidence suggested that environmental factors were largely or entirely to blame. Since then, studies have identified a clear genetic basis for two forms of PD that affect people younger than 50: one that affects a few families from Europe and another called autosomal recessive juvenile parkinsonism (ARJP) that affects some families in Japan. The first disorder is linked to a mutation in the gene for a protein called alpha-synuclein, and the second is linked to mutations in the gene for a protein called parkin. However, the role of genetics in the common, late-onset form of PD has remained controversial. In fact, several studies of twins have suggested that genes do not influence this form of PD. The new studies challenge that earlier work and suggest that multiple genes play a role in susceptibility to the disease.

One of the recent studies,[1] led by Margaret A. Pericak-Vance, Ph.D., of the Center for Human Genetics at Duke University Medical Center in Durham, North Carolina, and funded by the National Institute of Neurological Disorders and Stroke (NINDS), looked for a relationship between specific genetic markers and PD in 870 people from 174 families in which more than one person had been diagnosed with the disorder. They found evidence that five distinct regions, on chromosomes 5, 6, 8, 9, and 17, were associated with susceptibility to PD. The chromosome 6 region contains the parkin gene, which was previously associated only with early-onset PD. The familial link to chromosome 9 was found primarily in patients who do not respond to levodopa (a common treatment for PD) and the marker is located near a gene that is altered in another disorder called idiopathic torsion dystonia. This suggests that there may be a relationship between PD and dystonia. The strongest genetic association in families with late-onset PD was on chromosome 17, near the gene for a protein called tau. Tau is a component of neurofibrillary tangles, a specific brain abnormality found in other neurodegenerative diseases, including Alzheimer's disease, frontotemporal dementia with parkinsonism (FTDP), and progressive supranuclear palsy (PSP). Because people with PD do not have neurofibrillary tangles, researchers did not previously suspect tau as a factor in the disease. However, tau is important to normal cell function and it is possible that even minor abnormalities in how it works may lead to cell death, the researchers say.

A second NINDS-funded study,[2] led by Jeffrey M. Vance of Duke University, looked at specific variations within the tau gene and found evidence that three of the variations were linked to increased susceptibility for late-onset PD. A third study,[3] conducted by scientists at deCODE genetics, Inc., of Reykjavik, Iceland, looked at 51 Icelandic families with late-onset PD and linked the disease in these families to a region on chromosome 1.

Previous studies have suggested that other genes, including ubiquitin carboxy-terminal hydrolase (UCH-L1) and genes on chromosomes X, 1, 2, and 4, influence susceptibility to PD in some families. It also is possible that additional, still-unidentified genes may play a role in specific populations, the researchers say.

Knowledge of the genes that influence PD is potentially useful in a number of ways. For example, testing people for specific genes may help to identify subtypes of PD and lead to a better understanding of how to treat different groups of patients. "We could be talking about Parkinson's diseases—not just one disease," says William K. Scott, Ph.D., of Duke. Certain drugs and other treatments may be more or less effective in people with specific subtypes of PD.

The researchers stress that the genes linked to the late-onset form of PD are susceptibility genes—they do not cause the disorder all by themselves. Environmental factors probably interact with these genetic variations in ways that cause the disorder in some people.

While it is still unclear how the different genes may interact with the environment to cause PD, each identified factor represents an important piece in the puzzle, the researchers say. Parkinson's is a complex disease, and each genetic factor could have many effects and interactions with other genes that may influence the development and symptoms of the disorder. "We've got the outside of the puzzle—now we need to fill in the middle," says Dr. Pericak-Vance. Researchers think the various genes and environmental factors that influence PD may all affect a single pathway, or series of biochemical interactions, that lead to the disease. Understanding the steps of the pathway should help researchers develop strategies to interrupt the process and lead to new treatments or even ways to prevent the devastating disease.

References

1.   Scott WK, Nance MA, Watts RL, et. al. "Complete genomic screen in Parkinson disease: evidence for multiple genes." *Journal of the American Medical Association* 2001 Nov 14;286(18):2239-44.

2.   Martin ER, Scott WK, Nance MA, et. al. "Association of single-nucleotide polymorphisms of the tau gene with late-onset Parkinson disease." *Journal of the American Medical Association* 2001 Nov 14;286(18):2245-50.

3.   Hicks A, Petursson H, Jonsson T, et. al. "A susceptibility gene for late-onset idiopathic Parkinson's disease successfully mapped." *American Journal of Human Genetics* Oct 2001, 69, Abstract 123:200 (Supplement).

Who Gets Parkinson's Disease?

About 50,000 Americans are diagnosed with Parkinson's disease each year, with more than half a million Americans affected at any one time. Getting an accurate count of the number of cases may be impossible however, because many people in the early stages of the disease assume their symptoms are the result of normal aging and do not seek help from a physician. Also, diagnosis is sometimes difficult and uncertain because other conditions may produce some of the symptoms of Parkinson's disease. People with Parkinson's disease may be told by their doctors that they have other disorders or, conversely, people with similar diseases may be initially diagnosed as having Parkinson's disease.

Parkinson's disease strikes men and women in almost equal numbers and it knows no social, economic, or geographic boundaries. Some studies show that African-Americans and Asians are less likely than whites to develop Parkinson's disease. Scientists have not been able to explain this apparent lower incidence in certain populations. It is reasonable to assume, however, that all people have a similar probability of developing the disease.

Age, however, clearly correlates with the onset of symptoms. Parkinson's disease is a disease of late middle age, usually affecting people over the age of 50. The average age of onset is 60 years. However, some physicians have reportedly noticed more cases of early-onset Parkinson's disease in the past several years, and some have estimated that 5 to 10 percent of patients are under the age of 40.

What Are the Early Symptoms?

Early symptoms of Parkinson's disease are subtle and occur gradually. Patients may be tired or notice a general malaise. Some may feel a little shaky or have difficulty getting out of a chair. They may notice that they speak too softly or that their handwriting looks cramped and spidery. They may lose track of a word or thought, or they may feel irritable or depressed for no apparent reason. This very early period may last a long time before the more classic and obvious symptoms appear.

Friends or family members may be the first to notice changes. They may see that the person's face lacks expression and animation (known as masked face) or that the person remains in a certain position for a long time or does not move an arm or leg normally. Perhaps they see that the person seems stiff, unsteady, and unusually slow.

As the disease progresses, the shaking, or tremor, that affects the majority of Parkinson's patients may begin to interfere with daily activities. Patients may not be able to hold utensils steady or may find that the shaking makes reading a newspaper difficult. Parkinson's tremor may become worse when the patient is relaxed. A few seconds after the hands are rested on a table, for instance, the shaking is most pronounced. For most patients, tremor is usually the symptom that causes them to seek medical help.

What Are the Major Symptoms of the Disease?

Parkinson's disease does not affect everyone the same way. In some people the disease progresses quickly, in others it does not. Although some people become severely disabled, others experience only minor motor disruptions. Tremor is the major symptom for some patients, while for others tremor is only a minor complaint and different symptoms are more troublesome.

- **Tremor** associated with Parkinson's disease has a characteristic appearance. Typically, the tremor takes the form of a rhythmic back-and-forth motion of the thumb and forefinger at three beats per second. This is sometimes called pill rolling. Tremor usually begins in a hand, although sometimes a foot or the jaw is affected first. It is most obvious when the hand is at rest or when a person is under stress. In three out of four patients, the tremor may affect only one part or side of the body, especially during the early stages of the disease. Later it may become more general. Tremor is rarely disabling and it usually disappears during sleep or improves with intentional movement.

- **Rigidity,** or a resistance to movement, affects most parkinsonian patients. A major principle of body movement is that all muscles have an opposing muscle. Movement is possible not just because one muscle becomes more active, but because the opposing muscle relaxes. In Parkinson's disease, rigidity comes about when, in response to signals from the brain, the delicate balance of opposing muscles is disturbed. The muscles remain constantly tensed and contracted so that the person aches or feels stiff or weak. The rigidity becomes obvious when another person tries to move the patient's arm, which will move only in ratchet-like or short, jerky movements known as cogwheel rigidity.

- **Bradykinesia,** or the slowing down and loss of spontaneous and automatic movement, is particularly frustrating because it is unpredictable. One moment the patient can move easily. The next moment he or she may need help. This may well be the most disabling and distressing symptom of the disease because the patient cannot rapidly perform routine movements. Activities once performed quickly and easily—such as washing or dressing—may take several hours.

- **Postural instability,** or impaired balance and coordination, causes patients to develop a forward or backward lean and to fall easily. When bumped from the front or when starting to walk, patients with a backward lean have a tendency to step backwards, which is known as retropulsion. Postural instability can cause patients to have a stooped posture in which the head is bowed and the shoulders are drooped. As the disease progresses, walking may be affected. Patients may halt in mid-stride and freeze in place, possibly even toppling over. Or patients may walk with a series of quick, small steps as if hurrying forward to keep balance. This is known as festination.

106

Difficulty Walking in Parkinson Disease, by Alireza Minagar MD and Abraham Lieberman

Symptoms of Parkinson Disease

The main symptoms of Parkinson Disease (PD) are slowness and lack of movement (called bradykinesia), rigidity of the arms, legs, and trunk, tremor, difficulty walking, and poor balance. Difficulty walking and poor balance are the most disabling symptoms. Difficulty walking may occur with good balance. And difficulty walking may occur with poor balance. The parts of the brain that control walking and balance are separate each from the other—which is why difficulty walking and poor balance may or may not occur together. If difficulty walking and poor balance occur together then the difficulty walking is worse.

Difficulty Walking

In PD, difficulty walking may occur early or late in the illness. The difficulty walking consists of the person taking short steps, often the heel of one foot not clearing the toe of the other foot. Occasionally the short steps run together and the person runs forward (called antero-pulsion), or rarely, the person runs backward (called retropulsion). The short steps result from slowness and lack of movement of the legs.

The difficulty walking also consists of the person not swinging one or both arms. Swinging the arms helps maintain balance and aids in propelling the feet forward. The lack of arm swing results from rigidity of the arms and/or from loss of what are called associated movements. Associated movements are programmed into our brains so that when we put a foot forward the arm moves as well. These movements may be lost in Parkinson disease. The combination of short steps and lack of arm swing make walking worse than short steps alone. The short steps and lack of arm swing usually respond to Sinemet (levodopa/carbidopa) a long-acting dopamine agonist such as Mirapex or Permax.

Stooped Posture

Some people with PD develop a stooped posture. In a few people the stoop is so great they walk with their eyes glued to the floor. The stooped posture results from either:

1. The center-of-gravity being thrown forward with the person then stooping to catch-up.

2.   Or from a constant, uneven and powerful pull of the muscles of the front of the spine over those of the back of the spine.

The stooping itself may result in difficulty walking. The spine is a fulcrum around which the hip, thigh, and buttock muscles generate the power needed for walking. If the spine bends or stoops forward, the hip, thigh, and buttock muscles lose power. To demonstrate this:

1.   Stand and bend at the waist until your eyes stare at the floor.

2.   Walk while bending at the waist with your eyes on the floor. You'll find that you generate less power with your hip, thigh, and buttock muscles and that you're forced to walk with short steps.

The stooping may be partly corrected by Sinemet and/or a long-acting dopamine agonist such as Mirapex or Permax. The stooping must also be treated with corrective exercises tailored to each person and performed daily. The exercises may consist of the following:

1.   Reaching your hands over your head, grabbing and holding onto a "chinning" bar and slowing pulling yourself up without actually lifting your feet off the ground. This stretches the muscles of your spine. This exercise should be done 10 or more times at least twice a day. They should, initially, be done under the supervision of a physical therapist.

2.   Standing with your arms behind your back, your right hand grabbing your left wrist and pulling down. This movement forces your shoulders-up and straightens your spine. This downward pull of your right hand on your left wrist should be done 20 or more times. And should be done at least three times a day: a total of 60 for the day.

3.   Sitting on a stationery bicycle and pedaling (not fast) for 15 minutes a days while you fix your eyes on a picture or TV screen that's above eye level. This forces your shoulders up and straightens your spine.

Canes, Walkers, Walking Sticks

If you walk with a cane or a walker and the cane is too low, or the handlebars of the walker too low, this will force you to bend—causing you to take short steps. Whatever level of support you gain from the cane or walker is defeated by the bending your spine.

If you need a cane, try using a walking stick instead. The stick should be as high as your shoulder, you should hold the stick with your hand so there's a straight line from your shoulder, past your elbow to your hand. Holding a walking stick in this way forces your shoulders up and straightens your spine. Remember Moses, who was 120 years of age, used a walking stick not a cane, and he walked from Egypt, across the Sinai, around Jordan, and into Palestine. He could not have done it with a cane.

Be careful, a walking stick isn't for everyone, some people have less balance with a walking stick than a cane. Whatever they gain in walking is defeated by the loss of balance. If there's a question about using a walking stick or a cane, try both under the supervision of a physical therapist.

If you use a walker it should be high enough so that you don't stoop. If there's a question as to whether your walker's high enough, go to a supermarket and walk using a shopping cart. The handles of the cart are high, forcing you to walk straight. If you're more comfortable walking with a shopping cart than your walker, your walker isn't right for you:

1.   The walker may be too low.

2.   The wheels of the walker may be too small. The smaller the wheels the more effort you must make to push the walker. The more effort you make to push the walker, the more energy you spend, the more easily you tire.

3.   The walker may not be sturdy. Supermarket shopping carts are very sturdy.

Freezing

Freezing can be an inability to start walking, called start hesitation, or a sudden inability to continue walking, called stop hesitation, like a computer glitch that freezes the screen. The inability to start walking, start hesitation, may occur separate from or with the inability to continue walking, stop hesitation. These two types of freezing may involve different circuits or pathways in the brain. The inability to start walking, start hesitation, usually responds to Sinemet or a long acting dopamine agonist such as Mirapex or Permax. The sudden inability to continue walking, stop hesitation, may or may not respond to Sinemet or a dopamine agonist. The inability to continue walking usually occurs as a PD person turns, or comes to a door, or finds himself in a crowd of people.

Why PD people freeze is unclear. One theory is that the brain "sees" the length of our stride. We walk with a different stride length on level ground versus hilly ground, in open versus closed spaces. Once we start walking on level ground, our brain goes into autopilot and depending on what we see, one step automatically follows the next, each step about the same length as the one before. If we come to an obstacle: a hole in the ground, another person, a doorway, then we must change our stride length. The PD person is unable to switch from autopilot to another program, and like a faulty computer, he or she freezes. In some PD people even thinking of changing stride length as when approaching a door, or turning, is enough to cause them to freeze.

Anxiety and Freezing

Anxiety increases freezing. PD people who are anxious freeze more often and for longer times. Once a PD person freezes, his anxiety increases and he's even more likely to freeze. In some PD people freezing is like a panic attack: they sweat, their hearts beat fast, and they become short of breath. In some people, treating their anxiety, decreases their freezing. Treating anxiety may consist of:

1. Counseling—seeking to understand why they're anxious.

2. Identifying the circumstances and situations that cause freezing and avoiding them.

3. Relaxation techniques such as breathing exercises.

4. Medications including serotonin re-uptake inhibitors, SSRIs, such as Zoloft.

PD people who freeze learn a variety of tricks to get started or to restart walking after they freeze. The tricks include stepping over an imaginary line on the floor, taking several deep breaths, or waiting until the freeze unlocks. Almost all the tricks involve straightening the spine, so as to generate more power from the hip, thigh, and buttocks muscles. If a PD person learns a trick that more often than not breaks the freeze, the person becomes less anxious.

Freezing and Fluctuations

Some PD people on Sinemet fluctuate, they have on and off periods, and may freeze in an on or an off period. The freezing in the off period usually responds to additional medication: Sinemet or a long-acting dopamine agonist such as Mirapex or Permax. The freezing in the on period may or may not respond to additional medication. This further suggests there are different types of freezing episodes and different circuits and pathways in the brain are involved. Deep brain stimulation (DBS) is effective in treating some but not all freezing. Again suggesting several brain circuits and pathways are involved in freezing.

Difficulty Walking: More Than Parkinson Disease?

PD people who have difficulty walking and in whom the difficulty walking does not respond to medication should be studied for other causes of difficulty walking. Among these other causes are:

1. Arthritis of the hips and knees.

2. Diseases of the arteries to the legs.

3. Diseases of the nerves to the legs. These diseases called neuropathy, have many causes from diabetes to a B-vitamin deficiency, from alcohol abuse to toxic chemicals.

4. Diseases of the spinal cord. From a slipped disc in the lower (or lumbar) spine, to a bony spur compressing the upper (or cervical) spine. Disease of the upper (or cervical) spine is an overlooked cause of difficulty walking in PD people—especially when it occurs without pain.

5. Diseases of the brain other than PD. From multiple small and silent strokes to excess fluid on the brain, called hydrocephalus, to blood clots, and brain tumors.

The different diseases listed may be separated from PD and each from the other through a careful history, a detailed physical and neurological examination, a variety of blood tests, and an MRI of the upper spine and brain. The main thing, however, is to think of them and not assume only PD is responsible.

Are There Other Symptoms? (From Hope Through Research*)*

Various other symptoms accompany Parkinson's disease; some are minor, others are more bothersome. Many can be treated with appropriate medication or physical therapy. No one can predict which symptoms will affect an individual patient, and the intensity of the symptoms also varies from person to person. None of these symptoms is fatal, although swallowing problems can cause choking.

- **Depression**. This is a common problem and may appear early in the course of the disease, even before other symptoms are noticed. Depression may not be severe, but it may be intensified by the drugs used to treat other symptoms of Parkinson's disease. Fortunately, depression can be successfully treated with antidepressant medications.

- **Emotional changes.** Some people with Parkinson's disease become fearful and insecure. Perhaps they fear they cannot cope with new situations. They may not want to travel, go to parties, or socialize with friends. Some lose their motivation and become dependent on family members. Others may become irritable or uncharacteristically pessimistic. Memory loss and slow thinking may occur, although the ability to reason remains intact. Whether people actually suffer intellectual loss (also known as dementia) from Parkinson's disease is a controversial area still being studied.

- **Difficulty in swallowing and chewing.** Muscles used in swallowing may work less efficiently in later stages of the disease. In these cases, food and saliva may collect in the mouth and back of the throat, which can result in choking or drooling. Medications can often alleviate these problems.

- **Speech changes.** About half of all parkinsonian patients have problems with speech. They may speak too softly or in a monotone, hesitate before speaking, slur or repeat their words, or speak too fast. A speech therapist may be able to help patients reduce some of these problems.

- **Urinary problems or constipation.** In some patients bladder and bowel problems can occur due to the improper functioning of the autonomic nervous system, which is responsible for regulating smooth muscle activity. Some people may become incontinent while others have trouble urinating. In others, constipation may occur because the intestinal tract operates more slowly. Constipation can also be caused by inactivity, eating a poor diet, or drinking too little fluid. It can be a persistent problem and, in rare cases, can be serious enough to require hospitalization. Patients should not let constipation last for more than several days before taking steps to alleviate it.

- **Skin problems.** In Parkinson's disease, it is common for the skin on the face to become very oily, particularly on the forehead and at the sides of the nose. The scalp may become oily too, resulting in dandruff. In other cases, the skin can become very dry. These problems are also the result of an improperly functioning autonomic nervous system. Standard treatments for skin problems help. Excessive sweating, another common symptom, is usually controllable with medications used for Parkinson's disease.

- **Sleep problems.** These include difficulty staying asleep at night, restless sleep, nightmares and emotional dreams, and drowsiness during the day. It is unclear if these symptoms are related to the disease or to the medications used to treat Parkinson's disease. Patients should never take over-the-counter sleep aids without consulting their physicians.

What Are the Other Forms of Parkinsonism?

Other forms of parkinsonism include the following:

- **Postencephalitic parkinsonism.** Just after the first World War, a viral disease, encephalitis lethargica, attacked almost 5 million people throughout the world, and then suddenly disappeared in the 1920s. Known as sleeping sickness in the United States, this disease killed one-third of its victims and in many others led to post-encephalitic parkinsonism, a particularly severe form of movement disorder in which some patients developed, often years after the acute phase of the illness, disabling neurological disorders, including various forms of catatonia. (In 1973, neurologist Oliver Sacks published *Awakenings*, an account of his work in the late 1960s with surviving post-encephalitic patients in a New York hospital. Using the then-experimental drug levodopa, Dr. Sacks was able to temporarily awaken these patients from their statue-like state. A film by the same name was released in 1990.) In rare cases, other viral infections, including western equine encephalomyelitis, eastern equine encephalomyelitis, and Japanese B encephalitis, can leave patients with parkinsonian symptoms.

- **Drug-induced parkinsonism.** A reversible form of parkinsonism sometimes results from use of certain drugs—chlorpromazine and haloperidol, for example—prescribed for patients with psychiatric disorders. Some drugs used for stomach disorders

113

(metoclopramide) and high blood pressure (reserpine) may also produce parkinsonian symptoms. Stopping the medication or lowering the dosage causes the symptoms to abate.

- **Striatonigral degeneration.** In this form of parkinsonism, the substantia nigra is only mildly affected, while other brain areas show more severe damage than occurs in patients with primary Parkinson's disease. People with this type of parkinsonism tend to show more rigidity and the disease progresses more rapidly.

- **Arteriosclerotic parkinsonism.** Sometimes known as pseudo-parkinsonism, arteriosclerotic parkinsonism involves damage to brain vessels due to multiple small strokes. Tremor is rare in this type of parkinsonism, while dementia—the loss of mental skills and abilities—is common. Antiparkinsonian drugs are of little help to patients with this form of parkinsonism.

- **Toxin-induced parkinsonism.** Some toxins—such as manga-nese dust, carbon disulfide, and carbon monoxide—can also cause parkinsonism. A chemical known as MPTP (1-methyl-4-phenyl-1,2,5,6- tetrahydropyridine) causes a permanent form of parkin-sonism that closely resembles Parkinson's disease. Investigators discovered this reaction in the 1980s when heroin addicts in California who had taken an illicit street drug contaminated with MPTP began to develop severe parkinsonism. This discov-ery, which demonstrated that a toxic substance could damage the brain and produce parkinsonian symptoms, caused a dra-matic breakthrough in Parkinson's research: for the first time scientists were able to simulate Parkinson's disease in animals and conduct studies to increase understanding of the disease.

- **Parkinsonism-dementia complex of Guam.** This form occurs among the Chamorro populations of Guam and the Mariana Is-lands and may be accompanied by a disease resembling amyo-trophic lateral sclerosis (Lou Gehrig's disease). The course of the disease is rapid, with death typically occurring within 5 years. Some investigators suspect an environmental cause, perhaps the use of flour from the highly toxic seed of the cycad plant. This flour was a dietary staple for many years when rice and other food supplies were unavailable in this region, particularly during World War II. Other studies, however, refute this link.

- **Parkinsonism accompanying other conditions.** Parkinsonian symptoms may also appear in patients with other, clearly distinct neurological disorders such as Shy-Drager syndrome (sometimes

114

called multiple system atrophy), progressive supranuclear palsy, Wilson's disease, Huntington's disease, Hallervorden-Spatz syndrome, Alzheimer's disease, Creutzfeldt-Jakob disease, olivoponto-cerebellar atrophy, and post-traumatic encephalopathy.

How Do Doctors Diagnose Parkinson's Disease?

Even for an experienced neurologist, making an accurate diagnosis in the early stages of Parkinson's disease can be difficult. There are, as yet, no sophisticated blood or laboratory tests available to diagnose the disease. The physician may need to observe the patient for some time until it is apparent that the tremor is consistently present and is joined by one or more of the other classic symptoms. Since other forms of parkinsonism have similar features but require different treatments, making a precise diagnosis as soon as possible is essential for starting a patient on proper medication.

How Is the Disease Treated?

At present, there is no cure for Parkinson's disease. But a variety of medications provide dramatic relief from the symptoms.

When recommending a course of treatment, the physician determines how much the symptoms disrupt the patient's life and then tailors therapy to the person's particular condition. Since no two patients will react the same way to a given drug, it may take time and patience to get the dose just right. Even then, symptoms may not be completely alleviated. In the early stages of Parkinson's disease, physicians often begin treatment with one or a combination of the less powerful drugs—such as the anticholinergics or amantadine, saving the most powerful treatment, specifically levodopa, for the time when patients need it most.

Levodopa

Without doubt, the gold standard of present therapy is the drug levodopa (also called L-dopa). L-Dopa (from the full name L-3,4-dihydroxyphenylalanine) is a simple chemical found naturally in plants and animals. Levodopa is the generic name used for this chemical when it is formulated for drug use in patients. Nerve cells can use levodopa to make dopamine and replenish the brain's dwindling supply. Dopamine itself cannot be given because it doesn't cross the blood-brain barrier, the elaborate meshwork of fine blood vessels and cells that filters blood reaching the brain. Usually, patients are given levodopa combined with carbidopa. When added to levodopa, carbidopa delays the conversion of levodopa into dopamine until it reaches the brain, preventing or diminishing some of the side effects that often accompany levodopa therapy. Carbidopa also reduces the amount of levodopa needed.

Levodopa's success in treating the major symptoms of Parkinson's disease is a triumph of modern medicine. First introduced in the 1960s, it delays the onset of debilitating symptoms and allows the majority of parkinsonian patients—who would otherwise be very disabled—to extend the period of time in which they can lead relatively normal, productive lives.

Although levodopa helps at least three-quarters of parkinsonian cases, not all symptoms respond equally to the drug. Bradykinesia and rigidity respond best, while tremor may be only marginally reduced. Problems with balance and other symptoms may not be alleviated at all.

People who have taken other medications before starting levodopa therapy may have to cut back or eliminate these drugs in order to feel the full benefit of levodopa. Once levodopa therapy starts people often respond dramatically, but they may need to increase the dose gradually for maximum benefit.

Because a high-protein diet can interfere with the absorption of levodopa, some physicians recommend that patients taking the drug restrict protein consumption to the evening meal.

Levodopa is so effective that some people may forget they have Parkinson's disease. But levodopa is not a cure. Although it can diminish the symptoms, it does not replace lost nerve cells and it does not stop the progression of the disease.

Side Effects of Levodopa

Although beneficial for thousands of patients, levodopa is not without its limitations and side effects. The most common side effects are nausea, vomiting, low blood pressure, involuntary movements, and restlessness. In rare cases patients may become confused. The nausea and vomiting caused by levodopa are greatly reduced by the combination of levodopa and carbidopa which enhances the effectiveness of a lower dose. A slow-release formulation of this product, which gives patients a longer lasting effect, is also available.

Prolonging Levodopa Action

Recent studies revealed that when the drug tolcapone is added to the standard drug treatment for Parkinson's disease, levodopa-carbidopa, symptom relief is prolonged greatly. This promising new drug that blocks the breakdown of dopamine and levodopa would allow patients to take fewer doses and smaller amounts of levodopa-carbidopa and to decrease the problems of the wearing-off effect.

Dyskinesias, or involuntary movements such as twitching, nodding, and jerking, most commonly develop in people who are taking large doses of levodopa over an extended period. These movements may be either mild or severe and either very rapid or very slow. The only effective way to control these drug-induced movements is to lower the dose of levodopa or to use drugs that block dopamine, but these remedies usually cause the disease symptoms to reappear. Doctors and patients must work together closely to find a tolerable balance between the drug's benefits and side effects.

Other more troubling and distressing problems may occur with long-term levodopa use. Patients may begin to notice more pronounced symptoms before their first dose of medication in the morning, and they can feel when each dose begins to wear off (muscle spasms are a common effect). Symptoms gradually begin to return. The period of effectiveness from each dose may begin to shorten, called the wearing-off effect. Another potential problem is referred to as the on-off effect—sudden, unpredictable changes in movement, from normal to parkinsonian movement and back again, possibly occurring several times during the day. These effects probably indicate that the patient's response to the drug is changing or that the disease is progressing.

One approach to alleviating these side effects is to take levodopa more often and in smaller amounts. Sometimes, physicians instruct patients to stop levodopa for several days in an effort to improve the response to the drug and to manage the complications of long-term levodopa therapy. This controversial technique is known as a drug holiday. Because of the possibility of serious complications, drug holidays should be attempted only under a physician's direct supervision, preferably in a hospital. Parkinson's disease patients should never stop taking levodopa without their physician's knowledge or consent because of the potentially serious side effects of rapidly withdrawing the drug.

Are There Other Medications Available for Managing Disease Symptoms?

Levodopa is not a perfect drug. Fortunately, physicians have other treatment choices for particular symptoms or stages of the disease. Other therapies include the following:

117

- *Bromocriptine, pergolide, pramipexole, and ropinirole.* These four drugs mimic the role of dopamine in the brain, causing the neurons to react as they would to dopamine. They can be given alone or with levodopa and may be used in the early stages of the disease or started later to lengthen the duration of response to levodopa in patients experiencing wearing-off or on-off effects. They are generally less effective than levodopa in controlling rigidity and bradykinesia. Side effects may include paranoia, hallucinations, confusion, dyskinesias, nightmares, nausea, and vomiting.

- *Selegiline.* Studies supported by the NINDS have shown that the drug (also known as deprenyl) delays the need for levodopa therapy by an average of nine months. When selegiline is given with levodopa, it appears to enhance and prolong the response to levodopa and thus may reduce wearing-off fluctuations. Selegiline inhibits the activity of the enzyme monoamine oxidase B (MAO-B), the enzyme that metabolizes dopamine in the brain, delaying the breakdown of naturally occurring dopamine and of dopamine formed from levodopa and also provides mild symptomatic relief from parkinsonism in and of itself. Selegiline is an easy drug to take, although side effects may include nausea, orthostatic hypotension, or insomnia (when taken late in the day). Also, toxic reactions have occurred in some patients who took selegiline with fluoxetine (an antidepressant) and meperidine (used as a sedative and an analgesic).

- *Anticholinergics.* These drugs were the main treatment for Parkinson's disease until the introduction of levodopa. Their benefit is limited, but they may help control tremor and rigidity. They are particularly helpful in reducing drug-induced parkinsonism. Anticholinergics appear to act by blocking the action of another brain chemical, acetylcholine, whose effects become more pronounced when dopamine levels drop. Only about half the patients who receive anticholinergics respond, usually for a brief period and with only a 30 percent improvement. Although not as effective as levodopa or bromocriptine, anticholinergics may have a therapeutic effect at any stage of the disease when taken with either of these drugs. Common side effects include dry mouth, constipation, urinary retention, hallucinations, memory loss, blurred vision, changes in mental activity, and confusion.

- *Amantadine.* An antiviral drug, amantadine, helps reduce symptoms of Parkinson's disease. It is often used alone in the early stages of the disease or with an anticholinergic drug or levodopa. After several months amantadine's effectiveness wears off in a third to a half of the patients taking it, although effectiveness may return after a brief withdrawal from the drug. Amantadine has several side effects, including mottled skin, edema, confusion, blurred vision, and depression.

Is Surgery Ever Used to Treat Parkinson's Disease?

Treating Parkinson's disease with surgery was once a common practice. But after the discovery of levodopa, surgery was restricted to only a few cases. Currently, surgery is reserved for patients who have failed to respond satisfactorily to drugs. One of the procedures used, called cryothalamotomy, requires the surgical insertion of a supercooled metal tip of a probe into the thalamus (a relay station deep in the brain) to destroy the brain area that produces tremors. This and related procedures, such as thalamic stimulation, are coming back into favor for patients who have severe tremor or have the disease only on one side of the body. Investigators have also revived interest in a surgical procedure called pallidotomy in which a portion of the brain called the globus pallidus is lesioned. Some studies indicate that pallidotomy may improve symptoms of tremor, rigidity, and bradykinesia, possibly by interrupting the neural pathway between the globus pallidus and the striatum or thalamus. Further research on the value of surgically destroying these brain areas is currently being conducted. Restorative surgery, using nerve cell transplants to supplement the patient's own dopamine-producing nerve cells, is also under investigation.

Can Diet or Exercise Programs Help Relieve Symptoms?

Diet

Eating a well-balanced, nutritious diet can be beneficial for anybody. But for preventing or curing Parkinson's disease, there does not seem to be any specific vitamin, mineral, or other nutrient that has any therapeutic value. A high protein diet, however, may limit levodopa's effectiveness. Despite some early optimism, recent studies have shown that tocopherol (a form of vitamin E) does not delay Parkinson's disease. This conclusion came from a carefully conducted study supported by the NINDS called DATATOP (Deprenyl and Tocopherol Antioxidative Therapy for Parkinson's Disease) that examined, over 5 years, the effects of both deprenyl and vitamin E on early Parkinson's disease. While deprenyl was found to slow the early symptomatic progression of the disease and delay the need for levodopa, there was no evidence of therapeutic benefit from vitamin E.

Exercise

Because movements are affected in Parkinson's disease, exercising may help people improve their mobility. Some doctors prescribe physical therapy or muscle-strengthening exercises to tone muscles and to put underused and rigid muscles through a full range of motion. Exercises will not stop disease progression, but they may improve body strength so that the person is less disabled. Exercises also improve balance, helping people overcome gait problems, and can strengthen certain muscles so that people can speak and swallow better. Exercises can also improve the emotional well-being of parkinsonian patients by giving them a feeling of accomplishment. Although structured exercise programs help many patients, more general physical activity, such as walking, gardening, swimming, calisthenics, and using exercise machines, is also beneficial.

What Are the Benefits of Support Groups?

One of the most demoralizing aspects of the disease is how completely the patient's world changes. The most basic daily routines may be affected—from socializing with friends and enjoying normal and congenial relationships with family members to earning a living and taking care of a home. Faced with a very different life, people need encouragement to remain as active and involved as possible. That's when support groups can be of particular value to parkinsonian patients, their families, and their caregivers.

Glossary

Bradykinesia: gradual loss of spontaneous movement.

Corpus striatum: a part of the brain that helps regulate motor activities.

Cryothalamotomy: a surgical procedure in which a supercooled probe is inserted into a part of the brain called the thalamus in order to stop tremors.

Dementia: loss of intellectual abilities.

Dopamine: a chemical messenger, deficient in the brains of Parkinson's disease patients, that transmits impulses from one nerve cell to another.

Dyskinesias: abnormal involuntary movements that can result from long-term use of high doses of levodopa.

Festination: a symptom characterized by small, quick forward steps.

On-off effect: a change in the patient's condition, with sometimes rapid fluctuations between uncontrolled movements and normal movement, usually occurring after long-term use of levodopa and probably caused by changes in the ability to respond to this drug.

Pallidotomy: a surgical procedure in which a part of the brain called the globus pallidus is lesioned in order to improve symptoms of tremor, rigidity, and bradykinesia.

Parkinsonism: a term referring to a group of conditions that are characterized by four typical symptoms—tremor, rigidity, postural instability, and bradykinesia.

Postural instability: impaired balance and coordination, often causing patients to lean forward or backward and to fall easily.

Retropulsion: the tendency to step backwards if bumped from the front or upon initiating walking, usually seen in patients who tend to lean backwards because of problems with balance.

Rigidity: a symptom of the disease in which muscles feel stiff and display resistance to movement even when another person tries to move the affected part of the body, such as an arm.

Substantia nigra: movement-control center in the brain where loss of dopamine-producing nerve cells triggers the symptoms of Parkinson's disease; substantia nigra means black substance, so called because the cells in this area are dark.

Tremor: shakiness or trembling, often in a hand, which in Parkinson's disease is usually most apparent when the affected part is at rest.

Wearing-off effect: the tendency, following long-term levodopa treatment, for each dose of the drug to be effective for shorter and shorter periods.

Additional Information

Editor's Note: Please refer to Chapter 54 for a listing of organizations with additional information about Parkinson's disease.

Chapter 14

Dystonia

Chapter Contents

Section 14.1

Dystonia Overview from Definition to Prognosis

This section includes the following copyrighted documents from the Dystonia Medical Research Foundation: "Dystonia Defined," "Classification of Dystonia," "Causes of Dystonia," "Diagnosis of Dystonia," "Genetics," "Prognosis," and "Related Disorders," reprinted with permission from the Dystonia Medical Research Foundation. These documents are available online at www.dystonia-foundation.org; cited January 2002.

Dystonia Defined

Dystonia is a neurological movement disorder characterized by involuntary muscle contractions, which force certain parts of the body into abnormal, sometime painful, movements or postures. Dystonia can affect any part of the body including the arms and legs, trunk, neck, eyelids, face, or vocal cords.

If dystonia causes any type of impairment, it is because muscle contractions interfere with normal function. Features such as cognition, strength, and the senses, including vision and hearing are normal. While dystonia is not fatal, it is a chronic disorder and prognosis is difficult to predict.

It is the third most common movement disorder after Parkinson's Disease and Tremor, affecting more than 300,000 people in North America. Dystonia does not discriminate, it affects all races and ethnic groups.

Brief History of Dystonia

Dystonia, like many other chronic neurological disorders, was recognized as a distinct entity only relatively recently. Even before the term dystonia was coined, people with the syndrome were being reported explicitly in the literature.

In 1911, Hermann Oppenheim, an esteemed Berlin neurologist who wrote a leading textbook of neurology, was impressed with the variation in muscle tone seen in a neurologic syndrome that he had encountered in several young boys. He coined the term dystonia to indicate that "muscle tone was hypotonic at one occasion and in tonic muscle spasm at another, usually, but exclusively, elicited upon volitional movements." The term was widely accepted and has been used by neurologists ever since, even though throughout time, the definition changes. In addition to alteration of muscle tone, Oppenheim also described twisted postures associated with the muscle spasms affecting limbs and trunk, bizarre walking with bending and twisting of the torso, rapid and sometimes rhythmic jerking movements, and progression of symptoms leading eventually to sustained fixed postural deformities.

In 1944, Ernst Herz, from analysis of cinematographic and electromyographic recordings, regarded slow sustained postures as the best definition for dystonia.

In 1962, Derek Denny-Brown expanded upon this definition and defined dystonia as a fixed or relatively fixed attitude. One problem with using only sustained postures for the definition of dystonia is that it allows all types of abnormal postures to be called dystonia, such as fixed postures that could develop from a stroke. Another problem is that these definitions do not take into account the other types of abnormal movements seen in the disorder.

In February, 1984, a committee consisting of members of the Scientific Advisory Board of the Dystonia Medical Research Foundation met, deliberated, and developed the following definition: "dystonia is a syndrome of sustained muscle contractions, frequently causing twisting and repetitive movements, or abnormal postures." The committee consisted of Drs. André Barbeau, Donald B. Calne, Stanley Fahn, C. David Marsden, John H. Menkes, and G. Fred Wooten. This definition is still utilized.

This committee also proposed a classification scheme for all types of dystonia, recommending that there should be three classification schemes: by age at onset, by parts of body affected, and by etiology. With the advent of discovering different genetic types of dystonia, the etiologic classification was changed at the time of the 3rd International Dystonia Symposium in 1996. The main definition of dystonia will most likely remain the same, but the etiologic classification will change over time as new genetic forms are described.

Classification of Dystonia

Dystonia is classified in three ways: age of onset, body distribution of symptoms, and etiology or cause of the disorder.

Age of Onset

The symptoms of dystonia may begin during childhood (early-onset), in adolescence, or during adulthood.

Dystonia with either childhood-onset or adolescent-onset (<28) is usually associated with an inherited defect in a gene and begins in early childhood after a period of normal physical development. It often initially involves a limb, in particular the foot and leg. These symptoms may initially appear only during activities such as running or walking and may spread to involve other body areas.

The appearance of symptoms in adult-onset dystonia (>28) typically starts between ages 30 to 50 following decades of normal physical function. The symptoms tend to remain focal, affecting one particular part of the body.

Age of onset tends to be the best factor in determining the chance of progression. Generally, the earlier the onset of symptoms, the greater the chances are of progression of symptoms with age.

Body Distribution of Symptoms

Any body region may be affected by dystonia. Classification is done by the number and specific areas of the body that are affected:

- **Focal:** Most frequent type of dystonia; affects one single area of the body.

- **Segmental:** Affects at least two or more areas of the body that are adjacent.

- **Multi-focal:** Appears in two or more areas of the body that are not adjacent.

- **Generalized:** Involves several body areas on both sides of the body.

- **Hemi-dystonia:** Affects either the left or the right side of the body.

Etiology or Cause of the Dystonia

The classification of dystonia by causes uses broad categories: primary and secondary dystonia.

Primary dystonia is defined by the existence of dystonia alone without any underlying disorder. This category includes hereditary (classic) and sporadic (variant) forms of dystonia.

Early-onset generalized dystonia associated with the DYT1 gene is considered to be a classic form of primary form of dystonia because the movements and postures constitute the sole neurological abnormality.

Variant forms of dystonia are marked by atypical clinical features and may be etiologically distinct from the classic form. Dopa-Responsive, Paroxysmal, X-Linked Dystonia-Parkinsonian, Myoclonic, and Rapid-Onset Dystonia-Parkinsonian are all considered variant forms.

Secondary forms of dystonia arise from and can be attributed to numerous causes, such as birth injury, trauma, toxins, or stroke. Secondary dystonia can be symptomatic, and can also occur in association with other disorders such as Wilson's disease.

Causes of Dystonia

Primary dystonia is believed to be due to abnormal functioning of the basal ganglia which are deep brain structures involved with the control of movement. The basal ganglia assists in initiating and regulating movement. What goes wrong in the basal ganglia is still unknown. An imbalance of dopamine, a neurotransmitter in the basal ganglia, may underlie several different forms of dystonia, but much more research needs to be done for a better understanding of the brain mechanisms involved with dystonia.

Secondary forms of dystonia arise from and can be attributed to numerous causes, such as birth injury, trauma, toxins, or stroke. Secondary dystonia can be symptomatic and can also occur in association with other disorders such as Wilson's disease. When dystonia is secondary to certain injuries or small strokes, we often find lesions (areas of damage) in the putamen, one nucleus in the basal ganglia, as well as in certain nearby structures. Even though we can see no microscopic abnormalities of the brain in the great majority of cases of dystonia, including those with generalized dystonia, the evidence is so clear in the secondary dystonias that we believe the same part of the brain is involved in all types.

How Does Dystonia Work in the Brain?

Dystonia is a disorder that has to do with the way we move. The control of our movements is very complicated and involves many areas in the brain. The area of the brain that is involved in dystonia is called the basal ganglia. The basal ganglia is a deep region of the brain that controls the speed of movement and prevents unwanted movements.

If there is a small change in the way the basal ganglia works, it can cause movements to occur even if you don't want them to. This small change is not found by medical tests or pictures of the brain on a MRI scan. Even if this deep area of the brain is not working the right way and dystonia occurs, the areas of the brain that have to do with thinking and learning work normally. Once researchers understand what the problem is in this part of the brain, they will be able to come up with ways to allow persons with dystonia to control these unwanted movements.

Can Dystonia Come about Overnight? Are There Any Warning Signs?

Dystonia generally develops gradually. Occasionally the dystonia may occur suddenly, as in the acute dystonic reactions related to the administration of antipsychotic drugs. These attacks most commonly affect the head and neck muscles and are usually transient and readily treatable.

Some clinical features may precede the full clinical presentation of dystonia. Eye irritation, excessive sensitivity to bright light, and increased blinking may precede blepharospasm. Subtle facial or jaw spasms, difficulty chewing, changes in the cadence or pitch of speech may suggest early face, jaw, or voice dystonia. Mild jerky head movements, stiff neck, or local neck discomfort may occur in early torticollis. Cramping or fatiguing of the hands during writing, other manual activities, or walking may suggest limb dystonia. Sometimes a local dystonia may seem to arise directly following injury to a local body region.

Can Dystonia Affect Muscles Such as the Heart or Diaphragm?

Dystonia can affect breathing in several ways. Severe neck dystonia can cause difficulty breathing when the upper airway is partially closed off. Dystonia involving the vocal cords can potentially cause shortness of breath when the vocal cords close tight, but in general the tightness is present primarily when speaking. The act of breathing involves muscles between the ribs and a large muscle called the diaphragm. Dystonia can cause stiffness in the muscles between the ribs and can cause a sensation or shortness of breath. Occasionally, the diaphragm can also be affected. Finally, when a person with dystonia has involvement of the spine, twisting of the torso can limit how much the lungs can expand when breathing, and this can potentially cause shortness of breath. The heart muscle is not affected by dystonia.

Is It Possible to Have Focal Dystonia of the Back, Abdomen, Bladder, or Diaphragm?

Dystonia can involve muscles in almost all parts of the body. Although pure back dystonia is uncommon, it certainly does occur. The same applies to abdominal musculature although this is probably seen even less frequently. These forms of dystonia tend to result in the body being pulled to one side, backwards (in the case of back involvement), or forward (in the case of abdominal muscle involvement). The bladder proper is made up of a different type of muscles (smooth muscle) which are not affected by dystonia. On the other hand, the muscles around the opening of the bladder (the external sphincter) can be rarely involved, resulting in difficulty of passing urine. This, too, is an extremely rare phenomenon and probably occurs most often in forms of dystonia complicating other brain diseases such as Parkinson's disease and its treatment than in people with idiopathic or isolated dystonia.

Can You Die from Dystonia?

In the overwhelming majority of people with dystonia, it does not shorten life expectancy or result in death. In very severe, generalized dystonia, affecting all body areas, there can be problems that may arise secondary to the dystonia that can cause medical illnesses. However, these instances are quite rare and usually treatable.

What Role, If Any, Do Environmental Factors Play in Dystonia?

The role of environmental factors causing or contributing to dystonia remains uncertain. It is not clear why some individuals inheriting a specific gene develop a severe form of dystonia while many others who have inherited the same gene either never develop the problem or only demonstrate a very mild form (this is what is meant by variable penetrance in genetics parlance).

It is possible that unknown environmental factors could play a contributing role in determining whether or not a member of such a family might develop dystonia and, if so, whether it is a mild or severe form. On the other hand, numerous other unrecognized genetic factors may account for these differences. Where no genetic predisposition exists, it is also possible that environmental factors are an important cause of dystonia. However, at this time, the specific nature of such environmental factors is completely unknown.

Can Exposure to Toxins or Specific Chemicals Cause Dystonia?

The answer to this question is clearly yes. This is distinctly different from widespread environmental exposures to which large numbers of dystonic patients could be exposed. A number of uncommon toxins are capable of causing brain damage centered in the motor control region known as the basal ganglia. Dystonia may be one prominent feature experienced by patients with these exposures, but it is extremely uncommon for isolated dystonia to be seen in such patients. In other words, the vast majority of patients exposed to toxins (for example, manganeses) have additional neurological problems associated with the dystonia. Possibly the most common feature in such patients is the presence of a Parkinson's disease-like state.

A large number of drugs are capable of causing dystonia. In most cases, the dystonia is transient, but in some patients exposed to neuroleptics such as Haldol, the dystonia may be persistent. This disorder, known as tardive dystonia, in contrast to dystonia associated with other neurotoxins, commonly manifests isolated dystonia without additional neurological problems.

What Is the Chance of X-Ray Therapy Generating Dystonia?

There are no reports of radiotherapy generating dystonia in any parts of the body.

Can Childhood Illnesses, Such as Measles, Cause Dystonia?

Rarely is dystonia linked to the occurrence of a childhood illness. Dystonia can arise from birth injury, associated with a rare childhood metabolic disorder or following a brain infection such as encephalitis. Subacute sclerosing panencephalitis is a rare complication of measles that has been associated with dystonia. In most instances, however, uncomplicated measles does not cause dystonia. The disorders mentioned above usually have other associated features, including cognitive problems, seizures, or other neurologic abnormalities, and do not typically cause only dystonic symptoms.

Sometimes trauma to the head or neck area may cause slippage of the bony spine, particularly in a child. This is called atlantoaxial dislocation and may result in a picture which resembles spasmodic torticollis. This is not dystonia but is an orthopedic problem.

Is There Any Correlation between General Anesthetics and Dystonia?

There is not a causal link between general anesthetics and dystonia. Certain types of medication can cause dystonia. The medications most frequently implicated include antipsychotic agents and certain medications used to treat nausea and vomiting. These agents can cause acute and reversible symptoms of dystonia at the time of administration, most often involving the eyes, face, jaw, oral muscles, neck, and back, or can produce chronic dystonia following prolonged use, called tardive dystonia. Agents used as general anesthetics are not directly linked to dystonia.

Can the Prolonged Use of Antihistamines, Decongestants, or Headache Medicines Cause Dystonia?

The medications commonly used for the treatment of headache are not directly linked with dystonia. However, some of the medications used to treat the nausea and vomiting associated with migraine headaches, in particular, metoclopramide (Reglan), are known to cause acute reversible dystonic reactions and tardive dystonia. There have been rare, isolated instances in which antihistaminic agents have been associated with dystonia, which subsides following the discontinuation of the medication. Antihistaminic medications are actually used in some people to treat the symptoms of dystonia.

Could an Allergic Reaction to a Drug Cause Dystonia?

The term *allergic* refers to an idiosyncratic response to a drug in which the body recognizes the drug as a foreign substance, and the immune system is activated to eliminate the offending agent. Typical allergic reactions to drugs include rash, hives, shortness of breath, dizziness, and light-headedness. Dystonia does not result from allergy to drugs. Prudence in the use of medications is always wise. People should not take medicines unless they have been informed of the risks and benefits of the proposed therapy.

If Dystonia Is Not Genetically Caused (No Family History Known), What Is the Probable Cause of Childhood-Onset and Generalized Dystonia?

The absence of a clear family history of dystonia does not rule out a hereditary basis for childhood-onset generalized dystonia. Explanations for this phenomenon include mild undiagnosed dystonia in family members and certain types of inheritance (autosomal recessive, X-linked recessive, reduced penetrance of autosomal dominant genes). All these may result in skipped generations or indeed in a completely negative family history. It is possible that breakthroughs in genetics may soon allow the diagnosis of hereditary dystonia even in families without a clear family history.

Other conditions may cause childhood-onset generalized dystonia. Some of these conditions are hereditary as well. They are discussed separately from hereditary onset generalized dystonia because they also cause other signs of neurologic dysfunction such as seizures, mental retardation, weakness, coordination, and other difficulties.

These conditions are diagnosed with various tests such as brain scanning, blood, urine, and other tests. Lastly, childhood-onset generalized dystonia may result from brain damage resulting from head trauma, lack of brain oxygen, stroke, or exposure to toxin. Your doctor will determine to what extent testing should be performed to try to explain the occurrence of dystonia in childhood.

Can Neurofibromatosis Cause Dystonia?

Yes, neurofibromatosis is a condition of many small brain tumors that may cause dystonia.

If You Are Not Born with Dystonia, What Causes It to Manifest Itself Later in Life?

It is quite rare to see someone born with dystonia, manifesting symptoms at the time of birth. Childhood-onset dystonia associated with the inherited form of dystonia begins in early childhood after a period of normal physical development and often initially involves the leg and foot. In adult-onset dystonia, the onset is typically in the 40s following decades of normal physical function. The reason for the appearance of dystonia after initial normal development and function is not known. It is thought that in some people there are external factors that may trigger the dystonia, but specific triggers have not yet been identified.

Can Dystonia Be Caused by an Injury?

To date, there is some evidence to support a role of trauma including injury to the head or other body parts. It makes sense that if these factors can influence genetic forms of dystonia, they may also be important to other forms of primary dystonia where there is little or no genetic influence. Studies of these questions require accurate and detailed evaluations of the past histories of large numbers of patients as well as unaffected individuals or controls. One reason for pursuing these issues is that it is well established that trauma does occasionally result in some forms of well-established secondary dystonia.

For example, closed head injury can sometimes result in severe dystonia. Typically in these cases, the injury has been severe enough to result in damage to the basal ganglia, which can be visualized on brain imaging studies. Direct injury to a limb may also result in severe dystonic postures. The mechanisms underlying this peripheral injury-induced dystonia are poorly understood.

It appears from the literature that people who are carriers of the gene for dystonia may be more likely to have trauma as a triggering factor for the development of dystonia. When people have an injury and then develop dystonia in that body part, you are tempted to say, "There must be some relationship between the trauma and the dystonia." There are legal aspects of trauma-induced dystonia that have to be dealt with as well. It's a gray area at this point. It may be that there is a triggering factor, but we're really not clear as to why some people who have the gene manifest the symptoms and some do not.

Is Dystonia a Sensory Disorder?

On first appearance, dystonia is a movement disorder. It is characterized by abnormal postures and movements. Sensation seems normal. There are clues, however, that sensory function may not be completely normal and that sensory features are important. Since the sensory system is an important influence on the motor system, abnormalities of the sensory system could be relevant in causing motor dysfunction.

Sensory tricks can relieve a dystonic spasm. The most commonly noted is the *geste* in spasmodic torticollis where, for example, a finger placed lightly on the face will neutralize the spasm. Such tricks are seen in all forms of dystonia. Pressure on the eyelids might improve blepharospasm, a toothpick in the mouth might relieve tongue dystonia, and sensation applied to parts of the arm might improve a writer's cramp.

On the other hand, sensory stimulation might trigger dystonia. This might be called a reverse geste. Examples include a tart taste producing tongue dystonia or a loud noise producing spasmodic torticollis.

Sensory symptoms may well precede the appearance of dystonia. Common examples would be a gritty sensation in the eye preceding blepharospasm and irritation of the throat preceding spasmodic dysphonia. Photophobia is an example of distorted sensation.

Abnormal sensory input might well be a trigger for dystonia. Trauma to a body part is often a precedent to dystonia of that part. A blow to the head might precede torticollis, irritations of the eye are common in blepharospasm, and a deep cut of the hand might occur just before writer's cramp develops.

There may be an important problem with the processing of muscle spindle input. In patients with hand cramps, vibration can induce the patient's dystonia. Cutaneous input similar to that which produces the sensory trick can reverse the vibration-induced dystonia. Conversely, both action-induced and vibration-induced dystonia can be improved with lidocaine block of the muscle, which will reduce sensory input.

The brain response to somatosensory input is abnormal in dystonia. This can be demonstrated with PET studies and evoked potential studies using EEG. In addition, studies of sensory receptive fields of neurons in the thalamus in humans with dystonia show expanded regions where cells all respond to the same passive movement. Mapping of the location of cortical sensory areas of the different fingers is abnormal in dystonia, and this is potentially consistent with the idea that there is abnormal cortical plasticity.

Lastly, there is some evidence that there might, in fact, be subtle abnormalities of sensation in patients with dystonia. The best evidence is for an abnormality of proprioception, the sense of movement of body parts.

Diagnosis of Dystonia

How Do Doctors Diagnose Dystonia?

At this time, there is no test to confirm diagnosis of dystonia. Instead, the diagnosis of dystonia rests solely on the information from the affected individual and the physical and neurological examination. In order to correctly diagnose dystonia, doctors must be able to recognize the physical signs and be familiar with the symptoms. In certain instances, further tests may be ordered to be sure that there are not other problems associated with dystonia, but in many cases these tests will be normal.

When dystonia begins, often it may change significantly with different actions. For example, dystonia of the foot may occur when walking forward but disappear completely when walking backward or while sitting in a chair. In some people, dystonia involving the hand will only happen when writing and not with any other activity. The changeable nature of dystonia has led some physicians and even some dystonia-affected persons wondering if the cause of dystonia may be all in their head. This is not true. Dystonia is a neurologic condition that is not the result of a psychiatric problem. In order to diagnose dystonia, a doctor who is familiar with the disorder is necessary.

If dystonia is diagnosed it is important to remember that features such as cognition, strength, and the senses, including vision and hearing, are normal.

Is a normal MRI typical analysis for the diagnosis of dystonia? Yes, unless the dystonia is the result of some other problem. If it's idiopathic dystonia, the MRI is normal. Blood tests are normal, and electrophysiology is, to a large degree, also normal. As far as secondary dystonia, it depends upon the reason for having it.

Typically, if a large evaluation of someone with dystonia is done, that means it is thought that there is something atypical about the way the person looks that says, "We'd better make sure that there is nothing else going on."

The Genetics of Dystonia

Dystonia Genes

Genes that are defective in some way do not produce the correct protein and therefore either cause the disease directly or somehow influence the clinical features of the disease. Errors in genes are responsible for an estimated 3,000 to 4,000 clearly hereditary diseases, including certain forms of dystonia.

At present researchers have recognized multiple forms of inheritable dystonia and have identified at least ten genes or chromosomal locations responsible for the various manifestations including Early-Onset Generalized Dystonia, Dopa-Responsive Dystonia, Paroxysmal Dystonia, X-Linked Dystonia-Parkinsonism (Lubag), Myoclonic Dystonia, and Rapid-Onset Dystonia-Parkinsonism.

Identifying these defective genes is important because it gives researchers the first tool to unravel the complicated pathways involved in disease processes. For example, the realization that mutations in the gene encoding an enzyme (a protein that catalyzes a reaction) involved in the dopamine (a neurotransmitter in the brain) pathway causes dopa-responsive dystonia which has allowed researchers to understand why small doses of L-dopa can be used to treat affected persons and suggests that other genes involved in this pathway may cause variant form of this disorder.

DYT1 Gene

In 1997, researchers identified the DYT1 gene responsible for early-onset generalized dystonia. The DYT1 gene codes for a previously unknown protein, named torsinA, and it has significant similarities to the heat-shock proteins and chaperone proteins. Found in virtually all living organisms, the heat-shock proteins help cells recover from stresses including heat, traumatic injury, and chemical poisoning. Until now, no human disease has been associated with these proteins.

In people with early-onset dystonia, the DYT1 gene has a mutation that causes the deletion of three letters or nucleotides called GAG in the genetic code. This GAG deletion results in the loss of an amino acid, called glutamic acid, which is a component of the torsinA protein. This relatively minute change in the torsinA blueprint apparently causes critical changes in the function of the protein. The role of the torsinA protein is currently unknown, but somehow this defective protein disrupts communication among the neurons responsible for movement and muscle control, leading to the symptoms of the dystonia disorder.

Researchers believe that the same mutation in the DYT1 gene appeared independently in several ethnic populations throughout history and is possibly one of only a few mutations that result in early-onset dystonia. Exactly how the abnormal gene causes the dystonia is presently unknown.

Inheritance

The mode of inheritance for early-onset generalized dystonia is autosomal dominant, meaning only one copy of the DYT1 gene is needed to be a carrier. For reasons scientists do not yet understand, only 30 to 40% of those with the abnormal DYT1 gene develop symptoms of dystonia. Called variable penetrance, this means 60 to 70% of the people who carry this gene will not manifest symptoms. Even if a carrier of this gene does not develop symptoms, there is a 50% chance of passing it on to his/her children. There is no way yet to predict whether a person with the abnormal gene will develop symptoms of the disorder, and the severity of the illness may differ markedly within a family.

Testing

Until the discovery of the DYT1 gene, the only genetic test for early-onset dystonia was a linkage test. Direct molecular diagnostic testing is now available for anyone affected with early-onset or limb-onset dystonia, regardless of ethnic background or family history. A direct test looks for damage to the actual gene in question. It is more accurate than a linkage test which tests for chromosome differences usually linked to the disease gene.

Using DNA obtained from a small blood sample, this test analyzes for the presence of the known GAG deletion. It allows for diagnostic testing, confirmation of the diagnosis, carrier status, and prenatal testing. This test is unlikely to be positive for individuals with late-onset, primarily cervical or cranial dystonia, or blepharospasm, unless there is a family history of early-onset dystonia.

The decision to have a genetic test is a personal one and should not be made lightly. A genetic counselor can help you explore the benefits and downsides of getting tested as well as help you understand the implications of the test results. If you are thinking of getting tested, you should plan to talk with a genetic counselor, and most centers that do genetic testing, make it a requirement of performing the test.

Some insurance carriers reimburse for genetic counseling and testing; others do not, so individuals should check with their insurance companies before ordering this test. With any genetic test, there may be potential for insurance or employment discrimination. These issues should be explored as part of genetic counseling before choosing to undergo testing. U.S. legislation protecting privacy and preventing this potential discrimination has been developed and is pending.

Prognosis

Dystonia has a variable nature, therefore making it difficult to predict the prognosis of the disorder. Currently, no medication or therapy can prevent progression from happening. The dystonia (both generalized and focal forms) will usually stabilize within five years of onset, but symptoms may fluctuate—for example, stressful situations may make symptoms temporarily worse. The following questions provide an overview of the prognosis and effects of dystonia. More specific information about the various forms of dystonia can be found in the following sections 14.2, 14.3, and 14.4.

My dystonic symptoms have been stable with no change for five years. Can I expect them to remain the same, or will they progress to becoming more debilitating?

Often dystonia will stabilize and not progress. In some patients with cervical dystonia, there may even be a remission. As a general rule, the older one is when dystonia develops, the more likely it will not progress beyond a certain point but will plateau. The younger one is when dystonia develops, the more likely that it will progress over time, particularly if the dystonia begins in a leg. And in such patients, the disorder can stabilize eventually and not progress any further. However, dystonia should not be taken for granted. There is no guarantee that the disease will not progress even though it has stabilized itself for a number of years. There is always a degree of uncertainty that something may develop and that the dystonia will start to flair up in the future and become worse again.

Can childhood dystonia go into remission and reappear as an adult?

Yes. But this happens quite rarely The figure that used to be quoted was that as many as 10% of patients (child and adult onset combined) might have such a spontaneous remission. It is probably much less than that. More frequently, instead of a true remission, the severity of dystonic postures may become much less for months or years in a small minority of patients. Nearly everyone has some degree of day-to-day fluctuation in the severity of his or her symptoms For a few, the fluctuation may be so much better and for such a long time that it seems like a remission. However, a careful exam will still reveal some involuntary postures. Those who do seem to have a true remission are likely to again have symptomatic dystonia sometime later.

What are the chances of a child with generalized dystonia, affecting mainly the feet and legs, developing other types of dystonia, like cervical dystonia?

When dystonia begins in childhood involving the legs and the feet, it is quite common for it to progress to involve the trunk, the arms, and even the neck. This is particularly true for early-onset general-ized dystonia. In people with dopa-responsive dystonia, which also begins in the legs, the dystonia does not tend to become that severe in the upper body parts of the body.

Why do my symptoms improve at certain times of the day or during different seasons, and then become worse at other times?

It is fairly common for dopa-responsive dystonia to vary in sever-ity during the course of a day. In these patients, dystonia may be ab-sent when waking up in the morning or waking up after a nap and then worsening as the day progresses. Such diurnal variation is much less common in patients with idiopathic torsion dystonia, but some variation over long periods of time might develop. Dystonia, for ex-ample, tends to worsen with fatigue and after heavy exercise and tends to ameliorate with relaxation techniques. In most cases, dysto-nia tends to lessen and even disappear with deep sleep.

A child with generalized dystonia has progressed to a severe state. Medication is introduced and the child begins to respond and improve. What is the best that can be expected?

The medications that are currently available for treatment of gen-eralized dystonia do not cure this disorder. It is likely that over time, the signs of generalized dystonia will progress as part of the disease itself. Therefore, if medicines start to work, there should be cautious optimism that they will continue to help the patient, but they will have to be chronically administered and cannot be expected to solve the patient's problem completely.

In addition to medications, focal injections of botulinum toxin may help abate dystonia in a particular area of the body; for instance, in generalized dystonia, where the neck muscles are profoundly in spasm, injections of botulinum toxin into the neck can give added benefit which is already being obtained with medications.

Finally, surgical intervention in the form of an operation known as a thalamotomy can relieve signs of dystonia. Generally, surgery is reserved for patients with a disability that is not adequately con-trolled by medications. Again, cure is not possible and moderate abatement of symptoms is the most that can be hoped for. An ex-ample of a successful thalamotomy would be a patient who was formerly bed-ridden with severe spasms who now, after surgery, can stand and ambulate but still has significant dystonic spasms and voice problems.

Why do some patients have one dystonic symptom while others develop several?

Dystonia is highly variable in its manifestations, and this observation is one of the reasons that dystonia has been misunderstood for so long. Whereas one patient complains of painful cramps, another may find that the foot turns in unexpectedly during walking, but there is no pain or cramp at all. Scientists believe that the body area involved is determined by alteration in specific brain regions.

For example, in patients with dystonia on the left side of the body only, the chemical abnormality is thought to be predominantly or exclusively restricted to the right side of the brain. Further research is needed to determine exactly what portions of the brain relate to specific dystonic symptoms. One of the reasons that autopsy research is so important is the need to study individual symptoms and relate them to chemical and microscopic changes that occur in highly specific brain areas. Researchers hope that such efforts will lead to a clear understanding of the basis of dystonia and help scientists in their quest for treatment and cure.

Can dystonia cause difficulty swallowing or breathing?

Yes, sometimes. This depends primarily on the part(s) of the body affected. For instance, some people with dystonia involving the jaw or tongue may have chewing or swallowing difficulty. Occasionally, people with very severe cervical dystonia also may have some swallowing difficulty. Treatments, whether medications or botulinum toxin injections, can also potentially have swallowing side effects. Dystonia rarely affects breathing. Severe generalized dystonia may involve the diaphragm muscles (the primary breathing muscles) or cause enough truncal twisting to cause some problems with regular breathing.

After years of having dystonia, is the skeletal system affected in any way?

It may be, but not directly. Dystonia does not have a primary effect on bones. However, because of the abnormal postures that result from dystonic spasms, unusual mechanical stress may be placed on bones. For instance, if someone has a severe dystonia that involves a very sustained posture in one position, he/she may get a shortening of the ligaments and tendons so that the joint becomes contracted and can no longer move freely through a full range of motion. With time, this might be expected to cause excessive wear on the affected bones.

Even short of a contracture, some bones may experience excessive wear because of such abnormal mechanical stresses. Bone changes, however, are not usually symptomatically important to people with dystonia. It is more often the case that we are concerned about the effect on muscles and related supportive tissues as they influence posture.

Does dystonia cause nervousness?

No, not directly. Dystonia can cause varying amounts of disability. People's reactions to their disability vary widely and can include different degrees of anxiety or depression. When anxiety or depression are present enough to be clinically important, they can worsen the symptoms of dystonia. However, they do not worsen the underlying dystonia process. When anxiety or depression are prominent, they should be treated specifically as a separate problem with the usual options of treatment for those disorders.

Are there mood swings associated with dystonia?

There appear to be no particular mood problems associated directly with dystonia. However, sometimes the physical problems that occur with dystonia may lead to frustration and anxiety. Because dystonia tends to be a long-term disorder, this may lead to depression. Just as the symptoms of dystonia may vary from day to day, with good days and bad days, so may inner personal feelings. If emotional problems are prolonged, with feelings of sadness, hopelessness, and frustration, then advice should be sought from the doctor, and perhaps psychological counseling or suggested medications prescribed.

Is there anything helpful that can be done to ease my dystonia in a stressful situation?

Although clearly stress does not cause dystonia, many people with dystonia have reported that in a stressful situation, their symptoms worsen. This worsening is temporary and resolves when the stressful situation has passed. Unfortunately, getting rid of all stress in life is not possible. Therefore, techniques which result in a lessening of the stressful feelings may be beneficial. Relaxation techniques can be of considerable help. Although there are medications which can decrease anxiety, the effects of stress are best managed without additional medications. Healthcare professionals familiar with the techniques of stress reduction may be very helpful.

141

Why do the muscle contractions of dystonia stop during sleep?

The theory is that the origin of the problem comes from the basal ganglia, which is above the brain stem. In the brain stem there is a system called the reticular-activating system, which is important in sleep. Sleep seems to cut off all the impulses from the brain in the motor pathway so that all the muscles relax. And this result supports the theory that dystonia originates from above the brain stem.

Is there a correlation between dystonia and fatigue?

The constant movement of dystonia can be compared to working out 18 hours a day—and for people whose symptoms don't stop during sleep, 24 hours a day. This can definitely result in fatigue and diminished stamina and make it more difficult to get through the day. Fatigue may be confused with lack of energy or motivation that may be a sign of depression or other medical conditions

What's the best way to deal with pain?

Pain is difficult to treat if symptoms don't respond to oral medications or botulinum toxin injections—often by relieving dystonia contractions and spasms, you can relieve the pain caused by these symptoms. Botulinum toxin injection can be quite effective in this regard. Muscle relaxants may have the same effect. Over-the-counter pain medications (i.e. acetaminophen, ibuprofen, naproxen) should be tried first.

Physicians should ascertain whether the pain is due to the dystonia or to other secondary conditions such as arthritis or a compressed nerve. If it comes from degeneration of the neck spine or impingement and irritation of nerve roots, that pain is very difficult to get rid of. Frequently, patients with neck dystonia report a lot of headaches. The pain goes from the back of the head to the occipital region and it can go all the way to the front. That kind of headache can sometimes be relieved by botulinum toxin injections, but some of the stronger analgesics are sometimes needed.

What can be done to alleviate the pain in the hip area?

Dystonia, most of the time, is not associated with pain, except for cervical dystonia in which neck pain tends to be fairly common. When it comes to having joint pain, it may be that a joint developed arthritis from all of the actions of the dystonia working on that joint.

Hip pain, thus, could be due to an arthritic condition. This needs to be checked out by a physician; and, if it is due to arthritis, the arthritis should be treated. If pain is due to muscle spasms, then there would a need to try to eliminate the spasms with medication or injections of botulinum toxin.

How would you treat dystonia and depression?

There are two major classes of medications for dystonia. The first type of medication, called anticholinergics, affect acetylcholine which can result in both improved symptoms and improved mood.

Depression can aggravate dystonia symptoms and make them worse. If a person is affected by both depression and dystonia, treating the depression often results in an improvement in the dystonia. Drugs called selective serotonin re-uptake inhibitors affect the levels of serotonin in the brain, thereby affecting a person's mood. There are so many anti-depressants available that treatment can be highly personalized to fit the needs of the patient—family history alone is no longer a basis for prescribing depression medication.

Related Disorders

What is the difference between facial tic and blepharospasm?

The term facial tic is often used to describe involuntary movements that involve the face, particularly those around the eyes and the corner of the mouth. These movements are usually brief and not sustained. They are usually not associated with the squeezing that typically accompanies blepharospasm.

The common facial tic includes the condition hemifacial spasm, a condition characterized by very rapid, abnormal contractions of one side of the face. Sometimes hemifacial spasm may follow a Bell's palsy or be associated with facial weakness. Often the movements are provoked by eating, talking, or whistling. Some patients exhibit a response whereby when they move the lower part of the face, the upper face has spasms.

Another facial tic is the quick facial movements that occur in people who have the condition of chronic motor tics. Chronic motor tics may be unilateral or bilateral, and the movement is usually preceded by an urge to make the movements. After the movement is made, the urge is often relieved. The individual with chronic motor tics usually has the ability to suppress the movements if they concentrate on the movements.

143

Chronic motor tics may involve any part of the body including the face, arms, legs, or trunk.

The manifestation of blepharospasm is an involuntary movement that involves the upper face, and may also involve the lower face, tongue, pharynx, jaw, neck, or other body segments. However, these movements are usually not suppressible, because they are involuntary and not under the direct control of the person with them.

There is often a marked squeezing component as the condition may progress from quick movements to more sustained spasms. There is some overlap among how these conditions appear, so that even experts may disagree on whether a patient has chronic motor tics or blepharospasm. Most of the disagreement will occur when the symptoms are subtle, and they present with similar findings on examination. Taking a history will sometimes clarify the cause. Hemifacial spasm and blepharospasm are known to have an excellent response to botulinum toxin treatment. Facial tics may respond, too.

What is the difference between essential tremor and dystonia tremor?

Essential tremor is one of the most common movement disorders. It is ordinarily inherited. The tremor is not present when someone is relaxed but becomes evident when a body part assumes a posture or undertakes a specific action. The tremor is generally rhythmic and can vary from being only subtle to very severe and debilitating. The tremor affects the hands and arms and may affect the head and the voice. Dystonic tremors are quite variable in their presentation and on some occasions can look like essential tremor. They are, however, seldom seen in isolation and usually are associated with dystonic posturing. The tremors are also sometimes somewhat more irregular than what is seen with essential tremor. Because essential tremor and dystonia tremor may look the same, and both can be genetic, the question was recently asked whether patients with essential tremor might carry an abnormality at the DYT1 locus. This has been found not to be the case although the actual gene for essential tremor has not been identified.

Are you finding any relationship between Chronic Fatigue Syndrome and dystonia?

We are not aware of an increased incidence of chronic fatigue syndrome among dystonia patients. Most patients with idiopathic dystonia are otherwise in excellent medical health and suffer from the same conditions that other people have, too.

What is the difference between a Parkinson's patient with dystonia and a dystonia patient with Parkinson's symptoms?

Symptoms of dystonia and parkinsonism can sometimes run together in the same patient because both of these movement disorders seem to arise from involvement of the basal ganglia in the brain. Both parkinsonism and dystonia can be caused by a great many disorders, and some of these disorders actually have both features of parkinsonism and dystonia.

As examples, there are the disorders known as dopa-responsive dystonia (DRD) and x-linked dystonia-parkinsonism (known as Lubag). DRD commonly begins in children as a dystonia predominately affecting the feet and being first manifested by an abnormal gait. In these children, features of parkinsonism tend to develop such as slowness of movement and decreased amplitude of movement and also decreased muscle tone.

When DRD begins in adults, it usually appears first as parkinsonism and can be mistaken for Parkinson's disease. Lubag can also first develop as either dystonia or parkinsonism, and the symptoms of other disorder may join the clinical picture.

In the parkinsonian disorder known as Parkinson's disease, certain features of the disease can be thought of as a form of dystonia such as postural changes in the hands and feet and also in the neck.

These partial changes are so common that we consider them as part of Parkinson's disease and do not consider them to be a form of dystonia that has developed on top of parkinsonism. In parkinsonian syndromes such as progressive supranuclear palsy, certain features of dystonia may appear such as dystonia of the facial muscles or the neck muscles.

In generalized dystonia, the patient presents only as a pure dystonia without any features of parkinsonism. If parkinsonism were to develop in such a patient, it could be considered that this patient happens to have the misfortune of having two different disorders.

For example, a patient may have adult-onset cervical dystonia in which the neck is twisted and, after several years, develops features of parkinsonism. It is generally believed that cervical dystonia and Parkinson's disease are two separate entities occurring in the same patient.

Some medications might be helpful for both Parkinson symptoms and dystonia symptoms. For example, levodopa is the most effective drug to reverse Parkinson symptoms, and it is also very effective in treating DRD and in some patients with other forms of dystonia. Anticholinergic drugs, such as Artane, are often used to treat dystonia, but they can also help some of the symptoms of Parkinson's. Any of the drugs currently in use to treat dystonia were first utilized in the treatment of Parkinson's disease, and because of this factor were then tried in patients with dystonia.

Is tremor a symptom of dystonia?

Tremor is not a primary symptom of dystonia. Dystonia is primarily characterized by an involuntary sustained twisting or cramping posture. If someone began having a tremor, we would not necessarily expect dystonic postures as well. Having said that, tremor can sometimes be seen as a secondary symptom. For instance, many patients with cervical dystonia will also have an associated head tremor and some patients with writer's cramp will have an associated writing tremor of the hand.

Are cervical dystonia and fibromyalgia related?

No, but both can cause pain in the neck muscles, and therefore cervical dystonia can be misdiagnosed as fibromyalgia. Many with cervical dystonia complain of muscle aching and even more severe pain in the neck muscles. This appears to be due to the pain fibers present in these muscles. Sometimes the muscle contractions and twisting movements in the neck have resulted in arthritis of cervical spine. This can be dangerous in that the resulting thickening of tissue and narrowing of the spinal canal can, by pinching the nerve roots, cause pain and even impinge on the spinal cord to cause paralysis of the legs.

How is Hallervorden-Spatz disease related to dystonia?

Hallervorden-Spatz disease is a heredodegenerative disease of the brain, typically involving the basal ganglia., i.e., the deep brain structures in the brain related to abnormal movements. As a result of this degeneration, the clinical picture of Hallervorden-Spatz is often marked by pronounced dystonia. There is often some clinical features of parkinsonism in addition. An MRI scan of the brain is very helpful in making the diagnosis of Hallervorden-Spatz disease by depicting increased iron deposition in these deep brain regions. Hallervorden-Spatz disease is one of many disorders in which dystonia is a prominent but not an exclusive feature.

146

My child developed torticollis at age 2. Is this similar to adult-onset spasmodic torticollis?

Early childhood-onset of neck dystonia is generally different from adult-onset. Congenital torticollis most commonly presents during the first few weeks of life possibly related to restricted head movements of the fetus or to trauma to the neck muscles at or about the time of birth. Congenital torticollis usually improves with physical therapy; however, surgery may be needed. The onset of torticollis during early childhood is unusual. Causes may include hiatal hernia (with vomiting, feeding problems, and posturing of neck during feeding), double vision (producing head tilt), lack of oxygen or high bilirubin counts during the perinatal period (producing cerebral palsy), severe brain infection (encephalitis), head or neck trauma, toxin exposure, brain, or spinal tumors or vascular malformations, cysts of the third ventricle, and certain chemical disorders such as Leigh's disease. These conditions may generally be assessed with brain and neck imaging and blood and urine analysis

My daughter was first diagnosed with Cerebral Palsy, but then the doctors realized she had Dopa-Responsive Dystonia. Why is this?

Dopa-Responsive Dystonia (DRD) is also known as Segawa's dystonia named after Dr. Masaya Segawa of Japan, who first described it. DRD usually starts in childhood or adolescence with progressive difficulty in walking and, in some cases, spasticity.

Many symptoms of DRD do mimic cerebral palsy (CP) which may be the reason for the misdiagnosis. CP usually results from a brain injury before or during birth. Leg spasticity inhibiting the ability to walk occurs in both disorders. But DRD has several unusual characteristics that set it apart from cerebral palsy and other neurological disorders. Most unusual is that the symptoms are usually least severe in the morning and become worse through the course of the day. Because of this diurnal variation, DRD is often mistaken for an emotional problem.

The other major difference between DRD and cerebral palsy is that the former often runs in families while CP rarely does. Significant advances have taken place in the past two years in the genetics of Dopa-Responsive Dystonia. In 1993, the gene for DRD was mapped to chromosome 14 and then in 1994 that gene was located. Testing for the gene is available, and research continues to further understand the implications of these findings.

What is Wilson's Disease and how does it relate to dystonia?

Wilson's disease (hepatolenticular degeneration) is a hereditary disease resulting from excessive copper accumulation in the body. Normally, copper is excreted without any difficulties, but, in patients with Wilson's disease, the copper is deposited and accumulates in the liver, in the brain, and around the eye.

Dystonia is a prominent clinical feature in some patients with Wilson's disease. It may present itself as dystonia but is identifiable by an examination of the cornea for a Kayser-Fleisher ring, which is a brown or greenish ring of copper deposits around the cornea. Wilson's disease is treatable.

Is TMJ a form of dystonia?

Temporomandibular Joint disease is an arthritic condition, not a dystonia. Oromandibular dystonia may be misdiagnosed as TMJ.

How do overuse conditions and dystonia differ?

Problems with the hands due to overuse are much more common than writer's cramp. Overuse can be quite painful, but it is still unclear as to where the pain is coming from—the location of the pathology is unclear. Using different movements and muscles to perform a task may help. Stretching and maintaining good posture might also be helpful.

What is carpal tunnel syndrome?

In carpal tunnel syndrome it is very clear where the problem is, and the condition can be successfully treated. The nerve in the carpal tunnel of the hand is pinched—if a person has small carpal tunnels, he/she is more likely to develop a pinched nerve in that area. Most people with carpal tunnel syndrome develop symptoms in both hands.

Section 14.2

Inherited Forms of Dystonia

This section includes the following copyrighted documents from the Dystonia Medical Research Foundation's *Forms of Dystonia*: "Early-Onset Generalized Dystonia," "Dopa-Responsive Dystonia," "Paroxysmal Dystonia," and "Rapid-Onset Dystonia-Parkinsonism," reprinted with permission from the Dystonia Medical Research Foundation. These documents are available online at www.dystonia-foundation.org; cited January 2002.

Early-Onset Generalized Dystonia

What Is It?

Early-onset generalized dystonia, the most common hereditary form of dystonia, is characterized by the twisting of the limbs, specifically the foot/leg or hand/arm. The spasms may spread to involve twisting contractions of other parts of the body.

Symptoms

Symptoms in early-onset generalized dystonia can range from twisted postures, turning in of the foot or arm, muscle spasms, unusual walking with bending and twisting of the torso, rapid, sometimes rhythmic, jerking movements; and progression of symptoms leading to sustained or fixed postures. Because the legs and trunk are so commonly affected in early-onset generalized dystonia, abnormal gait may be common.

Factors such as age and site play a significant role in the progression of early-onset generalized dystonia. The younger the age of onset, the more likely the dystonic symptoms will begin in one of the legs, spread upward to other areas, and possibly become generalized.

Symptoms commonly begin with a specific action, that is, the abnormal movements appear with a specific action, and are not present at rest. For example, if it begins in one leg, the symptoms may only be present when walking and disappear when the child runs or walks backwards.

In generalized dystonia that begins in the arm, symptoms may be task-specific, apparent only during the act of writing or playing a musical instrument. If the disorder progresses, the symptoms of arm dystonia may appear when another part of the body is engaged in voluntary motor activity. If the dystonia spreads to involve parts of the body other than the limb of onset, it will first move to adjacent segments of the body, and then more distally.

Dystonia is usually present continually throughout the day whenever the affected body part is in use and may disappear with sleep.

The age of onset varies, but the peak period is between the ages of seven and ten with symptoms progressing then stabilizing within a five-year period. If early-onset generalized dystonia causes any type of impairment, it is because muscle contractions interfere with normal function. Features such as cognition, strength, and the senses, including vision and hearing, are normal. While dystonia is not fatal, it is a chronic disorder. Historically, early-onset generalized dystonia has also been referred to as idiopathic torsion dystonia and dystonia musculorum deformans.

Cause

Early-onset generalized dystonia is believed to be due to abnormal functioning of the basal ganglia which are deep brain structures involved with the control of movement. The basal ganglia assists in initiating and regulating movement. What goes wrong in the basal ganglia is still unknown. An imbalance of dopamine, a neurotransmitter in the basal ganglia, may underlie several different forms of dystonia.

The gene responsible for early-onset generalized dystonia, termed DYT1, was initially mapped to human chromosome 9q34 and this positional information was refined and used to identify the DYT1 gene.

The mode of inheritance for early-onset generalized dystonia is autosomal dominant. Only one copy of the DYT1 gene is needed to cause symptoms. For reasons scientists do not yet understand, only 30 to 40% of those with the abnormal DYT1 gene develop symptoms of dystonia. There is no way yet to predict whether a person with the abnormal gene will develop symptoms of the disorder and the severity of the illness may differ markedly within a family.

The DYT1 mutation that causes early-onset dystonia is a deletion of three nucleotides, called GAG. Nucleotides are the molecular building blocks of DNA. This relatively minute change in the torsinA blueprint apparently causes critical changes in the function of the protein, and in some cases, ultimately leads to the symptoms of dystonia. Therefore, individuals who have this mutation are carriers of the DYT1 GAG deletion.

Most cases of early-onset dystonia are not due to new mutations, but rather to accurate or faithful copying and inheritance of a gene mutation that occurred many generations in the past. Researchers believe that the same mutation in the DYT1 gene appeared independently in several ethnic populations throughout history and is possibly one of only a few mutations that result in early-onset generalized dystonia. Exactly how the abnormal gene causes dystonia is presently unknown.

Diagnosis

Diagnosis of early-onset generalized dystonia is based on information from the affected individual and the physical and neurological examination. Since this is a hereditary form of dystonia, a family history may be obtained.

Testing for the DYT1 gene may be helpful in confirming diagnosis of early-onset generalized dystonia. However, if the test is negative, this does not mean that the person does not have dystonia, but that he/she does not have this particular genetic subtype of dystonia.

Treatment

Please refer to Chapter 45 for information about dystonia treatments.

Related Questions

What kinds of special educational equipment and / or schooling strategies are appropriate for children with dystonia?

The most important thing is for school administrators and teachers to understand dystonia. It can be difficult for people to recognize that young people with significant muscle problems are just as bright as able-bodied children. Every child with dystonia will have different needs. Keyboards are sometimes helpful for those who can't write well. Access to an elevator instead of stairs is important for those have trouble walking. Students with generalized dystonia may also need a little more time for tests—for example, some have said that filling in the little circles on many standardized test sheets is difficult and takes time.

Is physical therapy appropriate for generalized dystonia?

In some cases stretching can be helpful to preserve a full range of motion. Strengthening exercises can also be beneficial if they are not too strenuous and are specifically suited for each individual case.

What's the best way to deal with pain?

Pain is difficult to treat if symptoms don't respond to oral medications or botulinum toxin injections. Muscle relaxants may have the same effect with such over-the-counter pain medications such as acetaminophen, ibuprofen, and naproxen. Physicians should be able to ascertain whether the pain is due to the dystonia or to other secondary conditions such as arthritis or a compressed nerve.

What should you do when extended family members won't accept your dystonia?

Fear, denial, and guilt among family members are pretty common. Don't hide away from these people—go to the holiday parties and family get-togethers. Most people will eventually adjust, and you have to shrug off those who don't. It is okay to let the extended family see how dystonia affects your everyday life.

Dopa-Responsive Dystonia

Dopa-Responsive Dystonia (DRD), a heredity form of dystonia, is characterized by progressive difficulty walking. Its symptoms may be similar to those of early-onset generalized dystonia.

Symptoms

DRD classically presents as a dystonic gait disorder in early childhood. Although symptoms usually present around age seven, clinical observations in several families have made it evident that manifestations of DRD may appear at any age. The most common complaint of people with DRD is having problems walking. Symptoms may appear minor (such as muscle cramps after exercise) or present later in life in a form that more closely resembles Parkinson's disease. The features of parkinsonism that may occur include slowness of movements, instability or lack of balance, and, less commonly, tremor of the hands at rest.

Symptoms of DRD are often worse later in the day (diurnal fluctuation) and may increase with exertion. They are almost always better in the morning after sleep.

Cause

DRD is believed to be due to abnormal functioning of the basal ganglia, which are deep brain structures involved with the control of movement. The basal ganglia assist in initiating and regulating move-ment. What goes wrong in the basal ganglia is still unknown. An im-balance of dopamine, a neurotransmitter in the basal ganglia, may underlie several different forms of dystonia, but much more research needs to be done for a better understanding of the brain mechanisms involved with dystonia.

Two genes responsive for DRD have been identified: one gene codes for the production of an enzyme called GTP cyclohydrolase and an-other codes for an enzyme called tyrosine hydroxylase. Both of these enzymes contribute to the production of dopamine. When these genes are affected so they cannot fully accomplish the task of producing dopamine and the level of dopamine in the body is reduced, people begin to have problems moving.

The most commonly identified form is termed dopa-responsive dystonia, which is a dominantly inherited condition cause by muta-tions in the GTP cyclohydrolase 1 gene (GTP-CH1). Another common form of DRD is caused by a mutation in the recessively inherited ty-rosine hydroxylase gene (hTH).

About 40% of DRD patients do not present a mutation in the GTP-CH1 or the hTH genes. Other known inherited metabolic conditions may cause DRD (including autosomal recessive deficiencies of GTP-CH1 and aromatic L-amino acid decarboxylase and other defects of tetrahydro-biopterin metabolism). These recessively inherited conditions often affect cognitive function, which is not associated with the dominantly inherited DRD. However, if the symptoms of dominantly inherited DRD affect a patient's speech, a cognitive problem may be presumed even though, in reality, the patient's cognitive function is normal.

Dr. Masaya Segawa of Japan first described this condition as "he-reditary progressive dystonia with marked diurnal variation." Dopa-Responsive Dystonia is the term used to describe the dystonias that respond to levodopa and is used broadly in journals.

Diagnosis

The diagnosis of DRD is not made by one definitive test, but by a series of clinical observations and specific biochemical assessments. Defining the exact etiology, or cause, may not be possible.

A therapeutic trial with levodopa remains the most practical ini-tial approach to diagnosis. However, dystonia that responds to levodopa may result from multiple conditions.

Not all DRD patients respond immediately to levodopa, and even an adverse reaction may help illuminate the etiology and warrant additional tests. Furthermore, not all individuals who are carriers will exhibit symptoms. A detailed family history is an important element of diagnosis.

Obtaining a cerebrospinal fluid sample (via lumbar puncture) is an important component of diagnosing DRD. This may be the easiest way to obtain a preliminary diagnosis and distinguish among the metabolic conditions mentioned above. There remains a chance that the cerebrospinal test will not provide a definitive diagnosis. It is crucial that the patient stop taking levodopa at least a week before the cerebrospinal fluid collection.

Many labs will not perform genetic tests to locate mutations in the GTP-CH1 or hTH genes without results from a previous lumbar puncture. Specific metabolic defects may be detected by an oral phenylalanine loading test, but the test is not 100% sensitive and the scope is limited. False negatives may occur with this test, detecting only about 80% of cases of DRD. Similarly, there are tests for very specific metabolic conditions that do not address the entire scope of possible deficiencies.

DRD also needs to be distinguished from other disorders with similar symptoms including cerebral palsy, early-onset generalized dystonia, spastic paraplegia, and disorders which cause childhood-onset parkinsonism.

A child diagnosed with early-onset generalized dystonia will often receive a trial prescription of levodopa to rule out DRD.

Many symptoms of DRD may mimic cerebral palsy (CP). Leg spasticity inhibiting the ability to walk occurs in both disorders, but DRD has several characteristics that set it apart from CP and other neurological disorders. Most noticeable are the diurnal variation of symptoms and the hereditary aspects of DRD. CP usually results from a brain injury before or during birth and rarely runs in families.

Patients and family members should realize that diagnosing DRD can be challenging, but that these are steps toward differentiating among the various types of dystonia that respond to levodopa.

Treatment

Please refer to Chapter 45 for information about dystonia treatments.

Paroxysmal Dystonia

Paroxysmal dystonia (PD) refers to relatively brief attacks of dystonic movements and postures with a return to normal posture between episodes. It is a form of paroxysmal dyskinesias.

The paroxysmal dyskinesias are movement disorders in which the abnormal movements are present only during the attacks. Between the attacks the person is generally neurologically normal, and there is no loss of consciousness during the attacks.

The paroxysmal dyskinesias are classified as action-induced (kinesigenic) or non-action induced (non-kinesigenic). The most common and best recognized paroxysmal dyskinesias are paroxysmal kinesigenic choreoathetosis (PKC) and paroxysmal dystonic non-kinesigenic choreoathetosis (PDC), also known as paroxysmal dystonia.

Symptoms

Paroxysmal kinesigenic choreoathetosis consists of debilitating attacks of abnormal movements that are triggered by sudden movements, startles, hyperventilation, and stress.

The movements may be choreoathetoid (a nervous disturbance marked by involuntary and uncontrollable movements characteristic of chorea and athetosis) with flowing, dancelike, or slow writhing features, or dystonic, sustained turning or twisting movements.

The attacks can even cause the person to fall. Speech can sometimes be affected due to dystonia, but there is never any alteration of consciousness. The attacks may vary in frequency but are generally brief, lasting seconds to five minutes. There can be as many as 100 attacks per day. A refractory period lasting about five minutes may occur after an attack, during which it is not possible to induce another attack. Approximately 50 percent of people with PKC experience a change in sensation, such as tightness, numbness, pins and needles, or tingling before the attack.

Paroxysmal dystonic choreoathetosis consists of debilitating attacks of primarily dystonic movements but can also involve choreoathetosis. The attacks range in length from minutes to several hours and may occur up to three or four times a day. Attacks in PDC can be precipitated by a number of factors, including alcohol, caffeine, fatigue, stress, or excitement. The attacks are often preceded by a sensory change such as tightness, numbness, pins and needles, or tingling in the affected region.

Cause

The majority of cases of PKC and PDC are idiopathic (of unknown cause) or familial (either autosomal dominant or occasionally sporadic).

155

The paroxysmal dyskinesias are usually dominantly inherited, but this is not always the case. When it is an autosomal dominant disorder, a child of one affected parent has a 50 percent chance of having the disorder. A child whose parents both have the autosomal dominant PKC or PDC will have a 75 percent chance of inheriting the gene for the disorder.

When it is a sporadic (recessive) inherited disorder, parents who both carry the disorder in their genes have a 25 percent chance of passing it on to their children. If only one parent is a carrier of the sporadic disorder, his or her child will have a 50 percent chance of becoming a carrier as well but will not actually have the disorder. Even if one does have the genes for this disorder, paroxysmal dystonia will not always express itself.

Secondary causes of the paroxysmal dyskinesias are abnormal blood sugars, overactive thyroid, parathyroid disorders, focal seizures, multiple sclerosis, encephalitis, head injury, cerebral anoxia, local basal ganglia, or thalamic lesions (such as strokes or tumors).

The most common conditions associated with symptomatic or secondary PKC are multiple sclerosis and head injury, whereas those with symptomatic PDC are multiple sclerosis, and perinatal encephalopathy (i.e., due to anoxia).

In extremely rare cases PDC may be a manifestation of a psychiatric disorder. This diagnosis should be made only by a qualified psychiatric professional. Unfortunately, PDC, as well as numerous other poorly understood movement disorders, have been too often inappropriately labeled psychogenic until the true cause is determined. Such a diagnosis not only causes unnecessary suffering but precludes appropriate treatment.

Age of onset of idiopathic (of unknown origin) cases of PKC and PDC is usually in childhood, between ages 6 and 16 years, although onset can range from a few months to 40 years old. Secondary cases may occur at any age. PKC and PDC occur more frequently in men than women.

The work-up for the paroxysmal dyskinesias can include an electroencephalogram (brain wave test), brain image (such as MRI or CT scan), blood chemistries, and calcium tests. In the idiopathic forms, these tests are generally normal whereas in the secondary forms a focal brain lesion may be found.

Treatment

Please refer to Chapter 45 for information on dystonia treatments.

Rapid-Onset Dystonia-Parkinsonism

Rapid-Onset Dystonia Parkinsonism (RDP), a rare hereditary form of dystonia, is characterized by the abrupt onset of slowness of movement (parkinsonism) and dystonic symptoms.

Symptoms

The classic features of RDP include involuntary dystonic spasms in the limbs, prominent involvement of the speech and swallowing muscles, slowness of movement, and poor balance.

Onset of the combined dystonic and parkinsonian symptoms can be sudden, occurring over hours to days. Symptoms usually stabilize in less then four weeks, after which, it is reported, there is little progression.

RDP usually occurs in adolescence or young adulthood (age range 15 to 45), but onset of mild dystonia-parkinsonism has been reported in individuals up to the age of 58.

Cause

The cause of RDP is not currently understood. Researchers do know that the mode of inheritance for RDP is autosomal dominant.

Genetic linkage studies have excluded RDP from the genomic region encoding for DYT1, the gene responsible for early-onset dystonia, as well as DYT5, the gene responsible for dopa-responsive dystonia. Low levels of the dopamine metabolite homovanillic acid in cerebrospinal fluid indicate a deficit in the dopaminergic system. Additional research needs to be conducted to determine if there is another internal trigger other than low dopamine metabolite levels that initiate the cascade of biochemical changes leading to the abrupt onset of dystonia and parkinsonian symptoms. Understanding this possible trigger may provide further insights into the mechanism of both dystonia and Parkinson's disease.

Diagnosis

Diagnosis is based on neurological examination. Tests such as CT or MRI are normal. A family history is required to distinguish the mild limb dystonia of RDP from early-onset dystonia.

To describe the severity of the symptoms, a scale of one to four has been developed based on the presence of parkinsonism and the ability to walk unassisted. The scale assigns 0 to those unaffected;

1. to those having limb dystonia only, including writer's cramp;

2. to those affected in the face, arm, and neck, and walking normally;

3. to those who are the same as 2 but affected in the legs and walk unassisted; and

4. to those who are the same as 3 but need a walker or use a wheelchair.

Treatment

Treatment for RDP at this time is limited. Levodopa/carbidopa or dopamine agonists may provide some mild improvement in some affected individuals.

Support

By educating yourself with information, you have taken the first step in dealing with dystonia. Dystonia and its emotional offshoots affect every aspect of a person's life—how we think, the way we act, and how we cope.

Stress is an inevitable part of life, and although it clearly does not cause dystonia, it can aggravate dystonia symptoms. Stress-reduction programs such as relaxation techniques, meditation, and journal writing may be beneficial.

Sometimes depression can be a byproduct of dystonia. It, too, can aggravate symptoms and make them worse, but, often, treating depression can result in an improvement of dystonia. It is important to remember that depression is a disease; it is treatable and not a reflection of one's self.

Thousands of people are experiencing similar symptoms, and you are not alone in coping with dystonia. Reassurance from family, friends, and others who have dystonia is beneficial. Support groups offer encouragement, camaraderie, and information about new treatments and medical advances.

Section 14.3

Focal Forms of Dystonia

This section includes the following copyrighted documents from the Dystonia Medical Research Foundation's *Focal Forms of Dystonia*: "Blepharospasm," "Oromandibular Dystonia," "Spasmodic Dystonia," "Cervical Dystonia," and "Writer's Cramp," reprinted with permission from the Dystonia Medical Research Foundation. These documents are available online at www.dystonia-foundation.org; cited January 2002.

Blepharospasm

Blepharospasm is a focal dystonia characterized by increased blinking and involuntary closing of the eyes. People with blepharospasm have normal vision. Visual disturbance is due solely to the forced closure of the eyelids.

Symptoms

Blepharospasm affects the eye muscles and usually begins gradually with excessive blinking and/or eye irritation. In the early stages it may only occur with specific precipitating stressors, such as bright lights, fatigue, and emotional tension. It is almost always present in both eyes.

As the condition progresses, it occurs frequently during the day. The spasms disappear in sleep, and some people find that after a good night of sleep, spasms do not appear for several hours after waking.

In a few cases, spasms may intensify so that the eyelids remain forcefully closed for several hours at a time.

Blepharospasm can occur with dystonia affecting the mouth and/ or jaw (oromandibular dystonia, Meige's syndrome). In such cases, spasms of the eyelids are accompanied by jaw clenching or mouth opening, grimacing, and tongue protrusion.

If blepharospasm causes any type of impairment, it is because muscle contractions interfere with normal function. Features such as cognition, strength, and the senses, including vision and hearing, are normal. While dystonia is not fatal, it is a chronic disorder and prognosis is difficult to predict.

Cause

Blepharospasm is believed to be due to abnormal functioning of the basal ganglia, which are deep brain structures involved with the control of movement. The basal ganglia assists in initiating and regulating movement. What goes wrong in the basal ganglia is still unknown. An imbalance of dopamine, a neurotransmitter in the basal ganglia, may underlie several different forms of dystonia, but much more research needs to be done for a better understanding of the brain mechanisms involved with dystonia.

Though a history of eye trauma may be obtained in some patients, the relationship between trauma and blepharospasm has not been established. In most people it develops spontaneously with no known precipitating factor.

Cases of inherited blepharospasm have been reported, usually in conjunction with early-onset generalized dystonia, which is associated with the DYT1 gene. Blepharospasm may be secondary or symptomatic, occurring in association with other disorders such as tardive dystonia, parkinsonian syndromes, and Wilson's disease.

Diagnosis

Diagnosis of blepharospasm is based on information from the affected individual and the physical and neurological examination. At this time, there is no test to confirm diagnosis of blepharospasm, and, in most cases, laboratory tests are normal.

Blepharospasm should not be confused with:

- Ptosis—drooping of the eyelids caused by weakness or paralysis of a levator muscle of the upper eyelid.

- Blepharitis—an inflammatory condition of the lids due to infection or allergies.

- Hemifacial spasm—a non-dystonic condition involving various muscles on one side of the face, often including the eyelid, and caused by irritation of the facial nerve. The muscle contractions are more rapid and transient than those of blepharospasm, and the condition is always confined to one side.

Treatment

Please refer to Chapter 45 for information on dystonia treatments.

Oromandibular Dystonia

Oromandibular dystonia is a focal dystonia characterized by forceful contractions of the jaw and tongue causing difficulty in opening and closing the mouth and often affecting chewing and speech.

Symptoms

Oromandibular is often associated with dystonia of the cervical muscles (cervical dystonia/spasmodic torticollis), eyelids (blepharospasm), or larynx (spasmodic Dysphonia). The combination of upper and lower dystonia is sometimes called cranial-cervical dystonia. When oromandibular is combined with blepharospasm, it may be referred to as Meige's Syndrome named after Henry Meige, the French neurologist who first described the symptoms in detail in 1910.

- The symptoms usually begin between the ages of 40 and 70 years old and appear to be more common in women than in men.

- Oromandibular dystonia may be a continuous disorder that persists even during sleep, or it may be task-specific, occurring only during activities such as speaking or chewing.

- Difficulty in swallowing is a common aspect of oromandibular dystonia if the jaw is affected, and spasms in the tongue can also make it difficult to swallow.

- If oromandibular dystonia causes any type of impairment, it is because muscle contractions interfere with normal function. Features such as cognition, strength, and the senses, including vision and hearing are normal.

- While dystonia is not fatal, it is a chronic disorder and prognosis is difficult to predict.

Cause

Oromandibular dystonia is believed to be due to abnormal functioning of the basal ganglia, which are deep brain structures involved with the control of movement. The basal ganglia assists in initiating and regulating movement. What goes wrong in the basal ganglia is still unknown. An imbalance of dopamine, a neurotransmitter in the basal ganglia, may underlie several different forms of dystonia, but much more research needs to be done for a better understanding of the brain mechanisms involved with dystonia.

Cases of inherited cranial dystonia have been reported, usually in conjunction with early-onset generalized dystonia which is associated with the DYT1 gene.

Oromandibular dystonia may be secondary, or symptomatic, occurring in association with other disorders such as tardive dystonia, Wilson's disease, Parkinson's disease, and X-linked dystonia-parkinsonian syndrome.

Diagnosis

Diagnosis of blepharospasm is based on information from the affected individual and the physical and neurological examination. At this time, there is no test to confirm diagnosis of oromandibular, and, in most cases, laboratory tests are normal.

Oromandibular dystonia should not be mistaken for Temporomandibular Joint Disease (TMJ) which is an arthritic condition, and not dystonia.

Treatment

For information on dystonia treatments, please refer to Chapter 45.

Related Questions

Can Meige's syndrome spread and/or cause headaches?

It's quite common for dystonia to spread from the face to the neck. In most cases, the dystonia will eventually plateau, and the progression will stop. Dystonia in the neck is more likely to cause pain in the neck, head, or shoulders. Pain is usually easier to treat than abnormal postures. Botulism toxin injections can lessen pain by reducing local spasms.

What is the difference between facial and oromandibular dystonias?

Different nerves are involved in the face than in the jaw. Both are forms of dystonia, but different pathways from the brain to the muscles are affected.

Spasmodic Dysphonia

Spasmodic dysphonia, a focal form of dystonia, involves involuntary spasms of the vocal cords causing interruptions of speech and affecting the voice quality.

Symptoms

Doctors recognize two types of spasmodic dysphonia. In the more common adductor type, speaking causes abnormal involuntary excessive contraction of the muscles that bring the vocal cords together. This causes a tight voice quality, often with abrupt initiation and termination of voicing resulting in a broken speech pattern and short breaks in speech.

In the abductor type, there is an overcontraction of the muscles that separate the vocal cords, resulting in a breathy, whispering voice pattern.

Three other sub-types of SD have been identified by clinicians. One is a combination of adductor and abductor symptoms in which an individual may demonstrate both types of spasms as he/she speaks. In a second subtype, SD symptoms are accompanied by a voice tremor. A third subtype involves a primary voice tremor that is so severe the patient experiences adductor voice stoppages during the tremor.

Symptoms may improve or disappear when whispering, laughing, or singing. Many of the symptoms vary during the day, become aggravated by certain speaking, especially talking on the phone, or increase during stressful situations.

Although it can start any time during a life, spasmodic dysphonia seems to begin frequently in the 40- to 50-year-old group.

SD may also be referred to as Laryngeal Dystonia.

If spasmodic dysphonia causes any type of impairment, it is because muscle contractions interfere with normal function. Features such as cognition, strength, and the senses, including vision and hearing, are normal.

Cause

In most cases the cause of spasmodic dysphonia is unknown. The general medical consensus is that SD is a central nervous system disorder and a focal form of dystonia.

Dystonia disorders are thought to be due to abnormal functioning in the area of the brain called the basal ganglia. The basal ganglia are structures situated deep in the brain.

Onset is usually gradual with no obvious explanation. Researchers are investigating possible mechanisms involved in the triggering of SD including familial factors, inflammation, and/or injury that may lead to central nervous system changes in laryngeal motor control.

SD may co-occur with other dystonias such as blepharospasm, oromandibular dystonia, or cervical dystonia.

Diagnosis

Spasmodic dysphonia is reported to be one of the most frequently misdiagnosed conditions in speech-language pathology. Because there is no definitive test for the SD, the diagnosis rests on the presence of characteristic clinical symptoms and signs in the absence of other conditions that may mimic spasmodic dysphonia.

It is important that an interdisciplinary team of professionals evaluate and provide accurate differential diagnosis. This team usually includes a speech-language pathologist who evaluates voice production and voice quality; a neurologist who carefully searches for other signs of dystonia or other neurological conditions; and an otolaryngologist who examines the vocal cords and their movements.

The excessive strain and misuse of muscle tension dysphonia, the harsh strained voice of certain neurological conditions, the weak voice symptoms of Parkinson's disease, certain psychogenic voice problems, and voice tremors are often confused with spasmodic dysphonia.

Related Questions

Is there a relationship between stuttering and dystonia?

Some people who are diagnosed with secondary stuttering do exhibit severe speech-triggered vocal cord spasms. Although secondary stuttering and spasmodic dysphonia may share some similar vocal symptoms, they are not causally related nor are they effectively treated in the same manner. Stuttering often affects multiple sites of the speech system (voice, articulation, and breathing), while SD only affects the vocal cords.

Do you recommend singing as a way of improving one's speaking voice?

Singing exercises can be very helpful. The motor programming for singing is different from that of speaking. Singing exercises can release some of the tension and stiffness that have crept into the neck and chest when one is getting ready to start talking, especially early in the morning.

Why is my voice better at some times and worse at others?

This phenomenon probably has to do with motor programming. We may program the muscles to move differently when we are experiencing emotional stress. The chemicals in the brain are probably functioning differently from when we are normally talking.

Cervical Dystonia

Cervical Dystonia, also known as spasmodic torticollis, is a focal dystonia characterized by neck muscles contracting involuntarily, causing abnormal movements and posture of the head and neck.

This term is used generally to describe spasms in any direction: forward (anterocollis), backwards (retrocollis), and sideways (torticollis). The movements may be sustained or jerky. Spasms in the muscles or pinching nerves in the neck can result in considerable pain and discomfort.

Symptoms

In cervical dystonia, the neck muscles contract involuntarily in various combinations. Sustained contractions cause abnormal posture of the head and neck, while periodic spasms produce jerky head movements. The severity may vary from mild to severe. Movements are often partially relieved by a gentle touch on the chin or other parts of the face.

If cervical dystonia causes any type of impairment, it is because muscle contractions interfere with normal function. Features such as cognition, strength, and the senses, including vision and hearing, are normal. While dystonia is not fatal, it is a chronic disorder and prognosis is difficult to predict.

Cause

Cervical dystonia is believed to be due to abnormal functioning of the basal ganglia, which are deep brain structures involved with the control of movement. The basal ganglia assists in initiating and regulating movement. What goes wrong in the basal ganglia is still unknown. An imbalance of dopamine, a neurotransmitter in the basal ganglia, may underlie several different forms of dystonia, but much more research needs to be done for a better understanding of the brain mechanisms involved with dystonia.

A history of head or neck injury may be obtained, but the relationship between trauma and dystonia is still unclear. Research to examine the role of trauma is being conducted, including whether there is evidence that trauma may precipitate dystonia in those who have genetic susceptibility. This remains a gray area. It is clear that the interval from trauma to the onset of dystonia can be years.

Cases of inherited cervical dystonia have been reported, usually in conjunction with early-onset generalized dystonia, which is associated with the DYT1 gene.

Diagnosis

Diagnosis of cervical dystonia is based on information from the affected individual and the physical and neurological examination. At this time, there is no test to confirm diagnosis of blepharospasm, and, in most cases, laboratory tests are normal.

Usually the torticollis reaches a plateau and remains stable within five years of onset. This form of focal dystonia is unlikely to spread or become generalized dystonia, though patients with generalized dystonia may also have cervical dystonia. Occasionally, there may be associated focal dystonia.

Cervical dystonia should not be confused with other conditions which cause a twisted neck such as local orthopedic, congenital problems of the neck, ophthalmologic conditions where the head tilts to compensate for double vision. It is sometimes misdiagnosed as stiff neck, arthritis, or wry neck.

Treatment

Please refer to Chapter 45 for dystonia treatment information.

Related Questions

What is selective peripheral denervation surgery?

Selective peripheral denervation, a technique pioneered by Professor Claude Bertrand, is now called the "Bertrand Procedure." This procedure is not a standard one; it is tailored for each patient. As there are different types of torticollis and different movements, it is essential to properly identify the muscles involved carefully, that is to say, the agonist (the muscle mainly responsible for a particular movement) and the antagonist (the muscle responsible for the opposite movement).

The purpose of the Bertrand Procedure is to abolish abnormal movements in all the muscles involved in producing the movement while preserving innervation of those that do not participate. That's what the word selective refers to. Peripheral refers to something that is outside of the brain and spinal canal while denervation is cutting the impulse to certain muscles.

Physiotherapy, starting very soon after surgery, is essential in order to recover a full range of motion, since the brain must relearn a new position.

What criteria is used to determine if a person with cervical dystonia is a candidate for the Bertrand Procedure (selective denervation surgery)?

The purpose of the Bertrand Procedure is to abolish abnormal movements in all the muscles involved while preserving innervation of those that do not participate.

The criteria used to determine if a person is eligible are the following:

1. The dystonia is mainly focalized to the neck;

2. The dystonia has been present for at least three years and is stabilized;

3. The patient had improvement with botulinum toxin injections, has become progressively resistant, and no longer responds to it;

4. Failure of botulinum toxin injections is not an absolute counter indication to the Bertrand Procedure;

5. Pure rotatory torticollis;

6. Rotatory torticollis with chin-up movements;

7. Superior retrocollis;

8. Pure laterocollis;

9. Laterocollis associated with other abnormal movements.

Are ramisectomy and rhizotomy surgeries still performed for cervical dystonia?

The rhizotomy procedure, in contrast to SPD, is inside the spine. That means the destruction of muscle is more generalized. There is also a greater degree of weakness. With selective peripheral denervation, patients don't have permanent weakness. Morbidity and complications are also greater with rhizotomy.

What is the difference between rhizotomy and selective peripheral denervation?

Ramisectomy and rhizotomy involve cutting the nerve or nerves supplying overactive muscles. These surgeries are also rarely performed today. Nonetheless, they may be effective in properly chosen patients.

They are most commonly performed for cervical dystonia patients who have developed resistance to botulinum toxin injections. Possible adverse effects include permanent weakness and difficulty swallowing.

What causes neck pain in cervical dystonia?

Pain in the neck (cervical) dystonia is very complicated. It can be generated by a lot of different structures in the neck. A dull ache results from muscle spasms. You can feel a tight band and some tenderness in the muscles, giving rise to the pain. Pain can also come from secondary contractions of other muscles, from nerves, and from degeneration of the neck spine, in which case arthritis produces pain. Shooting pain is more likely a nerve-generated pain. Neck dystonia can aggravate arthritis and make it get worse faster.

Is there a relationship between CD and arthritis?

Chronic torticollis can cause wear and tear to the neck and limit the range of motion. This may leave the joints more susceptible to arthritis. Oral medications can be used to relieve pain, but narcotics should be avoided. Over-the-counter analgesics (i.e. acetaminophen, ibuprofen, and naproxen) are the best options.

Is there a relationship between CD and headaches?

It is common for people with CD to experience headaches—these headaches are usually quite treatable. Many people have trouble with pressure on the occipital nerve at the back of the head that can cause severe pain. Nerve blocks with local anesthetic may be helpful.

In a person affected by CD, how does one determine if relatively new pain in the shoulder is the result of arthritis or a new focal dystonia?

An EMG (electromyography) can measure the amount of muscle activity—an increase in muscle activity would suggest the presence of dystonia. It's common for people with torticollis to have shoulder problems.

People with cervical dystonia can develop other problems in the spine such as arthritis, ruptured disks, or pinched nerves. People with cervical dystonia who need neck surgery need to be handled with care:

- Certain anesthetics such as droperidol or Compazine (prochlorperazine) should not be used.

- A botulinum toxin injection a few weeks before the surgery may reduce spasms during healing.

- Traction and other forms of physical therapy should be avoided.

- Both physician and patient should be aware that the pain of surgery may activate the dystonia.

What shouldn't people do to treat CD?

Neck manipulation of the neck by a chiropractor who is not very familiar with dystonia can really aggravate the condition. Traction, also, is not a good idea. Massage, however, can sometimes provide temporary relief. If it feels good, do it.

Are cervical dystonia and fibromyalgia related?

No, but both disorders can cause pain in the neck muscles, and therefore cervical dystonia can be misdiagnosed as fibromyalgia. Many with cervical dystonia complain of muscle aching and even more severe pain in the neck muscles. This appears to be due to the pain fibers present in these muscles. Sometimes the muscle contractions and twisting movements in the neck have resulted in arthritis of cervical spine. This can be dangerous in that the resulting thickening of tissue and narrowing of the spinal canal can, by pinching the nerve roots, cause pain and even impinge on the spinal cord to cause paralysis of the legs.

My child developed torticollis at age 2. Is this similar to adult on-set spasmodic torticollis?

Early childhood-onset of neck dystonia is generally different from adult-onset. Congenital torticollis most commonly presents during the first few weeks of life possibly related to restricted head movements of the fetus or to trauma to the neck muscles at or about the time of birth. Congenital torticollis usually improves with physical therapy; however, surgery may be needed. The onset of torticollis during early childhood is unusual. Causes may include hiatal hernia (with vomiting, feeding problems, and posturing of neck during feeding), double vision (producing head tilt), lack of oxygen or high bilirubin counts during the perinatal period (producing cerebral palsy), severe brain infection (encephalitis), head or neck trauma, toxin exposure, brain, or spinal tumors or vascular malformations, cysts of the third ventricle, and certain chemical disorders, such as Leigh's disease. These conditions may generally be assessed with brain and neck imaging and blood and urine analysis.

Writer's Cramp

Writer's cramp is a task-specific focal dystonia of the hand. Symptoms usually appear when a person is trying to do a task that requires fine motor movements. The symptoms may appear only during a particular type of movement, such as writing or playing the piano, but the dystonia may spread to affect many tasks.

Two types of writer's cramp have been described: simple and dystonic. People with simple writer's cramp have difficulty with only one specific task. For example, if writing activates the dystonia, as soon as the person picks up a pen or within writing a few words, dystonic postures of the hand begin to impede the speed and accuracy of writing. In dystonic writer's cramp, symptoms will be present not only when the person is writing, but also when performing other task specific activities, such as shaving, using eating utensils, or applying make-up.

Symptoms

Common manifestations of simple writer's cramp include excessive gripping of the pen, flexion, and sometimes deviation of the wrist, elevation of the elbow, and occasional extension of a finger or fingers causing the pen to fall from the hand. Sometimes the disorder progresses to include the elevation of shoulders or the retraction of arm while writing. Tremor is usually not a symptom of writer's cramp. The symptoms usually begin between the ages of 30 and 50 years old and affect both men and women.

Cramping or aching of the hand is not common. Mild discomfort may occur in the fingers, wrist, or forearm. A similar cramp may be seen in musicians as the violin is bowed, in certain athletes such as golfers, or in typists.

If writer's cramp causes any type of impairment, it is because muscle contractions interfere with normal function. Features such as cognition, strength, and the senses, including vision and hearing are normal. While dystonia is not fatal, it is a chronic disorder and prognosis is difficult to predict.

Cause

Writer's Cramp is believed to be due to abnormal functioning of the basal ganglia, which are deep brain structures involved with the control of movement. The basal ganglia assists in initiating and regulating movement. What goes wrong in the basal ganglia is still unknown. An imbalance of dopamine, a neurotransmitter in the basal ganglia, may underlie several different forms of dystonia, but much more research needs to be done for a better understanding of the brain mechanisms involved with dystonia.

Cases of inherited writer's cramp have been reported, usually in conjunction with early-onset generalized dystonia, which is associated with the DYT1 gene.

Diagnosis

Diagnosis of writer's cramp is based on information from the affected individual and the physical and neurological examination. At this time, there is no test to confirm diagnosis of blepharospasm, and in most cases, laboratory tests are normal.

Sometimes an electromyogram (EMG) will be done to show which muscles are overactive and to what degree.

The hands can be affected by many conditions. Arthritis, tendon problems, and muscle cramps can all cause pain in the hands. Carpal tunnel syndrome is the result of nerve compression.

Writer's cramp is often mistaken for overuse conditions, but they are separate problems. Overuse syndromes or repeated use syndromes are usually characterized by pain, whereas writer's cramp is more likely to cause problems with coordination.

Focal hand dystonia is responsible for only about 5% of all conditions affecting the hand.

Treatment

Please refer to Chapter 45 for information about dystonia treatments.

Related Questions

How do overuse conditions and dystonia differ?

Problems with the hands due to overuse are much more common than writer's cramp. Overuse can be quite painful, but it is still unclear as to where the pain is coming from—the location of the pathology is unclear. Using different movements and muscles to perform a task may help. Stretching and maintaining good posture might also be helpful.

What is carpal tunnel syndrome?

In carpal tunnel syndrome it is very clear where the problem is, and the condition can be successfully treated. The nerve in the carpal tunnel of the hand is pinched—if a person has small carpal tunnels, he/she is more likely to develop a pinched nerve in that area. Most people with carpal tunnel syndrome develop symptoms in both hands.

Is there a relationship between tremor and writer's cramp?

There is a condition called primary writing tremor in which the hand shakes (consistently in one direction) during writing. Whether this tremor is closer related to either writer's cramp or essential tremor is unclear.

Is writer's cramp likely to spread into the arms and shoulder?

Focal adult-onset dystonias usually stay isolated to one part of the body, but in some cases it will progress. It is unlikely, however, to become generalized.

Section 14.4

Secondary Dystonia

"Forms of Dystonia: Secondary Dystonia," available online at www.dystonia-foundation.org, cited January 2002, © Dystonia Medical Research Foundation, reprinted with permission; and excerpts from "The Dystonias," National Institute of Neurological Disorders and Stroke (NINDS), NIH Publication No. 00-717, June 2000.

The various forms of dystonia can be classified into two broad groups: primary dystonias and secondary dystonias. Primary dystonias are largely genetic in origin, whereas secondary dystonias result from an apparent outside factor and are usually attributed to a specific cause such as exposure to certain medications, trauma, toxins, infections, or stroke.

Secondary dystonia is defined as a dystonic disorder that develops mainly as the result of environmental factors that provide insult to the brain. Spinal cord injury, head, and peripheral injury are also recognized contributors to dystonia. Other examples of secondary dystonias include levodopa-induced dystonia in the treatment of parkinsonism;

acute and tardive dystonia due to dopamine receptor blocking agents; and dystonias associated with cerebral palsy, cerebral hypoxia, cerebrovascular disease, cerebral infections and postinfectious states, stroke, encephalitis, brain tumor, and toxicants such as manganese, cyanide, and 3-nitroproprionic acid.

A number of disorders in this group, such as infectious and toxicant-induced neurodegenerations, do not present as pure dystonia, but with a mixture of other neurologic features, often present parkinsonian features of bradykinesia and rigidity.

Many of the ascribed causes of secondary dystonia are based on historical information or subtle clinical findings, and have no diagnostic, radiologic, serologic, or other pathologic marker. One issue debated regarding secondary dystonias is the causal relationship with environmental factors, specifically neuroleptic exposure, perinatal asphyxia, and head and peripheral trauma. It is unclear whether these common insults alone are sufficient to cause dystonia or, as proposed in several studies, if they precipitate or exacerbate symptoms in genetically predisposed individuals. Research continues to better understand these various manifestations of dystonia.

Drug-Induced

A large number of drugs are capable of causing dystonia. In most cases, people develop an acute dystonic reaction resulting after a one-time exposure. The symptoms are usually transient and may be treated successfully with medications such as Benadryl.

Another type of drug-induced dystonia is called tardive dystonia. Tardive dystonia and tardive dyskinesia are neurologic syndromes caused by exposure to certain drugs, namely a class of medications called neuroleptics which are used to treat psychiatric disorders, some gastric conditions, and certain movement disorders. The amount of exposure to such drugs varies greatly among patients. Tardive dystonias and dyskinesias may also develop as a symptom of prolonged treatment with levodopa in some Parkinson's patients.

Drugs belonging to this class of neuroleptics include (trade name listed in parenthesis):

- Acetophenazine (Tindal®)
- Amoxapine (Asendin®)
- Chlorpromazine (Thorazine®)
- Fluphenazine (Permitil® or Prolixin®)
- Haloperidol (Haldol®)

- Loxapine (Loxitane®, Daxolin®)
- Mesoridazine (Serentil®)
- Metoclopramide (Reglan®)
- Molindone (Lidone® or Moban®)
- Perphenazine (Trilafon® or Triavil®)
- Piperacetazine (Quide®)
- Prochlorperazine (Compazine®)
- Promazine (Sparine®)
- Promethazine (Phenergan®)
- Thiethylperazine (Torecan®)
- Thioridazine (Mellaril®)
- Thiothixene (Navane®)
- Trifluoperazine (Stelazine®)
- Triflupromazine (Vesprin®)
- Trimeprazine (Temaril®)

The term tardive means late to indicate that the condition occurs after drug exposure, and the terms dyskinesia and dystonia describe the types of movements involved. These symptoms may develop after weeks or years of drug exposure. Both tardive dystonia and tardive dyskinesia typically involve (but are not necessarily limited to) the muscles of the face. Symptoms may also include muscle spasms of the neck, trunk, and/or arms.

The movements typical of tardive dystonia are generally slower and more sustained than dyskinesias, though the presence of a dystonic tremor in opposition to the main dystonia movement may cause a more rapid appearance of movement. Dyskinesias are usually characterized by quick, jerking movements that may include grimacing, tongue protrusion, lip smacking, puckering, and eye blinking. The arms, legs, and trunk may also be involved. Movements of the fingers may appear as though the individual is playing an invisible guitar or piano.

Both syndromes can occur simultaneously, and the frequency and pattern of movements may fluctuate. If both syndromes are present, the predominant condition will usually dictate the course of treatment.

The treatment of drug-induced dystonia will usually include a gradual withdrawal from the offending medication. If neuroleptics remain a crucial element of an individual's health, a class of newer, atypical neuroleptics (such as clozapine, olanzapine, and quetiapine) may be a suitable substitute. Anticholinergics (such as trihexyphenidyl and benztropine) and muscle relaxers used to treat other forms of dystonia may also be helpful. Baclofen and clonazepam are also sometimes used to treat tardive dystonia. Botulinum toxin injections to a particular muscle group are an additional option for treatment.

Like the treatment of tardive dystonia, the treatment of tardive dyskinesia is very specific to the individual patient. The first step may be to gradually minimize or discontinue the use of the offending medication. Substitute drugs may be recommended to replace neuroleptics. Other drugs such as benzodiazepines, adrenergic antagonists, and dopamine agonists may also be beneficial.

Researchers have yet to fully understand the causes and subsequent treatments of tardive dystonia and tardive dyskinesia. In many cases, discontinuing or lowering the dose of the causative drug will ease symptoms. In some cases, the symptoms will persist after use of the drug has been terminated but with careful management, symptoms may improve and/or disappear with time.

The National Institutes of Neurological Disorders and Stroke conducts and supports a broad range of research on movement disorders including tardive dystonias and dyskinesias. The National Institute of Mental Health is similarly committed to preventing further cases of drug-induced movement disorders in individuals who benefit from neuroleptic treatment.

Trauma

The link between trauma and dystonia is not yet fully understood. It appears from published studies that persons who are carriers of a gene for dystonia may be more likely to have trauma as a triggering factor for the development of dystonia. It is still a gray area at this point. It may be that trauma is a triggering factor, but researchers are not clear as to why some people who have a dystonia gene manifest symptoms and some to do not.

Toxins

A number of uncommon toxins are capable of causing brain damage centered in the motor control region known as the basal ganglia. Dystonia may be one prominent feature experienced by people with these exposures, but it is extremely uncommon for isolated dystonia to be seen in such patients. In other words, the vast majority of people exposed to toxins (for example, manganeses) have additional neurological problems associated with the dystonia. Possibly the most common feature in such patients is the presence of a Parkinson's disease-like state.

Environmental Factors

The role of environmental factors causing or contributing to dystonia remains uncertain. It is not clear why some individuals inheriting a specific gene develop a severe form of dystonia while many others who have inherited the same gene either never develop the problem or only demonstrate a very mild form (this is what is meant by variable penetrance in genetics parlance).

It is possible that unknown environmental factors could play a contributing role in determining whether a member of such a family might develop dystonia and, if so, whether it is a mild or severe form. On the other hand, numerous other unrecognized genetic factors may account for these differences. Where no genetic predisposition exists, it is also possible that environmental factors are an important cause of dystonia. However, at this time, the specific nature of such environmental factors is unknown.

Related Disorders

Secondary dystonias can accompany other disorders resulting in dystonic symptoms. Wilson's disease and Hallervorden-Spatz disease are examples of many disorders that can cause dystonia symptoms.

Wilson's disease (hepatolenticular degeneration) is a hereditary disease resulting from excessive copper accumulation in the body. Normally, copper is excreted without any difficulties, but in people with Wilson's disease the copper is deposited and accumulates in the liver, in the brain, and around the eye. Dystonia is a prominent clinical feature in some people with Wilson's disease. It may present itself as dystonia but is identifiable by an examination of the cornea for a Kayser-Fleisher ring, which is a brown or greenish ring of copper deposits around the cornea. Wilson's disease requires a very specific treatment; therefore in a case of secondary dystonia caused by Wilson's disease, the dystonia will be alleviated by treating the Wilson's disease.

Hallervorden-Spatz disease is a heredodegenerative disease of the brain, typically involving the basal ganglia. As a result of this degeneration, the clinical picture of Hallervorden-Spatz is often marked by pronounced dystonia. There are often some clinical features of parkinsonism in addition. A MRI scan of the brain is very helpful in making the diagnosis of Hallervorden-Spatz disease by depicting increased iron deposition in these deep brain regions. Hallervorden-Spatz disease is one of many disorders in which dystonia is a prominent but not an exclusive feature.

Additional Information

American Speech Language Hearing Association (ASHA)
10801 Rockville Pike
Rockville, MD 20852-3279
Toll-Free: 800-638-8255
Tel: 301-897-5700
Fax: 301-571-0457
Website: www.asha.org
E-mail: actioncenter@asha.org

Benign Essential Blepharospasm Research Foundation, Inc.
637 North 7th Street, Suite 102
P.O. Box 12468
Beaumont, TX 77726-2468
Tel: 409-832-0788
Fax: 409-832-0890
Website: www.blepharospasm.org
E-mail: bebrf@ih2000.net

Dystonia Medical Research Foundation
1 East Wacker Drive, Suite 2430
Chicago, IL 60601-1905
Toll-Free in Canada: 800-361-8061
Tel: 312-755-0198
Fax: 312-803-0138
Website: www.dystonia-foundation.org
E-mail: dystonia@dystonia-foundation.org

National Foundation for Jewish Genetic Diseases
250 Park Avenue c/o Suite 1000
New York, NY 10177
Tel: 212-371-1030
Website: www.nfjgd.org

National Spasmodic Torticollis Association
9920 Talbert Avenue, Suite 233
Fountain Valley, CA 92708
Toll-Free: 800-HURTFUL (487-8385)
Tel: 714-378-7837
Fax: 714-378-7830
Website: www.torticollis.org
E-mail: NSTAmail@aol.com

Tardive Dyskinesia/Tardive Dystonia National Association
P.O. Box 45732
Seattle, WA 98145-0732
Tel: 206-522-3166
Fax: 206-528-2117
E-mail: skjaer@halcyon.com

Worldwide Education & Awareness for Movement Disorders (WE MOVE)
204 West 84ᵗʰ Street
New York, NY 10024
Toll-Free: 800-437-MOV2 (6682)
Tel: 212-875-8312
Fax: 212-875-8389
Website: www.wemove.org
E-mail: wemove@wemove.org

Part Four

Early-Onset Neurological-Based Movement Disorders

Chapter 15

Causes of Children's Movement Disorders

Facts about Neurological Conditions

- Approximately 15 million children in the United States, between the ages of 0-19 years, experience neurological conditions that severely limit their quality of life and life span.

- Special education alone for these children costs society approximately 36 billion dollars annually. (These costs include more personnel for learning disabled classes, transportation to out of district placements, out of district schools for more involved children, equipment, aids, etc.). The advent of biomedical therapies has the potential for declining social costs as the impact of brain injuries is limited or reversed.

- There are no known cures and limited biomedical therapeutics. The majority of present and past research and fundraising dollars focus on saving lives and supportive services such as physical therapy, special education, and care giving.

This chapter includes "CSN Facts," "Areas of Research: Genetic/Metabolic Causes of Neurological Disease," "Areas of Research: Basic Cellular Developmental Neurobiology," and "Areas of Research: Acquired Neurological Dysfunction." Reprinted with permission from the Children's Neurobiological Solutions Foundation, © 2002 CNS Foundation. For additional information, contact the CNS Foundation at 1726 Franceschi Road, Santa Barbara, CA 93103, 866-267-5580 or 805-965-8838, or visit their website at www.cnsfoundation.org.

- Recent advances in biomedicine, particularly in the fields of developmental neurobiology, stem cell research, and genetics, have opened the gateway towards the discovery of brain repair therapies which can enhance mobility and cognition, giving quality of life and health to these children.

- Almost every disease in adulthood has a pediatric correlate. Or, to put it another way, most pediatric diseases have an adult version. Many direct parallels exist between pediatric diseases and their adult counterparts. Often the pediatric version of the disease, however, has a better-defined etiology—for example, an identified gene or cell-type abnormality—that makes it more amenable to a focused investigation. Information that might be gained from the pediatric diseases will undoubtedly contribute to our knowledge and treatment of the adult counterpart whose etiology might be more heterogeneous, complex, less understood and categorized, or vexed by many more confounding variables attributable to lifestyle and environment. This is particularly true for neurodegenerative and demyelinating diseases, spinal cord degenerations, movement disorders, and even stroke.

- Taking advantage of these exciting new fields, Children's Neurobiological Solutions has developed a world-renowned, cross-institutional Scientific Advisory Board of neuroscientists and clinicians, collaborating to achieve aggressive research goals. CNS research goals are focused on the discovery and development of therapeutics that will improve the functional abilities and health of these children, enhancing their quality of life, and reducing the burdens of their caretakers and society.

Genetic/Metabolic Causes of Neurological Disease

A significant number of neurological handicaps in children may be ascribed to defects in genes that then allow waste products to build up in the brain or that preclude useful proteins from being made. Other gene defects prevent newborn cells from finding their right locations in the brain or making proper connections. Other genetic defects cause cells to die prematurely. Although some of these diseases have names and their genes are known (e.g., Tay-Sachs disease), other diseases do not yet have their genes identified (e.g. certain forms of autism). In some, defective genes have been identified, but it is uncertain why that mutation should cause a neurological problem because the role of the gene is not yet well understood (e.g., Rett Syndrome). To know how to use genetic information therapeutically, one must know what that gene does and how to compensate for its absence or dysfunction. Sometimes, even when we think we understand a disease and we know the genetic defect involved and we believe we understand why that gene's defect should cause a neurological problem, we realize that we have an oversimplified view of the brain because simply replacing that gene or missing gene product (known as a protein) does not result in a cure (e.g., Krabbe's disease). In those cases we need to understand how the genes and the brain interact in order to design more effective therapies.

Basic Cellular Developmental Neurobiology

This category includes:

1. Studying neuronal and glial differentiation, i.e., how an immature cell knows what kind of brain cell it needs to become and how the wide variety of cell types in the nervous system come to exist.

2. Studying potential causes for subtle dysgenesis (i.e. how a cell of a given type knows where it is supposed to reside, what connections it is supposed to make, where it is supposed to make those connections and with whom, and why a cell might fail to do any of these things correctly.

3. Precursor cell biology and potential future cellular therapeutics (i.e., how one can study the most immature cells in the nervous system, understand the signals to which they respond, and mobilize such cells (either in the brain or grown in a dish for later reimplantation).

Acquired Neurological Dysfunction

Some neurological handicaps result from an injury or problem that happens to a fundamentally normal nervous system. These may include infections, trauma, inflammation, autoimmune attack, lack of blood flow and/or oxygen, (called hypoxia-ischemia—a stroke-like injury). Some forms of cerebral palsy (including periventricular leukomalacia) may fit into this category and may be amenable to cellular/molecular interventions. Interestingly, some problems may look to be acquired but really occur because the nervous system is not really normal but is somehow more susceptible to an insult that it should have normally been able to ward off or sustain without a problem.

Transitional Therapeutics

This category would include attempts to devise therapeutic interventions that might be regarded as stop-gap measures; i.e., treatments that might diminish the degree of a handicap, improve the quality of day-to-day living, or even buy time and prolong survival until a more definitive but longer-to-develop treatment has been devised. These transitional therapeutics might include bioengineering and/or combined biological-electronic approaches that might enhance communication or motor performance. Novel pharmacological therapies might also fit in this category.

Chapter 16

Acute Cerebellar Ataxia

Alternative names: Cerebellar ataxia; Ataxia–acute cerebellar; Cerebellitis; Acute cerebellar ataxia of childhood.

Definition

Acute cerebellar ataxia is the sudden onset of the movement disorder, ataxia, often following an infectious viral disease.

Causes and Risks

Acute cerebellar ataxia occurs most often in children, especially those younger than 3 years old. It often follows a viral infection by several weeks. Common predisposing infections include chickenpox and Coxsackie viral illnesses. In adults, the most common infections are Epstein-Barr virus and Mycoplasma infections.

Ataxia may be axial (trunk) or limb. Axial ataxia is characterized by a broad-based unsteady gait. When the child is sitting, the trunk may deviate side-to-side and back-to-front or any combination and return to the vertical in a jerky type motion. Jerky eye movements (nystagmus) and jerky explosive speech (dysarthria) may develop at the same time.

Limb ataxia manifests itself with poor fine motor control of the hands or legs and appears to lack coordination. The hand may sway back and forth when reaching for an object.

"Acute Cerebellar Ataxia," updated by Galit Kleiner-Fisman MD, FRCP(C), Department of Neurology, University of Toronto, Toronto, Ontario, Canada, © 2001 A.D.A.M, Inc. Reprinted with permission.

The condition usually subsides without treatment over a period of weeks to months. Occasionally, a child will be left with a persistent movement disorder or behavioral disorder.

Prevention

There is no known prevention.

Symptoms

- Sudden onset jerky body (trunk) movement
- Wide-based unsteady gait
- Inability to walk without support
- Jerky eye movements (nystagmus)
- Jerky speech pattern (dysarthria)
- Uncoordinated movements of the arms or legs

Other suggestive findings:

- Appears in child less than three years of age
- May follow a viral infection

Signs and Tests

The diagnosis of acute cerebellar ataxia is made by excluding other causes of ataxia, and by taking a history of a recent illness.
Tests may include:

- Cerebrospinal fluid studies (CSF total protein)
- CT or MRI scan of the head

Treatment

No treatment is generally attempted for acute cerebellar ataxia.

Prognosis

Full recovery usually occurs without treatment within a few months.

Complications

Movement or behavioral disorders may (rarely) persist. Call your health care provider if any symptoms of ataxia appear.

Chapter 17

Angelman Syndrome

In 1965, Dr. Harry Angelman, an English physician, first described three children with characteristics now known as the Angelman Syndrome (AS).[1] He noted that all had a stiff, jerky gait, absent speech, excessive laughter, and seizures. Other cases were eventually published [2-8] but the condition was considered to be extremely rare and many physicians doubted its existence. The first reports from North America appeared in the early 1980s [9-10] and within the last five years many new reports have appeared.[11-15] Dr. Angelman relates the following regarding his discovery of this syndrome.[16]

> "The history of medicine is full of interesting stories about the discovery of illnesses. The saga of Angelman's Syndrome is one such story. It was purely by chance that nearly thirty years ago three handicapped children were admitted at various times to my children's ward in England. They had a variety of disabilities and although at first sight they seemed to be suffering from different conditions, I felt that there was a common cause for their illness. The diagnosis was purely a clinical one because in spite of technical investigations, which today are more refined, I was unable to establish scientific proof that the three children all had the same handicap. In view of this I hesitated to write about them in the medical journals. However, when on holiday

in Italy I happened to see an oil painting in the Castelvecchio museum in Verona called, *A Boy with a Puppet*. The boy's laughing face and the fact that my patients exhibited jerky movements gave me the idea of writing an article about the three children with a title of *Puppet Children*. It was not a name that pleased all parents, but it served as a means of combining the three little patients into a single group. Later the name was changed to Angelman syndrome. This article was published in 1965 and after some initial interest lay almost forgotten until the early eighties."

The precise incidence of AS is unknown but in the United States and Canada, the Angelman Syndrome Foundation is aware of approximately 1000 individuals, so the disorder is not extremely rare. AS has been reported throughout the world among divergent racial groups. In North America, the great majority of known cases seem to be of Caucasian origin. Although the exact incidence of AS is unknown and estimate of between 1 in 15,000 to 1 in 30,000 seems reasonable.

Developmental and Physical Features

Angelman syndrome is usually not recognized at birth or in infancy since the developmental problems are nonspecific during this time. Parents may first suspect the diagnosis after reading about AS or meeting a child with the condition. The most common age of diagnosis is between three and seven years when the characteristic behaviors and features become most evident. A summary of the developmental and physical findings have recently been published[17] for the purpose of establishing clinical criteria for the diagnosis and these are listed. All of the features do not need to be present for the diagnosis to be made and the diagnosis is often first suspected when the typical behaviors are recognized.

Developmental History and Laboratory Findings

- Normal prenatal and birth history with normal head circumference; absence of major birth defects
- Developmental delay evident by 6–12 months of age
- Delayed but forward progression of development (no loss of skills)
- Normal metabolic, hematologic, and chemical laboratory profiles
- Structurally normal brain using MRI or CT (may have mild cortical atrophy or dysmyelination

Clinical Features

Consistent (100%)

- Developmental delay, functionally severe
- Speech impairment, none or minimal use of words; receptive and non-verbal communication skills higher than verbal ones
- Movement or balance disorder, usually ataxia of gait and/or tremulous movement of limbs
- Behavioral uniqueness: any combination of frequent laughter/smiling; apparent happy demeanor; easily excitable personality, often with hand flapping movements; hypermotoric behavior; short attention span

Frequent (more than 80%)

- Delayed, disproportionate growth in head circumference, usually resulting in microcephaly (absolute or relative) by age 2
- Seizures, onset usually < 3 years of age
- Abnormal EEC, characteristic pattern with large amplitude slow-spike waves

Associated (20–80%)

- Strabismus
- Hypopigmented skin and eyes
- Tongue thrusting; suck/swallowing disorders
- Hyperactive tendon reflexes
- Feeding problems during infancy
- Uplifted, flexed arms during walking
- Prominent mandible
- Increased sensitivity to heat
- Wide mouth, wide-spaced teeth
- Sleep disturbance
- Frequent drooling, protruding tongue
- Attraction to/fascination with water
- Excessive chewing/mouthing behaviors
- Flat back of head

Adapted from Williams CA, Angelman H, Clayton-Smith J, Driscoll DJ, Hendrickson JE, Knoll JHM, Magenis RE, Schinzel A, Wagstaff J, Whidden EM, Zori RT. Angelman Syndrome: Consensus for diagnostic criteria. *Am J Med Genet*. 1995;56:237.

Chromosome 15

For several decades the chromosome study of AS revealed no abnormalities, but with the development of improved methods a very small deleted area was found in chromosome 15. Newer molecular methods now demonstrate a deletion in about 70% of individuals with AS. The deleted area, although extremely small, is actually quite large when viewed at the molecular level. It is believed to be about 3.5 million molecules in length, enough of a distance to contain many genes.

The deleted region on chromosome 15 is known to contain genes that are activated or inactivated depending upon the chromosome's parent of origin (i.e., the 15 chromosome inherited from the mother might have a gene that is turned on but the same gene inherited from the father's 15 might be turned off). Because the deletions seen in AS only occur on the chromosome 15 given by the mother, it is believed the gene is turned on only on the maternal chromosome. No AS gene/s have yet been isolated although this may be forthcoming soon. Disruption of genes that are active on the paternally derived 15 is now known to cause another mental retardation disorder termed the Prader-Willi syndrome (PWS). The PWS gene/s are actually located close to the AS gene, but they are different.

After the discovery of the chromosome deletion, another rare cause of AS was discovered. This cause was due to the child having both 15 chromosomes inherited from the father, a condition termed paternal uniparental disomy (UPD). In this case, there is no deletion, but the child is still missing the active AS gene because the paternal-derived chromosomes 15 only have *turned off* AS genes on them.

Furthermore, there are also some families having two or more children with AS. In many of these families it was then shown that the AS children always inherited the same maternal chromosome 15s but inherited different paternal 15s indicating that the inherited maternal chromosome may have a mutation on it. Two genetic mechanisms have now been identified whereby AS can be inherited from the mother: mutations in Imprinting Control (IC) region and mutations in the putative AS gene which is called ubiquitin-protein ligase E3A (UBE3A).[18,19] The UBE3A gene is believed to be the causative gene in AS, and all of the other genetic mechanisms that are associated with

AS appear to cause inactivations or absence of this gene. UBE3A is an enzymatic component of a complex protein degradation system termed the ubiquitin-proteasome pathway.[20] This pathway is located in the cytoplasm of all cells. This pathway involves the action of a small protein molecule, ubiquitin, that can be attached to proteins thereby causing them to be degraded. However, we currently do not know what brain proteins the UBE3A enzyme is normally supposed to be degrading.

We also now know that there is an region on chromosome 15 that can control or turn on or off the action of the UBE3A gene. This control region is called the Imprinting Center (IC) and the small mutations have been identified in this area that can cause AS.[21] The IC appears to be able to exert its effect on UBE3A from a distant location, but how this regulation happens is not yet known.

All of these discoveries have now led to the realization that there are several genetic classes or mechanisms that cause AS and all generally lead to the typical clinical features observed in AS although minor differences may occur between groups. These mechanisms are summarized in Table 17.1.

Table 17.1. Genetic Classes of Angelman Syndrome

	Cause	Percent	Notes
1	Large common deletions	70-75%*	Includes deletion of the P gene, so hypopigmentation is common
2	Other chromosome abnormalities	2%	Unusual chromosome rearrangements can cause absence of the 15q11-13 region
3	Paternal uniparental disomy	4%	Inheritance of both paternal 15's, no maternal 15 present
4	Imprinting center mutation	1%	Rare occurrence
5	UBE3A mutation	3-5%	Newest identified mechanism. True incidence not yet established
6	Unknown	15%	All of the above mechanisms should be ruled out by genetic testing before assignment to this group.

* = estimated frequency of cases. These numbers vary slightly from study to study

Medical and Developmental Problems

Seizures

More than 90% are reported to have seizures, but this may be an overestimation because medical reports tend to dwell on the more severe cases. Less than 25% develop seizures before 12 months of age. Most have onset before 3 years, but occurrence in older children or in teenagers is not exceptional.[13] The seizures can be of any seizure type (i.e. major motor involving jerking of all extremities; absence type involving brief periods lack of awareness), and may require multiple anticonvulsant medications. Seizures may be difficult to recognize or distinguish from the child's usual tremulousness, hyperkinetic limb movements or attention deficits. The typical EEG is often more abnormal than expected and it may suggest seizures when in fact there are none.

There is no agreement as to the optimal seizure medication, but there are patterns of use that are more frequent. Anticonvulsant medications used for minor motor seizures (valproic acid, clonazepam, etc.) are more commonly prescribed than are ones for major motor seizures (diphenylhydantoin, phenobarbital, etc.). Single medication use is preferred, but seizure breakthrough is common. Some children with uncontrollable seizures have been placed on a ketogenic diet, but it is uncertain if this is beneficial. Children with AS are at risk for medication over-treatment because their movement abnormalities or attention deficits can be mistaken for seizures and because EEG abnormalities can persist even when seizures are controlled.

Gait and Movement Disorders

Hyperkinetic movements of the trunk and limbs have been noted in early infancy[19] and jitteriness or tremulousness may be present in the first 6 months of life. Voluntary movements are often irregular, varying from slight jerkiness to uncoordinated coarse movements that prevent walking, feeding, and reaching for objects. Gross motor milestones are delayed; sitting usually occurring after age 12 months and walking is often delayed until age 3 or 4 years.[13,15]

In early childhood, the mildly impaired child can have almost normal walking. There may be only mild toe-walking or an apparent prancing gait. This may be accompanied by a tendency to lean or lurch forward. The tendency to lean forward is accentuated during running and, in addition, the arms are held uplifted. For these children, balance and coordination does not appear to be a major problem. More severely affected children can be very stiff and robot-like or extremely shaky and jerky when walking. Although they can crawl fairly effectively, they may freeze up or appear to become anxious when placed in the standing position. The legs are kept wide based and the feet are flat and turned outward. This, accompanied by uplifted arms, flexed elbows, and downward turned hands, produces the characteristic gait of AS. Some children are so ataxic and jerky that walking is not possible until they are older and better able to compensate motorically for the jerkiness; about 10% may fail to achieve walking.[23] In situations where AS has not been diagnosed, the nonspecific diagnosis of cerebral palsy is often given to account for the abnormal walking. Physical therapy is usually helpful in improving ambulation and sometimes bracing or surgical intervention may be needed to properly align the legs.

Hyperactivity

Hyperactivity is probably the most typical behavior in AS. It is best described as hypermotoric with a short attention span. Essentially all young AS children have some component of hyperactivity[15] and males and females appear equally affected. Infants and toddlers may have seemingly ceaseless activity, constantly keeping their hands or toys in their mouth, moving from object to object. In extreme cases, the constant movement can cause accidental bruises and abrasions. Grabbing, pinching, and biting in older children have also been noted and may be heightened by the hypermotoric activity. Persistent and consistent behavior modification helps decrease or eliminate these unwanted behaviors.

Attention span can be so short that social interaction is prevented because the AS child cannot attend to facial and other social cues. In milder cases, attention may be sufficient enough to learn sign language and other communication techniques. For these children, educational and developmental training programs are much easier to structure and are generally more effective. Observations in young adults suggest that the hypermotoric state decreases with age. Most AS children do not receive drug therapy for hyperactivity although some may benefit from use of medications such as methylphenidate (Ritalin). Use of sedating agents such as phenothiazines is not recommended due to their potency and side effects.

Laughter and Happiness

It is not known why laughter is so frequent in AS. Even laughter in normal individuals is not well understood. Studies of the brain in

AS, using MRI or CT scans, have not shown any defect suggesting a site for a laughter-inducing abnormality. Although there is a type of seizure associated with laughter, termed gelastic epilepsy, this is not what occurs in AS. The laughter in AS seems mostly to be an expressive motor event; most reactions to stimuli, physical or mental, are accompanied by laughter or laughter-like facial grimacing. Although AS children experience a variety of emotions, apparent happiness predominates.

The first evidence of this distinctive behavior may be the onset of early or persistent social smiling at the age of 1-3 months. Giggling, chortling, and constant smiling soon develop and appear to represent normal reflexive laughter, but cooing and babbling are delayed or reduced. Later, several types of facial or behavioral expressions characterize the infant's personality. A few have pronounced laughing that is truly paroxysmal or contagious and bursts of laughter occurred in 70% in one study.[15] More often, happy grimacing and a happy disposition are the predominant behaviors. In rare cases, the apparent happy disposition is fleeting as irritability and hyperactivity are the prevailing personality traits; crying, shrieking, screaming, or short guttural sounds may then be the predominant behaviors.

Speech and Language

Some AS children seem to have enough comprehension to be able to speak, but in even the highest functioning, conversational speech does not develop. Clayton-Smith [23] reported that a few individuals spoke 1-3 words, and in a survey of 47 individuals, Buntirix et al.[15] reported that 39% spoke up to 4 words, but it was not noted if these words were used meaningfully. Children with AS caused by uniparental disomy or extremely small deletions may have higher verbal and cognitive skills; at times use of 10-20 words may occur, although pronunciation may be awkward.[16]

The speech disorder in AS has a somewhat typical evolution. Babies and young infants cry less often and have decreased cooing and babbling. A single apparent word, such as mama, may develop around 10-18 months but it is used infrequently and indiscriminately without symbolic meaning. By 2-3 years of age, it is clear that speech is delayed but it may not be evident how little the AS child is verbally communicating; crying and other vocal outbursts may also be reduced. By 3 years of age, higher functioning AS children are initiating some type of nonverbal language. Some point to body parts and indicate some of their needs by use of simple gestures, but they are much better at following and understanding commands. Others, especially those with severe seizures or extreme hyperactivity cannot be attentive enough to achieve the first stages of communication, such as establishing sustained eye contact. The nonverbal language skills of AS children vary greatly; with the most advanced ones able to learn some sign language and to use such aids as picture-based communication boards.

Mental Retardation and Developmental Testing

Developmental testing is compromised by the attention deficit, hyperactivity, and lack of speech and motor control. In such situations, test results are invariably in the severe range of functional impairment. More attentive children can perform in the moderate range and a minority can perform in some categories, like receptive social skills, in the mildly impaired range. As we learn more about the different genetic classes of AS it appears that patients with uniparental disomy have less severe clinical manifestations than those with large deletions.[24]

It is known that the cognitive abilities in AS are higher than indicated from developmental testing. The most striking area where this is evident is in the disparity between understanding language and speaking language. Because of their ability to understand language, AS children soon distinguish themselves from other severe mental retardation conditions. Young adults with AS are usually socially adept and respond to most personal cues and interactions. Because of their interest in people they establish rewarding friendships and communicate a broad repertoire of feelings and sentiments, enriching their relationship to families and friends. They participate in group activities, household chores, and in the activities and responsibilities of daily living. Like others, they enjoy most recreational activities such as TV, sports, going to the beach, etc.

There is a wide range however in the developmental outcome so that not all individuals with AS attain the above noted skills. A few will be more impaired in terms of their mental retardation and lack of attention, and this seems especially the case in those with difficult to control seizures or those with extremely pronounced ataxia and movement problems. Fortunately, most children with AS do not have these severe problems, but even for the less impaired child, inattentiveness and hyperactivity during early childhood often give the impression that profound functional impairment is the only outcome possible. However, with a secure home and consistent behavioral intervention and stimulation, the AS child begins to overcome these problems and developmental progress occurs.

Hypopigmentation

When AS is caused by the large deletion, skin and eye hypopigmentation usually results. This occurs because there is a pigment gene, located close to the AS gene, that is also missing. This pigment gene produces a protein (called the P protein) that is believed to be crucial in melanin synthesis. Melanin is the main pigment molecule in our skin. In some children with AS, this hypopigmentation can be so severe that a form of albinism is suspected. In those with uniparental disomy or very small deletions, this gene is not missing and normal skin and eye pigmentation is seen. AS children with hypopigmentation are sun sensitive, so use of a protective sunscreen is important. Not all AS children with deletions of the P gene are obviously hypopigmented, but may only have relatively lighter skin color than either parent.

Strabismus and Ocular Albinism

Surveys of AS patients demonstrate 30-60% incidence of strabismus. This problem appears to be more common in children with eye hypopigmentation, since pigment in the retina is crucial to normal development of the optic nerve pathways. Management of strabismus in AS is similar to that in other children: evaluation by an ophthalmologist, correction of any visual deficit, and where appropriate, patching and surgical adjustment of the extraocular muscles. The hypermotoric activities of some AS children will make wearing of patches or glasses difficult.

CNS Structure

The brain in AS is structurally normal although occasional abnormalities have been reported. The most common Mid or CT change, when any is detected, is mild cortical atrophy (i.e. a small decrease in the thickness of the cortex of the cerebrum) and/or mildly decreased myelination (i.e. the more central parts of the brain appear to have a slight degree of diminished white matter).[13,15] Several detailed microscopic and chemical studies of the brain in AS have been reported but the findings generally have been nonspecific or the number of cases has been to few to make meaningful conclusions.

Sleep Disorders

Parents report that decreased need for sleep and abnormal sleep/ wake cycles are characteristic of AS. Sleep disturbances have been reported in AS infants and abnormal sleep/wake cycles have been studied in one AS child who benefited from a behavioral treatment program. Many families construct safe but confining bedrooms to accommodate disruptive nighttime wakefulness. Use of sedatives such as chloral hydrate or diphenhydramine (Benadryl) may be helpful if wakefulness excessively disrupts home life. Administration of 0.3 mg melatonin one hour before bedtime, has been shown to be of help in some children, but should not be given in the middle of the night if the child awakens.[25] Nevertheless, most AS infants and children do not receive sleep medications and those who do usually do not require long-term use.

Feeding Problems and Oral-Motor Behaviors

Feeding problems, are frequent but not generally severe and usually manifest early as difficulty in sucking or swallowing.[13, 15, 22] Tongue movements may be uncoordinated with thrusting and generalized oral-motor uncoordination. There may be trouble initiating sucking and sustaining breast feeding, and bottle feeding may prove easier. Frequent spitting up may be interpreted as formula intolerance or gastroesophageal reflux. The feeding difficulties often first present to the physician as a problem of poor weight gain or as a failure to thrive concern. Infrequently, severe gastroesophageal reflux may require surgery.

AS children are notorious for putting everything in their mouths. In early infancy, hand sucking (and sometimes foot sucking) is frequent. Later, most exploratory play is by oral manipulation and chewing. The tongue appears to be of normal shape and size, but in 30-50%, persistent tongue protrusion is a distinctive feature. Some have constant protrusion and drooling while others have protrusion that is noticeable only during laughter. Some infants with protrusion eventually have no noticeable problem during later childhood (some seem to improve after oral-motor therapy). For the usual AS child with protruding tongue behavior, the problem remains throughout childhood and can persist into adulthood. Drooling is frequently a persistent problem, often requiring bibs. Use of medications, such as scopolamine to dry secretions usually does not provide an adequate long-term effect.

Physical Growth

Newborns appear to be physically well formed, but by 12 months of age some show a deceleration of cranial growth which may represent relative or absolute microcephaly (absolute microcephaly means having a head circumference in the lower 2.5 percentile). The prevalence of absolute microcephaly varies from 88%[13] to 34%[12] and may be as low as 25% when nondeletion cases are also included.[11] Most AS individuals however have head circumferences less than the 25th percentile by age 3 years, often accompanied by a flattened back of the head. Average height is lower than the mean for normal children but most AS children will plot within the normal range. Final adult height has ranged from 4 foot 9 inches to 5 foot 10 inches in a series of 8 adults with AS. Familial factors will influence growth so that taller parents have AS children that tend to be taller than the average AS child. During infancy weight gain may be slow due to feeding problems but by early childhood most AS children appear to have near normal subcutaneous fat. Obesity is rare but by late childhood some increased weight gain can occur.[23]

Education

The severe developmental delay in AS mandates that a full range of early training and enrichment programs be made available. Unstable or nonambulatory children may also benefit from physical therapy. Occupational therapy may help improve fine motor and oral-motor control. Special adaptive chairs or positioners may be required at various times, especially for hypotonic or extremely ataxic children. Speech and communication therapy is essential and should focus on nonverbal methods of communication. Augmentative communication aids, such as picture cards or communication boards, should be used at the earliest appropriate time.

Extremely active and hypermotoric AS children will require special provisions in the classroom and teacher aides or assistants may be needed to integrate the child into the classroom. AS children with attention deficits and hyperactivity need room to express themselves and to grapple with their hypermotoric activities. The classroom setting should be structured, in its physical design and its curricular program, so that the active AS child can fit in or adjust to the school environment. Individualization and flexibility are important factors. Consistent behavior modification in the school and at home can enable the AS child to be toilet trained (schedule-trained), and to perform most self-help skills related to eating, dressing, and performing general activities in the home.

Young Adulthood

During adolescence, puberty may be delayed by 1-3 years but sexual maturation occurs with development of normal secondary sexual characteristics. Some weight gain can be evident in this period but obesity is rare. Young AS adults continue to learn and are not known to have significant deterioration in their mental abilities. Physical health in AS appears to be remarkably good. For many, seizure medications can be discontinued in the early adolescent or adult years.[10,15] AS individuals with severe ataxia may lose their ability to walk if ambulation is not encouraged. Scoliosis can develop in adolescence and especially is a problem in those that are nonambulatory. Scoliosis is treated with early bracing to prevent progression and surgical correction or stabilization may be necessary for severe cases. Life span does not appear to be dramatically shortened. We are aware of a 58-year-old woman with AS and know of many in their third or fourth decades of life.

Laboratory Testing for AS

In the child in whom the diagnosis is suspected, a high resolution chromosome analysis is often first performed to insure that no other chromosome disorder is present, since features such as mental delay, microcephaly, or seizures can be seen in other chromosome abnormalities. Concurrent with the chromosome test, a fluorescent in situ hybridization (FISH) analysis is usually ordered. This is a newly developed test that uses molecular tags to detect the deletion on chromosome 15. The tags are directly applied to the chromosome and it is examined under a microscope after special stains are applied. The FISH test is far superior to the usual chromosome test. The child with AS should have their chromosomes 15 fully studied to insure that they are structurally normal; a maternal chromosome study as well provides additional confirmation that the maternal chromosome 15 is structurally normal. In the diagnostic testing for AS, some laboratories now offer a DNA methylation test in conjunction with chromosome and FISH testing. The methylation test can detect the large common deletion type of AS, as well as those with uniparental disomy or defects in the imprinting center (IC). Confirmation of uniparental disomy needs to be made by additional molecular testing (usually, study of parental sequencing in the IC area). About 80-85% of individuals with AS will be diagnosed by a combination of these tests, but there still remain 15-20% who will have some genetic testing. Some individuals in this latter group, perhaps less than 20%, will be found to have mutations in the UBE3A gene. At this time, molecular analysis for UBE3A and IC mutations is not commercially available, but is being performed in some research labs.

Genetic Counseling

About 70-75% of cases of AS are caused by spontaneously occurring large common deletions or by uniparental disomy. To our knowledge, recurrence has not been reported for these groups and recurrence risk is estimated to be less than 1%. Prenatal diagnosis is available by use of cytogenetic or molecular testing.

Individuals with AS due to IC mutations can have either inherited this mutation from a normal mother or have received the mutation spontaneously (i.e., not inherited). In the former case the theoretical recurrence risk is 50% and in the latter (i.e., spontaneous mutation) the risk is believed to be less than 1%.

Those with AS due to UBE3A mutations, as is the case with IC mutations, can have either received the mutation from a normal mother or acquired it by spontaneous mutation. Recurrence risk is felt to be 50% in the former and less than 1% in the latter. When IC or UBE3A mutations have been molecularly characterized, prenatal diagnosis is available via molecular testing. Cases of AS that are associated with a structurally abnormal chromosome 15 (i.e., a chromosome translocation) may have an increased risk for recurrence. In these instances, the recurrence risk must be based upon the specific chromosome abnormality and what is known about its risk of recurrence. Prenatal diagnosis by cytogenetic and/or molecular techniques is generally available in these instances.

Estimating recurrence risks is very difficult for individuals with AS who have normal genetic studies (i.e., have none of the above etiologies). Familial occurrence in this group does occur, so it is apparent that the recurrence risk for AS is higher than it is for those with, for example, a typical large common deletion. Until more is known about this group, caution is warranted during genetic counseling since the theoretical recurrence risk can be as high as 50% (if one assumes that undetected AS-causing mutations have been inherited from the mother).

It should be noted that the customary chromosome study, performed during routine prenatal diagnosis is often interpreted as normal in AS fetuses with deletions, since the small abnormalities on chromosome 15 would not be detected by this type of study. Specialized chromosome 15/FISH studies are needed for prenatal diagnosis in cases where the testing seeks to establish normal chromosome 15 structure. Also, fetal ultrasound offers no help in detecting physical abnormalities related to AS since the affected fetus is expected to be well formed. Amniotic fluid volume and alpha-fetoprotein levels also appear normal.

Because of the complexities of evaluating recurrence risk, genetic counseling from an expert familiar with AS is advised.

Acknowledgments

This document was developed by the Angelman Syndrome Foundation with assistance from the Raymond C. Philips Unit, Division of Genetics, Department of Pediatrics, University of Florida.

References

1. Angelman, H. "Puppet" children: A report on three cases. *Dev Med Child Neurol.* l965;7:681-688.

2. Bower BD, Jeavons PM. The "happy puppet" syndrome. *Arch Dis Child.* 1967;42:298-302.

3. Berg, JM and Pakula, Z. Angelman's ("happy puppet") syndrome. *Am J Dis Child.* 1972; 123:72-74.

4. Berggreen, S. "Happy puppet" syndrome. *Ugeskr Laeger.* 1972; 134:1174.

5. Kibel MA, Burness FR, The "happy puppet" syndrome. *Centr Afr J Med.* 1973; 19:91-93.

6. Mayo 0, Nelson MM, Townsend, HRA. Three more "happy puppets." *Dev Med Child Neural.* 1973;1S:63-74.

7. Moore JR, Jeavons PM. The "happy puppet" syndrome: Two new cases and a review of five previous cases. *Neuropaediatrie.* 1973;4: 172-179.

8. Elian M. Fourteen happy puppets. *Clin Pediatr.* 1975; 14:902-908.

9. Pashayan H, Singer W, Dove C, Eisenberg E, Seto B. The Angelman syndrome in two brothers. *Am J Med Genet.* 1982;13:295-298.

10. Williams CA, Frias IL. The Angelman ("happy puppet") syndrome. *Am J Med Genet.* 1982; 11:543-460.

11. Clayton-Smith J and Pembrey ME. Angelman syndrome. *J Med Genet.* l992;29(6):412-415.

12. Saitoh, S., Harada, N., Jinno, Y., et al. Molecular and clinical study of 61 Angelman syndrome patients. *Am J Med Genet.* 1994;52: 158-163.

13. Zori RT, Hendrickson J, Woolven S, Whidden EM, Gray B, Williams CA. Angelman syndrome: clinical profile. *J Child Neuro.* 1992;7(3):279-280.

14. Chan CTJ, Clayton-Smith J, Cheng XJ, et al. Molecular mechanisms in Angelman syndrome: a survey of 93 patients. *J Med Genet.* 1993;30:895-902.

15. Buntinx IM, Ilunnekam RCM, Brouwer OF, Stroink H, Beuten J, Mangelsehots K, Fryns JP. Clinical profile of Angelman syndrome at different ages. *Am J Med Genet.* 1995;56: 176-183.

16. Angelman H (1991): personal correspondence.

17. Williams CA, Angelman H, Clayton-Smith J, Driscoll DJ, Hendrickson JE, Knoll JHM, Magenis RE, Schinzel A, Wagstaff J, Whidden EM, Zori RT. Angelman syndrome: Consensus for diagnostic criteria. *Am J Med Genet.* 1995;56:237-238.

18. Kishino T, Lalande M, Wagstaff J. UBE3A/E6-AP mutations cause Angelman syndrome. *Nature Genet.* 1997;15:70-73.

19. Matsuura T, Sutcliffe JS, Fang P. et al. De novo truncations mutations in E6-AP ubiquitin-protein ligase gen (UBE3A) in Angelman syndrome. *Nature Genet.* 1997;15:74-77.

20. Mitch WE, Goldberg AL. Mechanisms of Muscle Wasting The Role of the Ubiquitin-Proteasome Pathway. *NEJM.* 1996;335: 58-64.

21. Saitoh S, Buiting K, Cassidy S, et al. Clinical Spectrum and Molecular Diagnosis of Angelman and Prader-Willi Syndrome Patients with an Imprinting Mutation. *Am J Med Genet.* 1997;68:195-206.

22. Fryburg JS, Breg WR, Lindgren V. Diagnosis of Angelman Syndrome in Infants. *Am J Med Genet.* 1991;38:58-64.

23. Clayton-Smith, J. Clinical research on Angelman syndrome in the United Kingdom: observations on 82 affected individuals. *Am J Med Genet.* l993;46(1): 12-15.

24.   Bottani A, Robinson VP, DeLozier-Blanchet CD, et al. Angelman syndrome due to paternal uniparental disomy of chromosome 15: A milder phenotype? *Am J Med Genet.* 1994;51:35-40.

25.   Wagstaff J. *Genetic and Clinical Studies of Angelman Syndrome.* Angelman Syndrome Foundation Medial and Scientific Symposium. July 3, 1997, Seattle, Washington.

Chapter 18

Ataxia-Telangiectasia (Louis-Bar Syndrome)

Definition

An inherited disorder that affects many tissues and systems in the body, characterized by the presence of multiple symptoms such as telangiectases, ataxic gait, proneness to infection, defective humoral/ cellular immunity, and increased risk of malignancies.

Causes and Risks

Ataxia-telangiectasia is transmitted as an autosomal recessive trait. The disease results from mutations in a gene called ATM. The most obvious symptoms of the disease are multiple telangiectases that are easily visible in the white of the eye and certain skin areas such as the ear and nose, graying of the hair, and irregular pigmentation of the skin in areas exposed to sunlight. In addition there is decreased coordination of movements, ataxia, in late childhood.

Prevention

Because these patients are very sensitive to radiation they should never be exposed to radiation therapy and no unnecessary x-rays should be done. Genetic counseling is of benefit to prospective parents

"Ataxia-Telangiectasia," updated 10/30/01 by David G. Brooks, M.D., Ph.D., Division of Medical Genetics, University of Pennsylvania Medical Center, Philadelphia, PA, © 2001 A.D.A.M., Inc. Reprinted with permission.

with a family history of ataxia-telangiectasia. Even parents of a child with this disorder may have a slight increased risk of cancer. They should have genetic counseling and more intensive screening for cancer.

Symptoms

- delayed walking
- unsteady, jerky gait, ataxic gait (cerebellar ataxia)
- dilated blood vessels in the whites of the eyes
- dilated blood vessels in skin of nose, ears, and flexion side of the elbow and knee
- severe recurrent respiratory infections
- decreasing mental development which slows or stops after age 10-12
- movement disorder (late)
- repetitive abnormal or jerky eye movements (nystagmus) (late)
- coffee-with-milk colored spots of the skin
- seizures

Signs

- mask-like face
- decreased to absent deep tendon reflexes
- multiple skin changes including pigmentary, eczematoid, and atrophic
- growth failure
- absence of pubertal development
- hypoplastic tonsils, lymph nodes, and spleen

Tests

- serum immunoglobulin levels (IgE, IgA)—especially decreased IgA and IgE levels
- decreased B and T cell screen
- elevated alpha fetoprotein (AFP)

- carcinoembryonic antigen (CEA)
- increased tendency of chromosomes to break on exposure to radiation
- genetic testing may be available for mutations in the ATM gene
- X-rays may show underdeveloped, small thymus in childhood
- abnormal glucose tolerance test

Treatment

There is no specific treatment for ataxia-telangiectasia. Treatment is directed at specific associated problems.

Support Groups

Ataxia Telangiectasia Children's Project
688 S. Military Trail
Deerfield Beach, FL 33442
Toll-Free: 800-543-5728
Website: www.atcp.org
E-mail: info@atcp.org

Prognosis

An early death is expected, commonly in early adolescence.

Complications

- severe recurrent pulmonary infections
- progressive movement disorder with confinement to a wheelchair
- malignant disease, especially lymphoma, that can result in death
- diabetes
- progressive scoliosis and kyphosis

Call your health care provider if signs or symptoms of the disease are present.

Chapter 19

Cerebral Palsy (CP)

In the 1860s, an English surgeon named William Little wrote the first medical descriptions of a puzzling disorder that struck children in the first years of life, causing stiff, spastic muscles in their legs and, to a lesser degree, their arms. These children had difficulty grasping objects, crawling, and walking. They did not get better as they grew up nor did they become worse. Their condition, which was called Little's disease for many years, is now known as spastic diplegia. It is just one of several disorders that affect control of movement and are grouped together under the term cerebral palsy.

Because it seemed that many of these children were born following premature or complicated deliveries, Little suggested their condition resulted from a lack of oxygen during birth. This oxygen shortage damaged sensitive brain tissues controlling movement, he proposed. But in 1897, the famous psychiatrist Sigmund Freud disagreed. Noting that children with cerebral palsy often had other problems such as mental retardation, visual disturbances, and seizures, Freud suggested that the disorder might sometimes have roots earlier in life, during the brain's development in the womb. "Difficult birth, in certain cases," he wrote, "is merely a symptom of deeper effects that influence the development of the fetus."

Despite Freud's observation, the belief that birth complications cause most cases of cerebral palsy was widespread among physicians,

---

"Cerebral Palsy: Hope Through Research," National Institute of Neurological Disorders and Stroke (NINDS), updated June 2000.

families, and even medical researchers until very recently. In the 1980s, however, scientists analyzed extensive data from a government study of more than 35,000 births and were surprised to discover that such complications account for only a fraction of cases—probably less than 10 percent. In most cases of cerebral palsy, no cause of the factors explored could be found. These findings from the NINDS perinatal study have profoundly altered medical theories about cerebral palsy and have spurred today's researchers to explore alternative causes.

At the same time, biomedical research has also led to significant changes in understanding, diagnosing, and treating persons with cerebral palsy. Risk factors not previously recognized have been identified, notably intrauterine exposure to infection and disorders of coagulation, and others are under investigation. Identification of infants with cerebral palsy very early in life gives youngsters the best opportunity to receive treatment for sensory disabilities and for prevention of contractures. Biomedical research has led to improved diagnostic techniques such as advanced brain imaging and modern gait analysis. Certain conditions known to cause cerebral palsy, such as rubella (German measles) and jaundice, can now be prevented or treated. Physical, psychological, and behavioral therapy that assist with such skills as movement and speech and foster social and emotional development can help children who have cerebral palsy to achieve and succeed. Medications, surgery, and braces can often improve nerve and muscle coordination, help treat associated medical problems, and either prevent or correct deformities.

Much of the research to improve medical understanding of cerebral palsy has been supported by the National Institute of Neurological Disorders and Stroke (NINDS), one of the federal government's National Institutes of Health. The NINDS is America's leading supporter of biomedical research into cerebral palsy and other neurological disorders. The NINDS hopes to help the more than 4,500 American babies and infants diagnosed each year, their families, and others concerned about cerebral palsy benefit from these research results.

What Is Cerebral Palsy?

Cerebral palsy is an umbrella-like term used to describe a group of chronic disorders impairing control of movement that appear in the first few years of life and generally do not worsen over time. The term cerebral refers to the brain's two halves, or hemispheres, and palsy describes any disorder that impairs control of body movement. Thus, these disorders are not caused by problems in the muscles or nerves. Instead, faulty development or damage to motor areas in the brain disrupts the brain's ability to adequately control movement and posture.

Symptoms of cerebral palsy lie along a spectrum of varying severity. An individual with cerebral palsy may have difficulty with fine motor tasks, such as writing or cutting with scissors; experience trouble with maintaining balance and walking; or be affected by involuntary movements, such as uncontrollable writhing motion of the hands or drooling. The symptoms differ from one person to the next, and may even change over time in the individual. Some people with cerebral palsy are also affected by other medical disorders, including seizures or mental impairment. Contrary to common belief, however, cerebral palsy does not always cause profound handicap. While a child with severe cerebral palsy might be unable to walk and need extensive, lifelong care, a child with mild cerebral palsy might only be slightly awkward and require no special assistance. Cerebral palsy is not contagious nor is it usually inherited from one generation to the next. At this time, it cannot be cured, although scientific research continues to yield improved treatments and methods of prevention.

How Many People Have This Disorder?

The United Cerebral Palsy Associations estimate that more than 500,000 Americans have cerebral palsy. Despite advances in preventing and treating certain causes of cerebral palsy, the number of children and adults it affects has remained essentially unchanged or perhaps risen slightly over the past 30 years. This is partly because more critically premature and frail infants are surviving through improved intensive care. Unfortunately, many of these infants have developmental problems of the nervous system or suffer neurological damage. Research is under way to improve care for these infants, as in ongoing studies of technology to alleviate troubled breathing and trials of drugs to prevent bleeding in the brain before or soon after birth.

What Are the Different Forms?

Spastic diplegia, the disorder first described by Dr. Little in the 1860s, is only one of several disorders called cerebral palsy. Today doctors classify cerebral palsy into four broad categories—spastic, athetoid, ataxic, and mixed forms—according to the type of movement disturbance.

Spastic cerebral palsy. In this form of cerebral palsy, which affects 70 to 80 percent of patients, the muscles are stiffly and permanently contracted. Doctors will often describe which type of spastic cerebral palsy a patient has based on which limbs are affected. The names given to these types combine a Latin description of affected limbs with the term plegia or paresis, meaning paralyzed or weak.

When both legs are affected by spasticity, they may turn in and cross at the knees. As these individuals walk, their legs move awkwardly and stiffly and nearly touch at the knees. This causes a characteristic walking rhythm, known as the scissors gait.

Individuals with spastic hemiparesis may also experience hemiparetic tremors, in which uncontrollable shaking affects the limbs on one side of the body. If these tremors are severe, they can seriously impair movement.

Athetoid, or dyskinetic, cerebral palsy. This form of cerebral palsy is characterized by uncontrolled, slow, writhing movements. These abnormal movements usually affect the hands, feet, arms, or legs and, in some cases, the muscles of the face and tongue, causing grimacing or drooling. The movements often increase during periods of emotional stress and disappear during sleep. Patients may also have problems coordinating the muscle movements needed for speech, a condition known as dysarthria. Athetoid cerebral palsy affects about 10 to 20 percent of patients.

Ataxic cerebral palsy. This rare form affects the sense of balance and depth perception. Affected persons often have poor coordination; walk unsteadily with a wide-based gait, placing their feet unusually far apart; and experience difficulty when attempting quick or precise movements, such as writing or buttoning a shirt. They may also have intention tremor. In this form of tremor, beginning a voluntary movement, such as reaching for a book, causes a trembling that affects the body part being used and that worsens as the individual gets nearer to the desired object. The ataxic form affects an estimated 5 to 10 percent of cerebral palsy patients.

Mixed forms. It is common for patients to have symptoms of more than one of the previous three forms. The most common mixed form includes spasticity and athetoid movements but other combinations are also possible.

What Other Medical Disorders Are Associated with Cerebral Palsy?

Many individuals who have cerebral palsy have no associated medical disorders. However, disorders that involve the brain and impair its motor function can also cause seizures and impair an individual's intellectual development, attentiveness to the outside world, activity and behavior, and vision and hearing. Medical disorders associated with cerebral palsy include:

- **Mental impairment.** About one-third of children who have cerebral palsy are mildly intellectually impaired, one-third are moderately or severely impaired, and the remaining third are intellectually normal. Mental impairment is even more common among children with spastic quadriplegia.

- **Seizures or epilepsy.** As many as half of all children with cerebral palsy have seizures. During a seizure, the normal, orderly pattern of electrical activity in the brain is disrupted by uncontrolled bursts of electricity. When seizures recur without a direct trigger, such as fever, the condition is called epilepsy. In the person who has cerebral palsy and epilepsy, this disruption may be spread throughout the brain and cause varied symptoms all over the body—as in tonic-clonic seizures—or may be confined to just one part of the brain and cause more specific symptoms—as in partial seizures.

  Tonic-clonic seizures generally cause patients to cry out and are followed by loss of consciousness, twitching of both legs and arms, convulsive body movements, and loss of bladder control.

  Partial seizures are classified as simple or complex. In simple partial seizures, the individual has localized symptoms, such as muscle twitches, chewing movements, and numbness or tingling. In complex partial seizures, the individual may hallucinate, stagger, perform automatic and purposeless movements, or experience impaired consciousness or confusion.

- **Growth problems**. A syndrome called *failure to thrive* is common in children with moderate-to-severe cerebral palsy, especially those with spastic quadriparesis. Failure to thrive is a general term physicians use to describe children who seem to lag behind in growth and development despite having enough food. In babies, this lag usually takes the form of too little weight gain; in young children, it can appear as abnormal shortness; in teenagers, it may appear as a combination of shortness and lack of sexual development. Failure to thrive probably has several causes, including, in particular, poor nutrition and damage to the brain centers controlling growth and development. In addition, the muscles and limbs affected by cerebral palsy tend to be smaller than normal. This is especially noticeable in some patients with spastic hemiplegia, because limbs on the affected side of the body may not grow as quickly or as large as those on the more normal side. This condition usually affects the hand and foot most severely. Since the involved foot in hemiplegia is often smaller than the unaffected foot even among patients who walk, this size difference is probably not due to lack of use. Scientists believe the problem is more likely to result from disruption of the complex process responsible for normal body growth.

- **Impaired vision or hearing**. A large number of children with cerebral palsy have strabismus, a condition in which the eyes are not aligned because of differences in the left and right eye muscles. In an adult, this condition causes double vision. In children, however, the brain often adapts to the condition by ignoring signals from one of the misaligned eyes. Untreated, this can lead to very poor vision in one eye and can interfere with certain visual skills, such as judging distance. In some cases, physicians may recommend surgery to correct strabismus. Children with hemiparesis may have hemianopia, which is defective vision or blindness that impairs the normal field of vision of one eye. For example, when hemianopia affects the right eye, a child looking straight ahead might have perfect vision except on the far right. In homonymous hemianopia, the impairment affects the same part of the visual field of both eyes. Impaired hearing is also more frequent among those with cerebral palsy than in the general population.

- **Abnormal sensation and perception**. Some children with cerebral palsy have impaired ability to feel simple sensations like touch and pain. They may also have stereognosia, or difficulty perceiving and identifying objects using the sense of touch. A child with stereognosia, for example, would have trouble identifying a hard ball, sponge, or other object placed in his hand without looking at the object.

What Causes Cerebral Palsy?

Cerebral palsy is not one disease with a single cause, like chicken pox or measles. It is a group of disorders with similar problems in control of movement, but probably with different causes. When physicians try to uncover the cause of cerebral palsy in an individual child, they look at the form of cerebral palsy, the mother's and child's medical history, and onset of the disorder.

In the United States, about 10 to 20 percent of children who have cerebral palsy acquire the disorder after birth. (The figures are higher in underdeveloped countries.) Acquired cerebral palsy results from brain damage in the first few months or years of life and can follow brain infections, such as bacterial meningitis or viral encephalitis, or results from head injury—most often from a motor vehicle accident, a fall, or child abuse.

Congenital cerebral palsy, on the other hand, is present at birth, although it may not be detected for months. In most cases, the cause of congenital cerebral palsy is unknown. Thanks to research, however, scientists have pinpointed some specific events during pregnancy or around the time of birth that can damage motor centers in the developing brain. Some of these causes of congenital cerebral palsy include:

- **Infections during pregnancy.** German measles, or rubella, is caused by a virus that can infect pregnant women and, therefore, the fetus in the uterus, to cause damage to the developing nervous system. Other infections that can cause brain injury in the developing fetus include cytomegalovirus and toxoplasmosis. There is relatively recent evidence that placental and perhaps other maternal infection can be associated with cerebral palsy.

- **Jaundice in the infant.** Bile pigments, compounds that are normally found in small amounts in the bloodstream, are produced when blood cells are destroyed. When many blood cells are destroyed in a short time, as in the condition called Rh incompatibility, the yellow-colored pigments can build up and cause jaundice. Severe, untreated jaundice can damage brain cells.

- **Rh incompatibility.** In this blood condition, the mother's body produces immune cells called antibodies that destroy the fetus's blood cells, leading to a form of jaundice in the newborn.

- **Severe oxygen shortage in the brain or trauma to the head during labor and delivery.** The newborn infant's blood is specially equipped to compensate for low levels of oxygen, and asphyxia (lack of oxygen caused by interruption in breathing or poor oxygen supply) is common in babies during the stresses of labor and delivery. But if asphyxia severely lowers the supply of oxygen to the infant's brain for lengthy periods, the child may develop brain damage called hypoxic-ischemic encephalopathy. A significant proportion of babies with this type of brain damage die, and others may develop cerebral palsy, which is then often accompanied by mental impairment and seizures.

In the past, physicians and scientists attributed most cases of cerebral palsy to asphyxia or other complications during birth if they could not identify another cause. However, extensive research by NINDS scientists and others has shown that very few babies who experience asphyxia during birth develop encephalopathy soon after birth. Research also shows that a large proportion of babies who experience asphyxia do not grow up to have cerebral palsy or other neurological disorders. Birth complications including asphyxia are now estimated to account for about 6 percent of congenital cerebral palsy cases.

- **Stroke.** Coagulation disorders in mothers or infants can produce stroke in the fetus or newborn baby. Bleeding in the brain has several causes—including broken blood vessels in the brain, clogged blood vessels, or abnormal blood cells—and is one form of stroke. Although strokes are better known for their effects on older adults, they can also occur in the fetus during pregnancy or the newborn around the time of birth, damaging brain tissue and causing neurological problems. Ongoing research is testing potential treatments that may one day help prevent stroke in fetuses and newborns.

What Are the Risk Factors?

Research scientists have examined thousands of expectant mothers, followed them through childbirth, and monitored their children's early neurological development. As a result, they have uncovered certain characteristics, called risk factors, that increase the possibility that a child will later be diagnosed with cerebral palsy:

- **Breech presentation.** Babies with cerebral palsy are more likely to present feet first, instead of head first, at the beginning of labor.

- **Complicated labor and delivery.** Vascular or respiratory problems of the baby during labor and delivery may sometimes be the first sign that a baby has suffered brain damage or that a baby's brain has not developed normally. Such complications can cause permanent brain damage.

- **Low Apgar score.** The Apgar score (named for anesthesiologist Virginia Apgar) is a numbered rating that reflects a newborn's condition. To determine an Apgar score, doctors periodically check the baby's heart rate, breathing, muscle tone, reflexes, and skin color in the first minutes after birth. They then assign points; the higher the score, the more normal the baby's condition. A low score at 10-20 minutes after delivery is often considered an important sign of potential problems.

- **Low birthweight and premature birth.** The risk of cerebral palsy is higher among babies who weigh less than 2500 grams (5 lbs., 7 1/2 oz.) at birth and among babies who are born less than 37 weeks into pregnancy. This risk increases as birthweight falls.

- **Multiple births.** Twins, triplets, and other multiple births are linked to an increased risk of cerebral palsy.

- **Nervous system malformations.** Some babies born with cerebral palsy have visible signs of nervous system malformation, such as an abnormally small head (microcephaly). This suggests that problems occurred in the development of the nervous system while the baby was in the womb.

- **Maternal bleeding or severe proteinuria late in pregnancy.** Vaginal bleeding during the sixth to ninth months of pregnancy and severe proteinuria (the presence of excess proteins in the urine) are linked to a higher risk of having a baby with cerebral palsy.

- **Maternal hyperthyroidism, mental retardation, or seizures.** Mothers with any of these conditions are slightly more likely to have a child with cerebral palsy.

- **Seizures in the newborn.** An infant who has seizures faces a higher risk of being diagnosed, later in childhood, with cerebral palsy.

Knowing these warning signs helps doctors keep a close eye on children who face a higher risk for long-term problems in the nervous system. However, parents should not become too alarmed if their child has one or more of these factors. Most such children do not have and do not develop cerebral palsy.

Can Cerebral Palsy Be Prevented?

Several of the causes of cerebral palsy that have been identified through research are preventable or treatable:

- Head injury can be prevented by regular use of child safety seats when driving in a car, wearing helmets during bicycle rides, and elimination of child abuse. In addition, common sense measures around the household—like close supervision during bathing and keeping poisons out of reach—can reduce the risk of accidental injury.

- Jaundice of newborn infants can be treated with phototherapy. In phototherapy, babies are exposed to special blue lights that break down bile pigments, preventing them from building up and threatening the brain. In the few cases in which this treatment is not enough, physicians can correct the condition with a special form of blood transfusion.

- Rh incompatibility is easily identified by a simple blood test routinely performed on expectant mothers and, if indicated, expectant fathers. This incompatibility in blood types does not usually cause problems during a woman's first pregnancy, since the mother's body generally does not produce the unwanted antibodies until after delivery. In most cases, a special serum given after each childbirth can prevent the unwanted production of antibodies. In unusual cases, such as when a pregnant woman develops the antibodies during her first pregnancy or antibody production is not prevented, doctors can help minimize problems by closely watching the developing baby and, when needed, performing a transfusion to the baby while in the womb or an exchange transfusion (in which a large volume of the baby's blood is removed and replaced) after birth.

- Rubella, or German measles, can be prevented if women are vaccinated against this disease before becoming pregnant.

In addition, it is always good to work toward a healthy pregnancy through regular prenatal care and good nutrition and by eliminating smoking, alcohol consumption, and drug abuse. Despite the best efforts of parents and physicians, however, children will still be born with cerebral palsy. Since in most cases the cause of cerebral palsy is unknown, little can currently be done to prevent it. As investigators learn more about the causes of cerebral palsy through basic and clinical research, doctors and parents will be better equipped to help prevent this disorder.

What Are the Early Signs?

Early signs of cerebral palsy usually appear before 3 years of age, and parents are often the first to suspect that their infant is not developing motor skills normally. Infants with cerebral palsy are frequently slow to reach developmental milestones, such as learning to roll over, sit, crawl, smile, or walk. This is sometimes called developmental delay.

Some affected children have abnormal muscle tone. Decreased muscle tone is called hypotonia; the baby may seem flaccid and relaxed, even floppy. Increased muscle tone is called hypertonia, and the baby may seem stiff or rigid. In some cases, the baby has an early period of hypotonia that progresses to hypertonia after the first 2 to 3 months of life. Affected children may also have unusual posture or favor one side of their body.

Parents who are concerned about their baby's development for any reason should contact their physician, who can help distinguish normal variation in development from a developmental disorder.

How Is Cerebral Palsy Diagnosed?

Doctors diagnose cerebral palsy by testing an infant's motor skills and looking carefully at the infant's medical history. In addition to checking for those symptoms described above—slow development, abnormal muscle tone, and unusual posture—a physician also tests the infant's reflexes and looks for early development of hand preference.

Reflexes are movements that the body makes automatically in response to a specific cue. For example, if a newborn baby is held on its back and tilted so the legs are above its head, the baby will automatically extend its arms in a gesture, called the Moro reflex, that looks like an embrace. Babies normally lose this reflex after they reach 6 months, but those with cerebral palsy may retain it for abnormally long periods. This is just one of several reflexes that a physician can check.

Doctors can also look for hand preference—a tendency to use either the right or left hand more often. When the doctor holds an object in front and to the side of the infant, an infant with hand preference will use the favored hand to reach for the object, even when it is held closer to the opposite hand. During the first 12 months of life, babies do not usually show hand preference. But infants with spastic hemiplegia, in particular, may develop a preference much earlier, since the hand on the unaffected side of their body is stronger and more useful.

The next step in diagnosing cerebral palsy is to rule out other disorders that can cause movement problems. Most important, doctors must determine that the child's condition is not getting worse. Although its symptoms may change over time, cerebral palsy by definition is not progressive. If a child is continuously losing motor skills, the problem more likely springs from elsewhere—including genetic diseases, muscle diseases, disorders of metabolism, or tumors in the nervous system. The child's medical history, special diagnostic tests, and, in some cases, repeated check-ups can help confirm that other disorders are not at fault.

The doctor may also order specialized tests to learn more about the possible cause of cerebral palsy. One such test is computed tomography, or CT, a sophisticated imaging technique that uses x-rays and a computer to create an anatomical picture of the brain's tissues and structures. A CT scan may reveal brain areas that are underdeveloped, abnormal cysts (sacs that are often filled with liquid) in the brain, or other physical problems. With the information from CT scans, doctors may be better equipped to judge the long-term outlook for an affected child.

Magnetic resonance imaging, or MRI, is a brain imaging technique that is rapidly gaining widespread use for identifying brain disorders. This technique uses a magnetic field and radio waves, rather than x-rays. MRI gives better pictures of structures or abnormal areas located near bone than CT.

A third test that can expose problems in brain tissues is ultrasonography. This technique bounces sound waves off the brain and uses the pattern of echoes to form a picture, or sonogram, of its structures. Ultrasonography can be used in infants before the bones of the skull harden and close. Although it is less precise than CT and MRI scanning, this technique can detect cysts and structures in the brain, is less expensive, and does not require long periods of immobility.

Finally, physicians may want to look for other conditions that are linked to cerebral palsy, including seizure disorders, mental impairment, and vision or hearing problems.

When the doctor suspects a seizure disorder, an electroencephalogram, or EEG, may be ordered. An EEG uses special patches called electrodes placed on the scalp to record the natural electrical currents inside the brain. This recording can help the doctor see telltale patterns in the brain's electrical activity that suggest a seizure disorder.

Intelligence tests are often used to determine if a child with cerebral palsy is mentally impaired. Sometimes, however, a child's intelligence may be underestimated because problems with movement, sensation, or speech due to cerebral palsy make it difficult for him or her to perform well on these tests.

If problems with vision are suspected, the doctor may refer the patient to an ophthalmologist for examination; if hearing impairment seems likely, an otologist may be called in.

Identifying these accompanying conditions is important and is becoming more accurate as ongoing research yields advances that make diagnosis easier. Many of these conditions can then be addressed through specific treatments, improving the long-term outlook for those with cerebral palsy.

How Is Cerebral Palsy Managed?

Cerebral palsy cannot be cured, but treatment can often improve a child's capabilities. In fact, progress due to medical research now means that many patients can enjoy near-normal lives if their neurological problems are properly managed. There is no standard therapy that works for all patients. Instead, the physician must work with a team of health care professionals first to identify a child's unique needs and impairments and then to create an individual treatment plan that addresses them.

Some approaches that can be included in this plan are drugs to control seizures and muscle spasms, special braces to compensate for muscle imbalance, surgery, mechanical aids to help overcome impairments, counseling for emotional and psychological needs, and physical, occupational, speech, and behavioral therapy. In general, the earlier treatment begins, the better chance a child has of overcoming developmental disabilities or learning new ways to accomplish difficult tasks.

The members of the treatment team for a child with cerebral palsy should be knowledgeable professionals with a wide range of specialties. A typical treatment team might include:

- a physician, such as a pediatrician, a pediatric neurologist, or a pediatric physiatrist, trained to help developmentally disabled children. This physician, often the leader of the treatment team, works to synthesize the professional advice of all team members into a comprehensive treatment plan, implements treatments, and follows the patient's progress over a number of years.

- an orthopedist, a surgeon who specializes in treating the bones, muscles, tendons, and other parts of the body's skeletal system. An orthopedist might be called on to predict, diagnose, or treat muscle problems associated with cerebral palsy.

- a physical therapist, who designs and implements special exercise programs to improve movement and strength.

- an occupational therapist, who can help patients learn skills for day-to-day living, school, and work.

- a speech and language pathologist, who specializes in diagnosing and treating communication problems.

- a social worker, who can help patients and their families locate community assistance and education programs.

- a psychologist, who helps patients and their families cope with the special stresses and demands of cerebral palsy. In some cases, psychologists may also oversee therapy to modify unhelpful or destructive behaviors or habits.

- an educator, who may play an especially important role when mental impairment or learning disabilities present a challenge to education.

Individuals who have cerebral palsy and their family or caregivers are also key members of the treatment team, and they should be intimately involved in all steps of planning, making decisions, and applying treatments. Studies have shown that family support and personal determination are two of the most important predictors of which individuals who have cerebral palsy will achieve long-term goals.

Too often, however, physicians and parents may focus primarily on an individual symptom—especially the inability to walk. While mastering specific skills is an important focus of treatment on a day-to-day basis, the ultimate goal is to help individuals grow to adulthood and have maximum independence in society. In the words of one physician, "After all, the real point of walking is to get from point A to point B. Even if a child needs a wheelchair, what's important is that they're able to achieve this goal."

What Specific Treatments Are Available?

Physical, Behavioral, and Other Therapies

Therapy—whether for movement, speech, or practical tasks—is a cornerstone of cerebral palsy treatment. The skills a 2-year-old needs to explore the world are very different from those that a child needs in the classroom or a young adult needs to become independent. Cerebral palsy therapy should be tailored to reflect these changing demands.

Physical therapy usually begins in the first few years of life, soon after the diagnosis is made. Physical therapy programs use specific sets of exercises to work toward two important goals: preventing the weakening or deterioration of muscles that can follow lack of use (called disuse atrophy) and avoiding contracture, in which muscles become fixed in a rigid, abnormal position.

Contracture is one of the most common and serious complications of cerebral palsy. Normally, a child whose bones are growing stretches the body's muscles and tendons through running and walking and other daily activities. This ensures that muscles will grow at the same rate. But in children with cerebral palsy, spasticity prevents this stretching and, as a result, muscles do not grow fast enough to keep up with lengthening bones. The resulting contracture can disrupt balance and trigger loss of previous abilities. Physical therapy alone, or in combination with special braces (sometimes called orthotic devices), works to prevent this complication by stretching spastic muscles. For example, if a child has spastic hamstrings (tendons located behind the knee), the therapist and parents should encourage the child to sit with the legs extended to stretch them.

A third goal of some physical therapy programs is to improve the child's motor development. A widespread program of physical therapy that works toward this goal is the Bobath technique, named for a husband and wife team who pioneered this approach in England. This program is based on the idea that the primitive reflexes retained by many children with cerebral palsy present major roadblocks to learning voluntary control. A therapist using the Bobath technique tries to counteract these reflexes by positioning the child in an opposing movement. So, for example, if a child with cerebral palsy normally keeps his arm flexed, the therapist would repeatedly extend it.

A second such approach to physical therapy is patterning, which is based on the principle that motor skills should be taught in more or less the same sequence that they develop normally. In this contro-versial approach, the therapist guides the child with movement prob-lems along the path of normal motor development. For example, the child is first taught elementary movements like pulling himself to a standing position and crawling before he is taught to walk—regard-less of his age. Some experts and organizations, including the Ameri-can Academy of Pediatrics, have expressed strong reservations about the patterning approach, because studies have not documented its value.

Physical therapy is usually just one element of an infant develop-ment program that also includes efforts to provide a varied and stimu-lating environment. Like all children, the child with cerebral palsy needs new experiences and interactions with the world around him in order to learn. Stimulation programs can bring this valuable ex-perience to the child who is physically unable to explore.

As the child with cerebral palsy approaches school age, the empha-sis of therapy shifts away from early motor development. Efforts now focus on preparing the child for the classroom, helping the child mas-ter activities of daily living, and maximizing the child's ability to com-municate.

Physical therapy can now help the child with cerebral palsy pre-pare for the classroom by improving his or her ability to sit, move independently or in a wheelchair, or perform precise tasks, such as writing. In occupational therapy, the therapist works with the child to develop such skills as feeding, dressing, or using the bathroom. This can help reduce demands on caregivers and boost self-reliance and self-esteem. For the many children who have difficulty communicat-ing, speech therapy works to identify specific difficulties and overcome them through a program of exercises. For example, if a child has dif-ficulty saying words that begin with "b," the therapist may suggest daily practice with a list of "b" words, increasing their difficulty as each list is mastered. Speech therapy can also work to help the child learn to use special communication devices, such as a computer with voice synthesizers.

Behavioral therapy provides yet another avenue to increase a child's abilities. This therapy, which uses psychological theory and techniques, can complement physical, speech, or occupational therapy. For example, behavioral therapy might include hiding a toy inside a box to reward a child for learning to reach into the box with his weaker hand. Likewise, a child learning to say his "b" words might be given a balloon for mastering the word. In other cases, therapists may try to discourage unhelpful or destructive behaviors, such as hair-pulling or biting, by selectively presenting a child with rewards and praise during other, more positive activities.

As a child with cerebral palsy grows older, the need for and types of therapy and other support services will continue to change. Continuing physical therapy addresses movement problems and is supplemented by vocational training, recreation and leisure programs, and special education when necessary. Counseling for emotional and psychological challenges may be needed at any age, but is often most critical during adolescence. Depending on their physical and intellectual abilities, adults may need attendant care, living accommodations, transportation, or employment opportunities.

Regardless of the patient's age and which forms of therapy are used, treatment does not end when the patient leaves the office or treatment center. In fact, most of the work is often done at home. The therapist functions as a coach, providing parents and patients with the strategy and drills that can help improve performance at home, at school, and in the world. As research continues, doctors and parents can expect new forms of therapy and better information about which forms of therapy are most effective for individuals with cerebral palsy.

Drug Therapy

Physicians usually prescribe drugs for those who have seizures associated with cerebral palsy, and these medications are very effective in preventing seizures in many patients. In general, the drugs given to individual patients are chosen based on the type of seizures, since no one drug controls all types. However, different people with the same type of seizure may do better on different drugs, and some individuals may need a combination of two or more drugs to achieve good seizure control.

Drugs are also sometimes used to control spasticity, particularly following surgery. The three medications that are used most often are diazepam, which acts as a general relaxant of the brain and body; baclofen, which blocks signals sent from the spinal cord to contract the muscles; and dantrolene, which interferes with the process of muscle contraction. Given by mouth, these drugs can reduce spasticity for short periods, but their value for long-term control of spasticity has not been clearly demonstrated. They may also trigger significant side effects, such as drowsiness, and their long-term effects on the developing nervous system are largely unknown. One possible solution to avoid such side effects may lie in current research to explore new routes for delivering these drugs.

Patients with athetoid cerebral palsy may sometimes be given drugs that help reduce abnormal movements. Most often, the prescribed drug belongs to a group of chemicals called anticholinergics that work by reducing the activity of acetylcholine. Acetylcholine is a chemical messenger that helps some brain cells communicate and that triggers muscle contraction. Anticholinergic drugs include trihexyphenidyl, benztropine, and procyclidine hydrochloride.

Occasionally, physicians may use alcohol washes—or injections of alcohol into a muscle—to reduce spasticity for a short period. This technique is most often used when physicians want to correct a developing contracture. Injecting alcohol into a muscle that is too short weakens the muscle for several weeks and gives physicians time to work on lengthening the muscle through bracing, therapy, or casts. In some cases, if the contracture is detected early enough, this technique may avert the need for surgery.

Surgery

Surgery is often recommended when contractures are severe enough to cause movement problems. In the operating room, surgeons can lengthen muscles and tendons that are proportionately too short. First, however, they must determine the exact muscles at fault, since lengthening the wrong muscle could make the problem worse.

Finding problem muscles that need correction can be a difficult task. To walk two strides with a normal gait, it takes more than 30 major muscles working at exactly the right time and exactly the right force. A problem in any one muscle can cause abnormal gait. Furthermore, the natural adjustments the body makes to compensate for muscle problems can be misleading. A new tool that enables doctors to spot gait abnormalities, pinpoint problem muscles, and separate real problems from compensation is called gait analysis. Gait analysis combines cameras that record the patient while walking, computers that analyze each portion of the patient's gait, force plates that detect when feet touch the ground, and a special recording technique that detects muscle activity (known as electromyography). Using these data, doctors are better equipped to intervene and correct significant problems. They can also use gait analysis to check surgical results.

Because lengthening a muscle makes it weaker, surgery for contractures is usually followed by months of recovery. For this reason, doctors try to fix all of the affected muscles at once when it is possible, or if more than one surgical procedure is unavoidable, they may try to schedule operations close together.

A second surgical technique, known as selective dorsal root rhizotomy, aims to reduce spasticity in the legs by reducing the amount of stimulation that reaches leg muscles via nerves. In the procedure, doctors try to locate and selectively sever overactivated nerves controlling leg muscles. Although there is scientific controversy over how selective this technique actually is, recent research results suggest it can reduce spasticity in some patients, particularly those who have spastic diplegia. Ongoing research is evaluating this surgery's effectiveness.

Experimental surgical techniques include chronic cerebellar stimulation and stereotaxic thalamotomy. In chronic cerebellar stimulation, electrodes are implanted on the surface of the cerebellum—the part of the brain responsible for coordinating movement—and are used to stimulate certain cerebellar nerves. While it was hoped that this technique would decrease spasticity and improve motor function, results of this invasive procedure have been mixed. Some studies have reported improvements in spasticity and function, others have not.

Stereotaxic thalamotomy involves precise cutting of parts of the thalamus, which serves as the brain's relay station for messages from the muscles and sensory organs. This has been shown effective only for reducing hemiparetic tremors. (see glossary at the end of the chapter).

Mechanical Aids

Whether they are as humble as Velcro shoes or as advanced as computerized communication devices, special machines and gadgets in the home, school, and workplace can help the child or adult with cerebral palsy overcome limitations.

The computer is probably the most dramatic example of a new device that can make a difference in the lives of those with cerebral palsy. For example, a child who is unable to speak or write but can make head movements may be able to learn to control a computer using a special light pointer that attaches to a headband. Equipped with a computer and voice synthesizer, this child could communicate with others. In other cases, technology has led to new versions of old devices, such as the traditional wheelchair and its modern offspring that runs on electricity.

Many such devices are products of engineering research supported by private foundations and other groups.

What Other Major Problems Are Associated with Cerebral Palsy?

Poor control of the muscles of the throat, mouth, and tongue sometimes leads to drooling. Drooling can cause severe skin irritation and, because it is socially unacceptable, can lead to further isolation of affected children from their peers. Although numerous treatments for drooling have been tested over the years, there is no one treatment that always helps. Drugs called anticholinergics can reduce the flow of saliva but may cause significant side effects, such as mouth dryness and poor digestion. Surgery, while sometimes effective, carries the risk of complications, including worsening of swallowing problems. Some patients benefit from a technique called biofeedback that can tell them when they are drooling or having difficulty controlling muscles that close the mouth. This kind of therapy is most likely to work if the patient has a mental age of more than 2 or 3 years, is motivated to control drooling, and understands that drooling is not socially acceptable.

Difficulty with eating and swallowing—also triggered by motor problems in the mouth—can cause poor nutrition. Poor nutrition, in turn, may make the individual more vulnerable to infections and cause or aggravate failure to thrive—a lag in growth and development that is common among those with cerebral palsy. To make swallowing easier, the caregiver may want to prepare semisolid food, such as strained vegetables and fruits. Proper position, such as sitting up while eating or drinking and extending the individual's neck away from the body to reduce the risk of choking, is also helpful. In severe cases of swallowing problems and malnutrition, physicians may recommend tube feeding, in which a tube delivers food and nutrients down the throat and into the stomach, or gastrostomy, in which a surgical opening allows a tube to be placed directly into the stomach.

A common complication is incontinence, caused by faulty control over the muscles that keep the bladder closed. Incontinence can take the form of bed-wetting (also known as enuresis), uncontrolled urination during physical activities (or stress incontinence), or slow leaking of urine from the bladder. Possible medical treatments for incontinence include special exercises, biofeedback, prescription drugs, surgery, or surgically implanted devices to replace or aid muscles. Specially designed undergarments are also available.

What Research Is Being Done?

Investigators from many arenas of medicine and health are using their expertise to help improve treatment and prevention of cerebral palsy. Much of their work is supported through the National Institute of Neurological Disorders and Stroke (NINDS), the National Institute of Child Health and Human Development, other agencies within the Federal Government, nonprofit groups such as the United Cerebral Palsy Research Foundation, and private institutions.

The ultimate hope for overcoming cerebral palsy lies with prevention. In order to prevent cerebral palsy, however, scientists must first understand the complex process of normal brain development and what can make this process go awry.

Between early pregnancy and the first months of life, one cell divides to form first a handful of cells, and then hundreds, millions, and, eventually, billions of cells. Some of these cells specialize to become brain cells. These brain cells specialize into different types and migrate to their appropriate site in the brain. They send out branches to form crucial connections with other brain cells. Ultimately, the most complex entity known to us is created: a human brain with its billions of interconnected neurons.

Mounting evidence is pointing investigators toward this intricate process in the womb for clues about cerebral palsy. For example, a group of researchers has recently observed that more than one-third of children who have cerebral palsy also have missing enamel on certain teeth. This tooth defect can be traced to problems in the early months of fetal development, suggesting that a disruption at this period in development might be linked both to this tooth defect and to cerebral palsy.

As a result of this and other research, many scientists now believe that a significant number of children develop cerebral palsy because of mishaps early in brain development. They are examining how brain cells specialize, how they know where to migrate, how they form the right connections—and they are looking for preventable factors that can disrupt this process before or after birth.

Scientists are also scrutinizing other events—such as bleeding in the brain, seizures, and breathing and circulation problems—that threaten the brain of the newborn baby. Through this research, they hope to learn how these hazards can damage the newborn's brain and to develop new methods for prevention.

Some newborn infants, for example, have life-threatening problems with breathing and blood circulation. A recently introduced treatment to help these infants is extracorporeal membrane oxygenation, in which blood is routed from the patient to a special machine that takes over the lungs' task of removing carbon dioxide and adding oxygen. Although this technique can dramatically help many such infants, some scientists have observed that a substantial fraction of treated children later experience long-term neurological problems, including developmental delay and cerebral palsy. Investigators are studying infants through pregnancy, delivery, birth, and infancy, and are tracking those who undergo this treatment. By observing them at all stages of development, scientists can learn whether their problems developed before birth, result from the same breathing problems that made them candidates for the treatment, or spring from errors in the treatment itself. Once this is determined, they may be able to correct any existing problems or develop new treatment methods to prevent brain damage.

Other scientists are exploring how brain insults like hypoxic-ischemic encephalopathy (brain damage from a shortage of oxygen or blood flow), bleeding in the brain, and seizures can cause the abnormal release of brain chemicals and trigger brain damage. For example, research has shown that bleeding in the brain unleashes dangerously high amounts of a brain chemical called glutamate. While glutamate is normally used in the brain for communication, too much glutamate overstimulates the brain's cells and causes a cycle of destruction. Scientists are now looking closely at glutamate to detect how its release harms brain tissue and spreads the damage from stroke. By learning how such brain chemicals that normally help us function can hurt the brain, scientists may be equipped to develop new drugs that block their harmful effects.

In related research, some investigators are already conducting studies to learn if certain drugs can help prevent neonatal stroke. Several of these drugs seem promising because they appear to reduce the excess production of potentially dangerous chemicals in the brain and may help control brain blood flow and volume. Earlier research has linked sudden changes in blood flow and volume to stroke in the newborn.

Low birthweight itself is also the subject of extensive research. In spite of improvements in health care for some pregnant women, the incidence of low birthweight babies born each year in the United States remains at about 7 1/2 percent. Some scientists currently investigating this serious health problem are working to understand how infections, hormonal problems, and genetic factors may increase a woman's chances of giving birth prematurely. They are also conducting more applied research that could yield: 1) new drugs that can safely delay labor, 2) new devices to further improve medical care for premature infants, and 3) new insight into how smoking and alcohol consumption can disrupt fetal development.

While this research offers hope for preventing cerebral palsy in the future, ongoing research to improve treatment brightens the outlook for those who must face the challenges of cerebral palsy today. An important thrust of such research is the evaluation of treatments already in use so that physicians and parents have the information they need to choose the best therapy. A good example of this effort is an ongoing NINDS-supported study that promises to yield new information about which patients are most likely to benefit from selective dorsal root rhizotomy, a recently introduced surgery that is becoming increasingly in demand for reduction of spasticity.

Similarly, although physical therapy programs are a popular and widespread approach to managing cerebral palsy, little scientific evidence exists to help physicians, other health professionals, and parents determine how well physical therapy works or to choose the best approach among many. Current research on cerebral palsy aims to provide this information through careful studies that compare the abilities of children who have had physical and other therapy with those who have not.

As part of this effort, scientists are working to create new measures to judge the effectiveness of treatment, as in ongoing research to precisely identify the specific brain areas responsible for movement may yield one such approach. Using magnetic pulses, researchers can locate brain areas that control specific actions, such as raising an arm or lifting a leg, and construct detailed maps. By comparing charts made before and after therapy among children who have cerebral palsy, researchers may gain new insights into how therapy affects the brain's organization and new data about its effectiveness.

Investigators are also working to develop new drugs—and new ways of using existing drugs—to help relieve cerebral palsy's symptoms. In one such set of studies, early research results suggest that doctors may improve the effectiveness of the anti-spasticity drug called baclofen by giving the drug through spinal injections, rather than by mouth. In addition, scientists are also exploring the use of tiny implanted pumps that deliver a constant supply of anti-spasticity drugs into the fluid around the spinal cord, in the hope of improving these drugs' effectiveness and reducing side-effects, such as drowsiness.

Other experimental drug development efforts are exploring the use of minute amounts of the familiar toxin called botulinum. Ingested in large amounts, this toxin is responsible for botulism poisoning, in which the body's muscles become paralyzed. Injected in tiny amounts, however, this toxin has shown early promise in reducing spasticity in specific muscles.

231

A large research effort is also directed at producing more effective, nontoxic drugs to control seizures. Through its Antiepileptic Drug Development Program, the NINDS screens new compounds developed by industrial and university laboratories around the world for toxicity and anticonvulsant activity and coordinates clinical studies of efficacy and safety. To date, this program has screened more than 13,000 compounds and, as a result, five new antiepileptic drugs—carbamazepine, clonazepam, valproate, clorazepate, and felbamate—have been approved for marketing. A new project within the program is exploring how the structure of a given antiseizure medication relates to its effectiveness. If successful, this project may enable scientists to design better antiseizure medications more quickly and cheaply.

As researchers continue to explore new treatments for cerebral palsy and to expand our knowledge of brain development, we can expect significant medical advances to prevent cerebral palsy and many other disorders that strike in early life.

Research Update June 2000

Magnesium Sulfate and Decreased Risk of Cerebral Palsy

Research conducted and supported by the National Institute of Neurological Disorders and Stroke (NINDS) continuously seeks to uncover new clues about cerebral palsy (CP). Investigators from the NINDS and the California Birth Defects Monitoring Program (CBDMP) presented data suggesting that very low birthweight babies have a decreased incidence of CP when their mothers are treated with magnesium sulfate soon before giving birth. The results of this study, which were based on observations of a group of children born in four Northern California counties, were published in the February 1995 issue of *Pediatrics*.*

Low birthweight babies are 100 times more likely to develop CP than normal birthweight infants. If further research confirms the study's findings, use of magnesium sulfate may prevent 25 percent of the cases of CP in the approximately 52,000 low birthweight babies born each year in the United States.

Magnesium is a natural compound that is responsible for numerous chemical processes within the body and brain. Obstetricians in the United States often administer magnesium sulfate, an inexpensive form of the compound, to pregnant women to prevent preterm labor and high blood pressure brought on by pregnancy. The drug, administered intravenously in the hospital, is considered safe when given under medical supervision.

Scientists speculate that magnesium may play a role in brain development and possibly prevent bleeding inside the brains of preterm infants. Previous research has shown that magnesium may protect against brain bleeding in very premature infants. Animal studies have demonstrated that magnesium given after a traumatic brain injury can reduce the severity of brain damage.

Despite these encouraging research findings, pregnant women should not change their magnesium intake because the effects of high doses have not yet been studied and the possible risks and benefits are not known.

Researchers caution that more research will be required to establish a definitive relationship between the drug and prevention of the disorder. Clinical trials now underway, one of them a collaboration between the NINDS and the National Institute of Child Health and Human Development, are evaluating magnesium for the prevention of cerebral palsy in prematurely born babies.

*Nelson KB, and Grether JK. Can magnesium sulfate reduce the risk of cerebral palsy in very low birthweight infants? *Pediatrics*, February 1995, vol. 95, no. 2, page 263.

Glossary

Apgar score. A numbered score doctors use to assess a baby's physical state at the time of birth.

Apraxia. Impaired ability to carry out purposeful movements in an individual who does not have significant motor problems.

Asphyxia. Lack of oxygen due to trouble with breathing or poor oxygen supply in the air.

Bile pigments. Yellow-colored substances produced by the human body as a by-product of digestion.

Cerebral. Relating to the two hemispheres of the human brain.

Computed tomography (CT). An imaging technique that uses x-rays and a computer to create a picture of the brain's tissues and structures.

Congenital. Present at birth.

Contracture. A condition in which muscles become fixed in a rigid, abnormal position causing distortion or deformity.

Dysarthria. Problems with speaking caused by difficulty moving or coordinating the muscles needed for speech.

Electroencephalogram (EEG). A technique for recording the pattern of electrical currents inside the brain.

Electromyography. A special recording technique that detects muscle activity.

Failure to thrive. A condition characterized by lag in physical growth and development.

Gait analysis. A technique that uses camera recording, force plates, electromyography, and computer analysis to objectively measure an individual's pattern of walking.

Gastrostomy. A surgical procedure to create an artificial opening in the stomach.

Hemianopia. Defective vision or blindness that impairs half of the normal field of vision.

Hemiparetic tremors. Uncontrollable shaking affecting the limbs on the spastic side of the body in those who have spastic hemiplegia.

Hypertonia. Increased tone.

Hypotonia. Decreased tone.

Hypoxic-ischemic encephalopathy. Brain damage caused by poor blood flow or insufficient oxygen supply to the brain.

Jaundice. A blood disorder caused by the abnormal buildup of bile pigments in the bloodstream.

Magnetic resonance imaging (MRI). An imaging technique which uses radio waves, magnetic fields, and computer analysis to create a picture of body tissues and structures.

Neonatal hemorrhage. Bleeding of brain blood vessels in the newborn.

Orthotic devices. Special devices, such as splints or braces, used to treat problems of the muscles, ligaments, or bones of the skeletal system.

Paresis or plegia. Weakness or paralysis. In cerebral palsy, these terms are typically combined with another phrase that describes the distribution of paralysis and weakness, e.g., paraparesis.

Palsy. Paralysis, or problems in the control of voluntary movement.

Reflexes. Movements that the body makes automatically in response to a specific cue.

Rh incompatibility. A blood condition in which antibodies in a pregnant woman's blood can attack fetal blood cells, impairing the fetus's supply of oxygen and nutrients.

Rubella. Also known as German measles, rubella is a viral infection that can damage the nervous system in the developing fetus.

Selective dorsal root rhizotomy. A surgical procedure in which selected nerves are severed to reduce spasticity in the legs.

Spastic diplegia. A form of cerebral palsy in which both arms and both legs are affected, the legs being more severely affected.

Spastic hemiplegia (or hemiparesis). A form of cerebral palsy in which spasticity affects the arm and leg on one side of the body.

Spastic paraplegia (or paraparesis). A form of cerebral palsy in which spasticity affects both legs but the arms are relatively or completely spared.

Spastic quadriplegia (or quadriparesis). A form of cerebral palsy in which all four limbs are affected equally.

Stereognosia. Difficulty perceiving and identifying objects using the sense of touch.

Strabismus. Misalignment of the eyes.

Ultrasonography. A technique that bounces sound waves off of tissues and structures and uses the pattern of echoes to form an image, called a sonogram.

Additional Information

Brain Resources and Information Network (BRAIN)
P.O. Box 5801
Bethesda, MD 20824
Toll-Free: 800-352-9424

Brain Resources and Information Network (BRAIN) continued
TTY: 301-468-5981
Website: www.ninds.nih.gov

Epilepsy Foundation
4351 Garden City Drive, Suite 500
Landover, MD 20785-2267
Toll-Free: 800-EFA-1000 (332-1000)
Tel: 301-459-3700
Fax: 301-577-2684
Website: www.epilepsyfoundation.org
E-mail: postmaster@efa.org

This foundation sponsors programs for patient and public education, legal and government affairs, and employment training and placement. The foundation also supports research, maintains the National Epilepsy Library (800-EFA-4050), publishes a variety of patient/family and professional education materials, and sponsors affiliates.

March of Dimes Birth Defects Foundation
1275 Mamaroneck Avenue
White Plains, NY 10605
Toll-Free: 888-MODIMES (663-4637)
Tel: 914-428-7100
Fax: 914-428-8203
Website: www.modimes.org
E-mail: resourcecenter@modimes.org

This foundation funds research, medical services, public education, and genetic counseling. Resources include fact sheets, brochures, educational kits, and audiovisual materials.

Easter Seals
230 West Monroe Street, Suite 1800
Chicago, IL 60606-4802
Toll-Free: 800-221-6827
Tel: 312-726-6200
Fax: 312-726-1494
TTY: 312-726-4258
Website: www.easter-seals.org
E-mail: info@easterseals.org

This organization includes state and local affiliates and operates facilities and programs across the country. They offer a range of rehabilitation services, research and public education programs, and assistive technology services. Their programs also include therapy, counseling, training, social clubs, camping, transportation, and referrals. In addition, the society sponsors a grants program for research on disabling conditions and rehabilitation, provides low-cost booklets and pamphlets to the public, and publishes a bimonthly journal.

United Cerebral Palsy Associations, Inc. and The United Cerebral Palsy Research and Educational Foundation
1660 L Street, NW, Suite 700
Washington, DC 20036
Toll-Free: 800-USA-5UCP (872-5827)
Tel: 202-776-0406
Fax: 202-776-0414
Website: www.ucp.org
E-mail: webmaster@ucp.org

This coalition of associations provide family support, legislative advocacy, public information and education, and training, specifically for issues of importance to those who have cerebral palsy. It also publishes newsletters and various brochures and pamphlets. The UCP Research and Educational Foundation supports research to prevent cerebral palsy and develop therapies to improve the quality of life for those affected by this disorder.

Children's Hemiplegia and Stroke Association (CHASA)
4101 West Green Oaks Blvd.
Suite 305, PMB #149
Arlington, TX 76016
Tel: 817-492-4325
Website: www.hemikids.org
E-mail: info@chasa.org

Non-profit 501(c)(3) corporation that offers support and information for families of children who have hemiplegia due to stroke or other causes. Also provides information regarding research and causes of any type of pediatric stroke.

Chapter 20

Congenital Myasthenic Syndromes

What Is a Congenital Myasthenic Syndrome (CMS)?

A CMS is an inherited disorder that causes muscle weakness (myasthenia) by affecting the connection between nerve cells and muscle cells, called the neuromuscular junction (NMJ). The origins and symptoms of CMS sometimes resemble those of two other NMJ disorders, myasthenia gravis and Lambert-Eaton syndrome. While these disorders occur when the immune system attacks the NMJ, CMS is caused by defects in genes that are essential at the NMJ.

As the name implies, those genetic defects typically cause muscle weakness from the time of birth, but sometimes the onset of weakness is delayed until childhood or even adulthood. It's likely that CMS is often misdiagnosed as myasthenia gravis or other neuromuscular disorders.

How Does the NMJ Normally Work?

The neuromuscular junction is a type of synapse, a site of cell-to-cell communication, where a nerve cell can stimulate a muscle cell to contract and produce movement. The nerve cell, sometimes called the presynaptic side of the NMJ, stimulates the muscle cell by releasing a chemical signal called acetylcholine (ACh).

239

The ACh travels across a synaptic space to reach the postsynaptic surface of the muscle cell, where it acts like a key to open pores (or channels) called ACh receptors (AChRs). Opening of the AChRs allows electrolytes to flow into the muscle cell and trigger contraction. To shut off the signaling process, an enzyme called acetylcholinesterase (AChE) breaks down ACh in the synaptic space.

What Happens to the Neuromuscular Junction in CMS?

There are at least three major types of congenital myasthenic syndrome, based on genetic defects that affect the presynaptic, synaptic, or postsynaptic parts of the neuromuscular junction.

Presynaptic CMS is caused by decreased production or release of ACh at the NMJ.

In **synaptic CMS**, a deficiency of AChE leads to excessive muscle stimulation, which ultimately damages the muscle.

Postsynaptic CMS is caused by deficiencies or mechanical changes in the AChRs. Some mechanical changes cause extended opening of AChRs and overstimulation of muscles, a condition called slow-channel CMS, while others cause short-lived opening of AChRs and understimulation, a condition called fast-channel CMS. Postsynaptic CMS (which accounts for about 75 percent of all CMS) and at least one presynaptic CMS can closely resemble myasthenia gravis, which occurs when the immune system directs antibodies against the AChRs.

What Are the Symptoms of CMS?

The exact symptoms vary with the type of CMS and the specific genetic defect. But in general, CMS has its onset in infancy, and causes muscle weakness and unusual fatigue (increased weakness upon sustained exertion). Often, the weakness is most pronounced in muscles of the eyes and face, causing partial paralysis of eye movements (ophthalmoparesis), droopy eyelids (ptosis), and an open-mouthed expression. Weakness in the mouth and throat can also cause feeding difficulties, which might require use of a feeding tube.

Severe forms of CMS can weaken the respiratory muscles, requiring at least occasional use of a ventilator to support breathing. Also, severe weakness in the limbs and trunk sometimes delays the achievement of motor milestones (sitting, crawling, and walking). Mild CMS during infancy can progress during childhood or adulthood, leading to respiratory problems and a loss of mobility later in life. When CMS has its onset in childhood or adulthood, it causes relatively mild symptoms—such as ptosis, facial and limb weakness, and a tendency toward fatigue—that can progress over time. Slow-channel and fast-channel syndromes tend to be less severe than other types of CMS.

How Is CMS Inherited?

Although it's unknown for a few types of CMS, the inheritance pattern for most types is autosomal recessive. This means that it takes two copies of the defective gene—one from each parent—to cause the disease. However, because slow-channel CMS is caused by a gain of function in the AChR, it's inherited in an autosomal dominant manner. This means that one copy of a defective AChR gene is enough to cause the disease, so an affected parent has a 50 percent chance of passing the disease on to a child.

How Is CMS Diagnosed?

An important part of CMS diagnosis is a physical examination that reveals fatigable weakness in the eye, face, and/or limb muscles, especially during infancy. Likewise, electromyography (EMG) usually (but not always) reveals a declining muscle response to repeated stimulation. A negative test for anti-AChR antibodies in the serum (blood) can help distinguish CMS from myasthenia gravis, but doesn't rule out seronegative types of myasthenia gravis.

A family history with a similarly affected relative is supportive, but not necessary. Genetic testing for CMS is done on a research basis, but isn't available for general clinical practice. Finally, special physiological studies on muscle biopsies, also on a research basis, are needed to define the origins of some CMS.

How Is CMS Treated?

Many people with congenital myasthenic syndrome have been given treatments used for myasthenia gravis, such as immunosuppressants, or cholinesterase inhibitors—drugs that boost ACh levels by blocking the action of AChE. Immunosuppressants aren't effective for CMS, but a dose of cholinesterase inhibitor (most commonly Mestinon) can help restore near-normal NMJ function and alleviate symptoms for several hours in both presynaptic and postsynaptic CMS.

Often, the most effective treatment for fast-channel syndrome and AChR deficiency is a combination of cholinesterase inhibitor with 3,4-DAP, a drug that stimulates ACh release. Slow channel syndrome can be worsened by 3,4-DAP and Mestinon, but responds very well to quinidine, which plugs open AChRs. Synaptic CMS (AChE deficiency) is worsened by cholinesterase inhibitors and 3,4-DAP, and currently has no effective treatment.

Chapter 21

Hallervorden-Spatz Syndrome

What Is Hallervorden-Spatz Syndrome?

Hallervorden-Spatz syndrome (HSS) is a rare, inherited, neurological movement disorder characterized by the progressive degeneration of the nervous system (neurodegenerative disorder). Recently, one of the genetic causes was identified; however, there are probably other causative genes that exist that have not yet been found. Approximately 50% of individuals with a clinical diagnosis of HSS have gene mutations in PANK2, which helps to metabolize vitamin B5.

The common feature among all individuals with HSS is iron accumulation in the brain along with a progressive movement disorder. Individuals can plateau for long periods of time and then undergo intervals of rapid deterioration. Symptoms may vary greatly from case to case, partly because the genetic cause may differ between families. There are likely different genes that that cause HSS; and furthermore, different mutations within a gene could lead to a more or less severe presentation. The factors that influence disease severity and the rate of progression are still unknown.

Common features include slow writhing and distorting muscle contractions (dystonia—an abnormality in muscle tone), muscular rigidity,

---

"What Is Hallervorden-Spatz Syndrome," reprinted with permission from the Hallervorden-Spatz Syndrome Association (HSSA). © 2002. Hallervorden-Spatz Syndrome Association. For additional information contact HSSA at 2082 Monaco Ct., El Cajon, CA 92019-4235, (619) 588-2315, or visit their website at www.hssa.org.

and sudden involuntary muscle spasms (spasticity). These features can result in clumsiness, gait (walking) problems, difficulty controlling movement, and speech problems. Another common feature is degeneration of the retina resulting in progressive night blindness and loss of peripheral (side) vision. In general, symptoms are progressive and become worse over time.

It has been suggested that the disorder should be renamed because of the unethical activities of Dr. Hallervorden (and perhaps also Dr. Spatz) related to involving euthanasia of mentally ill patients during World War II. The emerging name of NBIA (Neurodegeneration with Brain Iron Accumulation) reflects the continuing discoveries about the underlying cause of the disorder. The term NBIA is already used by some and is general enough to cover all conditions previously categorized as Hallervorden-Spatz syndrome. The largest subgroup of NBIA observed so far is PKAN (pantothenate kinase associated neurodegeneration). It is a defect of the gene PANK2, which causes a deficiency of the enzyme pantothenate kinase. As the terminology changes, one may notice the terms NBIA and PKAN being used interchangeably with HSS.

Symptoms

There are several descriptive terms for the neuromuscular symptoms associated with all forms of Hallervorden-Spatz syndrome. Dystonia is a group of disorders characterized by involuntary muscle contractions that may force certain body parts into unusual, and sometimes painful, movements and positions. Choreoathetosis is a condition characterized by involuntary, rapid, jerky movements (chorea) occurring in association with relatively slow, sinuous, writhing motions (athetosis). In addition, there may be stiffness in the arms and legs because of continuous resistance to muscle relaxing (spasticity) and abnormal tightening of the muscles (muscular rigidity). Spasticity and muscle rigidity usually begin in the legs and later develop in the arms. As affected individuals age, they may eventually lose control of voluntary movements. Muscle spasms combined with decreased bone mass can result in bone fractures (not caused by trauma or accident).

Dystonia affects the muscles in the mouth and throat, which may cause poor articulation and slurring (dysarthria) and difficulty swallowing (dysphagia). The progression of dystonia in these muscles can result in loss of speech as well as tongue biting.

Specific forms of dystonia that may occur in association with Hallervorden-Spatz syndrome include blepharospasm and torticollis.

Blepharospasm is a condition in which the muscles of the eyelids do not function properly resulting in excessive blinking and involuntary closing of the eyelids. Torticollis is a condition in which there are involuntary contractions of neck muscles resulting in abnormal movements and positions of the head and neck.

Many of the delays in development pertain to motor skills (movement), although a small subgroup may have intellectual delays. Although intellectual impairment has often been described as a part of the condition in the past, it is unclear if this is a true feature. Intellectual testing may be hampered by the movement disorder; therefore, newer methods of studying intelligence are necessary to determine if there are any cognitive features of this condition.

The symptoms and physical findings associated with Hallervorden-Spatz syndrome usually develop during childhood before the age of 10 and can be distinguished between classical or atypical disease. However, cases of the disorder developing during adolescence and adulthood have been reported. Individuals with classical disease have a more rapid progression of symptoms. In most cases, atypical disease progresses slowly over several years. The symptoms and physical findings vary widely from case to case and some researchers believe that there are different forms of the disorder. Affected individuals will not have all of the symptoms.

Classical PKAN develops in the first ten years of life (average age for developing symptoms is 3 1/2 years). These children may initially be perceived as clumsy and later develop more noticeable problems with walking. Eventually, falling becomes a frequent feature. Because of the limited ability to protect themselves during falls, children may have repeated injury to the face and chin. Many individuals with the classic form of PKAN require a wheelchair by their mid-teens (in some cases earlier). Most lose the ability to move/walk independently between 10-15 years after the beginning of symptoms.

The most common neuromuscular symptoms associated with Hallervorden-Spatz syndrome are choreoathetosis and dystonia. Choreoathetosis is a condition characterized by involuntary, rapid, jerky movements (chorea) occurring in association with relatively slow, sinuous, writhing motions (athetosis). Dystonia is a group of disorders characterized by involuntary muscle contractions that may force certain body parts into unusual, and sometimes painful, movements and positions (dystonia). Additional conditions associated with choreoathetosis and dystonia include involuntary muscle spasms that result in slow, stiff movements of the arms and legs (spasticity); abnormal tightening of the muscles (muscular rigidity); and the inability to coordinate voluntary movements (ataxia). Spasticity and muscle rigidity usually begins in the legs and spreads to affect the arms. As affected individuals age, they may eventually lose control of voluntary movements, resulting in an inability to walk, talk, or use their arms.

Affected individuals may also develop additional symptoms including confusion, disorientation, and/or deterioration of intellectual abilities (dementia); difficulty speaking (dysarthria); difficulty swallowing (dysphagia); seizures; and individuals with Hallervorden-Spatz syndrome (classical PKAN) are more likely to have specific eye problems. Approximately 2/3 of these patients will have symptoms including involuntary, rapid, rhythmic eye movements (nystagmus); visual impairment due to the gradual deterioration of the nerves of the eyes (optic atrophy); or retinal degeneration. This is a progressive degeneration of the nerve-rich membrane lining the eyes (retina), resulting in tunnel vision, night blindness, and loss of peripheral vision. Loss of this peripheral vision may contribute to the more frequent falls and gait disturbances in the early stages. Optic atrophy, a vision impairment caused by gradual degeneration of the nerves of the eyes, is only found in 3% of patients.

The atypical form of PKAN usually occurs after the age of ten years and progresses more slowly. The average age for developing symptoms is 13 years. Loss of independent ambulation (walking) often occurs 15-40 years after the initial development of symptoms. The initial presenting symptoms usually involve speech. Common speech problems are repetition of words or phrases (palilalia), rapid speech (tachylalia), and poor articulation/slurring (dysarthria). Psychiatric symptoms are more commonly observed and include impulsive behavior, violent outbursts, depression, or a tendency to rapid mood swings. While the movement disorder is a very common feature, it usually develops later. In general, atypical disease is less severe and more slowly progressive than early-onset PKAN.

In cases of neurodegeneration with brain iron accumulation (NBIA) that are not caused by PKAN, the movement-related symptoms (such as dystonia) may be very similar. The symptoms in NBIA are more varied because there are probably several different causes of neurodegeneration in this group. There is a subgroup of patients with moderate to severe mental retardation. Also, seizure disorders are more common among non-PKAN individuals.

Causes

Individuals with Hallervorden-Spatz syndrome often have abnormal accumulation of iron in certain areas of the brain. This is especially seen in regions of the basal ganglia called the globus pallidus and the substantia nigra. The basal ganglia is a collection of structures deep within the base of the brain that assist in regulating movements. The exact relationship between iron accumulation and the symptoms of Hallervorden-Spatz syndrome is not fully understood.

Genetics

Hallervorden-Spatz syndrome (PKAN) is inherited as an autosomal recessive trait, although sporadic cases have also been described in the literature condition. Many other cases of NBIA are presumed to be autosomal recessive as well. In autosomal recessive disorders, a person has received a non-working gene from both parents. Human traits, including the classic genetic diseases, are the product of the interaction of two genes, one received from the father and one from the mother.

PKAN is due to disruptions or changes (mutations) on a gene located on the short arm (p) of chromosome 20 (20p13). The gene is known as the PANK2 gene on chromosome 20. This gene encodes the enzyme pantothenate kinase. Dysfunction of this gene may lead to the accumulation of the amino acid cysteine, resulting in damage to cells and the accumulation of iron deposits within certain areas of the brain. Current research is investigating how this missing enzyme results in damage to neurons in the brain as well as the characteristic iron buildup. It is hypothesized that some cysteine-containing chemicals accumulate in high levels causing damage to the neurons in the basal ganglia. No genes have been found for other forms of NBIA. It is possible that other genes will be found that also cause Hallervorden-Spatz syndrome in other cases.

Chromosomes are found in the nucleus of all body cells. They carry the genetic characteristics of each individual. Pairs of human chromosomes are numbered from 1 through 22, with an unequal 23rd pair of X and Y chromosomes for males, and two X chromosomes for females. Each chromosome has a short arm designated as "p" and a long arm identified by the letter "q." Chromosomes are further subdivided into bands that are numbered. For example, "chromosome 20p13" refers to band 13 on the short arm of chromosome 20.

Hallervorden-Spatz syndrome affects males and females in equal numbers. The symptoms typically develop during childhood, although occasionally they begin during late adolescence or adulthood.

The frequency of Hallervorden-Spatz syndrome in the general population is unknown, but is estimated between 1-3/1,000,000 individuals. Because rare disorders like Hallervorden-Spatz syndrome often go unrecognized, these disorders may be under diagnosed, or misdiagnosed, making it difficult to determine the true frequency of Hallervorden-Spatz syndrome in the general population and the accuracy of these estimates.

Diagnosis

The diagnosis of Hallervorden-Spatz syndrome is made based upon a detailed patient history, a thorough clinical evaluation, and a variety of specialized tests. The diagnosis is confirmed by specialized imaging techniques (CT scan and magnetic resonance imaging). This imaging technique shows the characteristic iron accumulation of large amounts of pigmented material in certain areas of the brain (globus pallidus and pars reticulata of the substantia nigra). Individuals with PKAN have a characteristic feature called the eye-of-the-tiger sign. This is not seen in other forms of NBIA. MRI should be useful in distinguishing PKAN and non-PKAN individuals and may also help to determine which families should have DNA testing for PKAN. When viewed with these imaging techniques, these areas of the brain appear to have a brownish discoloration due to excessive iron accumulation. Localized swelling of tissue is also evident, especially in those areas that affect the function of the central nervous system. One test that may be useful for the diagnosis of Hallervorden-Spatz syndrome measures the uptake of radioactive iron (ferrous citrate) into certain areas of the brain. Unusually high uptake is characteristic of this disease.

Treatment

There is no specific treatment for individuals with Hallervorden-Spatz syndrome. Treatment is directed towards the specific symptoms that appear in each individual. Research is focusing on a better understanding of the underlying cause of this disorder, which may eventually help to find a more comprehensive treatment. It is hoped that the location of the responsible gene, which was published in 2001, will encourage research that may ultimately help in the search for therapies.

Treatment may require the coordinated efforts of a team of specialists. Physicians that the family may work with include the pediatrician or internist, neurologist, ophthalmologist, and geneticist. A team approach to supportive therapy may include physical therapy, exercise physiology, occupation therapy, and speech pathology. In addition, many families may benefit from genetic counseling.

One of the most consistent forms of relief from disabling dystonia is baclofen. This medication has been taken orally, although recently a baclofen pump has been used to administer regular doses automatically into the nervous system.

Drugs that reduce the levels of iron in the body (iron chelation) have been attempted to treat individuals with Hallervorden-Spatz syndrome. These agents have proven ineffective. However, new drugs are being developed that researchers hope may be more yield better results.

Levodopa, bromocriptine, or trihexyphenidyl can often improve the dystonia, though they do not appear to help patients with PKAN. However, their overall effectiveness is unknown and the responsiveness in individual cases is unpredictable. In some cases, botulinum toxin injections may help. Baclofen can be used to treat spasticity, and seizures may respond to either carbamazepine or phenytoin.

Pallidotomy and thalamotomy have been investigational attempts at controlling dystonia. These are both surgical techniques which destroy (ablate) very specific regions of the brain, the pallidus and thalamus, respectively. Some families have reported some immediate and temporary relief.

However, most patients return to their pre-operative level of dystonia within one year of the operation. Pallidotomy is used for the treatment of disorders that are characterized by changes in muscle tone, postural disturbances, abnormalities in conducting certain voluntary movements, and the development of abnormal involuntary movements (i.e., extrapyramidal disorders). Thalamotomy is usually only used in cases of severe, progressive dystonia that fails to respond to other treatments (intractable).

Individuals experiencing seizures usually benefit from standard anti-convulsive drugs. In addition, standard approaches to pain management are generally recommended where there is no identifiable treatment for the underlying cause of pain.

With the recent discovery of the association between pantothenate kinase and NBIA, there is a new potential therapy that focuses on the underlying chemical defect. Supplemental pantothenate (pantothenic acid, calcium pantothenate) can be taken orally. Pantothenate is another name for vitamin B5, a water-soluble vitamin. Theoretically, this is most likely to assist individuals with very low levels of pantothenate kinase activity. It is hypothesized that classical disease results from complete absence of the enzyme pantothenate kinase, whereas atypical disease results from a severe deficiency, although the individuals still may have some level of enzyme activity. Clinical trials will soon be underway to investigate the effectiveness of this treat-ment with various forms of NBIA.

The benefits and limitations of any of the above treatments should be discussed in detail with a physician. Genetic counseling may be of benefit for affected individuals and their families. Other treatment is symptomatic and supportive.

Chapter 22

Rett Syndrome

Overview of Rett Syndrome

Rett Syndrome (RS) is a neurological disorder seen almost exclusively in females, and found in a variety of racial and ethnic groups worldwide. It is now known that RS can occur in males, but is usually lethal, causing miscarriage, stillbirth, or early death. First described by Dr. Andreas Rett, RS received worldwide recognition following a paper by Dr. Bengt Hagberg and colleagues in 1983.

The child with RS usually shows an early period of apparently normal or near normal development until 6-18 months of life. A period of temporary stagnation or regression follows during which the child loses communication skills and purposeful use of the hands. Soon, stereotyped hand movements, gait disturbances, and slowing of the rate of head growth become apparent. Other problems may include seizures and disorganized breathing patterns which occur when awake.

Apraxia (dyspraxia), the inability to program the body to perform motor movements, is the most fundamental and severely handicapping

This chapter includes "Overview," "People Ask about Rett Syndrome," "Stages of Rett Syndrome," and "Revised Diagnostic Criteria for Rett Syndrome" © 2002 International Rett Syndrome Association. This information is excerpted from "What Is Rett Syndrome?" by the International Rett Syndrome Association. The complete text is available on the IRSA website at www.rettsyndrome.org. Also included are excerpts from "Rett Syndrome Fact Sheet," National Institute of Neurological Disorders and Stroke (NINDS), NIH Publication No. 01-4863, reviewed July 1, 2001.

251

aspect of RS. It can interfere with every body movement, including eye gaze and speech, making it difficult for the girl with RS to do what she wants to do.

Due to apraxia and lack of verbal communication skills, an accurate assessment of intelligence is difficult. Most traditional testing methods require use of the hands and/or speech, which may be impossible for the girl with RS.

RS is most often misdiagnosed as autism, cerebral palsy, or nonspecific developmental delay. While many health professionals may not be familiar with RS, it is a relatively frequent cause of neurological dysfunction in females. The prevalence rate in various countries is from 1:10,000 to 1:23,000 live female births.

Most researchers now agree that RS is a developmental disorder rather than a progressive, degenerative disorder as once thought. In October of 1999, the discovery of a genetic mutation (MECP2) on the X chromosome (Xq28) revealed significant insight into the cause of Rett syndrome. This mutation has now been found in up to 75% of typical and atypical cases of RS. Continued research will focus on other still unidentified genetic factors that contribute to RS. Researchers agree that the severity of RS is probably not linked to the exact location of individual mutations on MECP2, but to the X inactivation patterns in each affected girl. Barring illness or complications, survival into adulthood is expected.

The young girl with RS is well known for her attractive features, and as she grows older, her especially penetrating eyes. She typically sits independently and finger feeds at the expected time. Most girls do not crawl typically, but may bottom scoot or combat crawl without using their hands. Some children start to use single words and word combinations before they lose this ability.

Predicting the severity of RS in any individual is difficult. Many girls begin independent walking within the normal age range, while others show significant delay or inability to walk independently. Some begin walking and lose this skill, while others continue to walk throughout life. Still others do not walk until late childhood or adolescence.

Seizures can range from non-existent to severe, but do tend to lessen in their intensity in later adolescence. Breathing abnormalities may occur and also tend to decrease with age. While scoliosis is a prominent feature of RS, it can range from mild to severe. Despite these difficulties, girls and women with RS can continue to learn and enjoy family and friends well into middle age and beyond. They experience a full range of emotions and show their engaging personalities as they take part in social, educational and recreational activities at home and in the community. The ICD-9 code for RS is 330.8 (294.1)

Frequently Asked Questions

I Have Never Heard of Rett Syndrome. Why?

Most people have never heard of Rett syndrome because it has only recently been formally recognized. In fact, it wasn't until 1983 that the condition known as Rett syndrome first appeared in medical literature. Those with Rett syndrome were likely once misdiagnosed with autism or cerebral palsy.

What Causes Rett Syndrome?

Rett syndrome is a condition caused by a gene mutation (MECP2) that occurs before birth. The discovery of the Rett syndrome gene was announced on October 1, 1999 by researchers at Baylor College of Medicine in Houston, Texas.

Why Is It Called Rett Syndrome?

Rett syndrome is named for Dr. Andreas Rett, of Vienna, Austria, who first recognized the disorder at his clinic in 1965. A syndrome is the term for a group of symptoms that identify a special condition.

Why Is Rett Syndrome Seen Mainly in Females?

Females have two X chromosomes (XX) and males have one X chromosome and one Y chromosome (XY). The mutation which causes Rett syndrome (MECP2) is on the X chromosome. So, if the mutation causing Rett syndrome appears on one X, females are able to survive because they still have another X. Males, on the other hand, have only one X (XY). If the mutation appears on a male's X chromosome, he would most likely not survive to birth.

This has led researchers to speculate that a male fetus that survives to birth with the MECP2 mutation would have far more severe symptoms than a female fetus—to the point that the condition would probably not even be recognized as Rett syndrome.

How Many People Have Rett Syndrome?

Before the gene discovery, Rett syndrome was found to occur about once in 15,000 female births. New findings suggest that milder forms of Rett syndrome may exist in much higher numbers. There may be hundreds of thousands of girls and women with Rett syndrome throughout the world who are misdiagnosed or unidentified.

When Is Rett Syndrome First Noticed?

The genetic mutation is there before birth, but it takes some time for enough problems to develop to be able to notice that something is wrong. A girl with Rett syndrome is usually born healthy and exhibits normal or near-normal development until 6-18 months of life.

What Are the Symptoms of Rett Syndrome?

Again, Rett syndrome almost always affects girls as opposed to boys. At some point in the years following the first 6-18 months of life, the child experiences an overall regression. Below are the criteria for the diagnosis of Rett syndrome that must be present in combination with a positive test result for the MECP2 gene:

- Decreased head growth from 4 months to 4 years of age.

- Loss of the ability to use hands functionally.

- Loss of the ability to speak.

- Repetitive hand movements such as clapping, tapping, or wringing. Individuals with Rett syndrome often move their hands in a characteristic washing motion and/or repeatedly put their hands into their mouth.

- If the child is able to walk, movement is stiff with the legs wide apart. As the child gets older, moving and walking may become increasingly difficult.

Other symptoms may include:

- Unusual breathing patterns: either holding the breath (apnea), or over-breathing (hyperventilation).

- Seizures, which take place when the brain unexpectedly creates extra powerful electrical signals, affecting behavior and movement. Seizures aren't usually harmful in and of themselves.

- Scoliosis, a curvature of the spine, may cause the child to lean to either side, or toward the front.

- Some girls frequently grind their teeth.

- Foot size is small, and poor circulation may make their feet very cold and/or swollen.

- Girls are usually small in both height and weight for their age.

- Girls may also be irritable and have trouble sleeping, have difficulty chewing and swallowing, and/or tremble and shake when upset or scared.

Does Rett Syndrome Occur More Than Once in a Family?

99.5% of the time, Rett syndrome occurs only once in a family. The spontaneous mutation that causes Rett syndrome happens after conception (not inherited from the parents). In a very small number of cases, less than .5%, the Rett syndrome gene is inherited, passing from one generation to the next or occurring more than once in a family.

What Is the Most Difficult Challenge for Someone with Rett Syndrome?

The individual with Rett syndrome has a number of problems that affect her in different ways. The biggest problem is apraxia, or the inability to program (usually automatic) the planning done by the brain to execute movements. Apraxia affects all aspects of motor functioning: the ability to walk, move, talk, etc.

What Kind of Therapies Are Used as Treatment?

- Physical therapy is used to help with flexibility and to improve movement/walking.

- Occupational therapy helps with use of hands for everyday activities like eating and drinking, brushing teeth, and playing with toys or games.

- Speech therapy and music therapy are used to teach alternative ways of communicating. (Apraxia makes talking very difficult).

- Through hydrotherapy, individuals are able to perform basic exercises/movements more easily.

- Hippotherapy (horseback riding) helps strengthen muscles and improves balance.

How Can I Help?

In everyday interactions, patience is key. Individuals with Rett syndrome need extra time to respond—it may take several minutes before a girl can give an answer or make a movement to show understanding.

Is There a Treatment for Rett Syndrome?

Right now, the treatments available for Rett syndrome are to improve symptoms, such as medications to control seizures or to help motor coordination or breathing. However, scientific studies of medications based on the gene mutation are now underway, and the future holds promise that more effective treatments can be found.

What Is the Life Expectancy of Someone with Rett Syndrome?

An individual with Rett syndrome has a 95% chance of surviving to 20-25 years of age (compared to 98% in the general female population). From age 25-40, life expectancy decreases to 69% (compared to 97% in the general female population). The average life expectancy in Rett syndrome is estimated at 47 years.

Stages of Rett Syndrome

Stage I: Early Onset

Age: 6 months to 1 1/2 years
Duration: months

This stage is usually overlooked, as the symptoms of RS are just emerging and are somewhat vague. The infant may show less eye contact and have reduced interest in toys. She is often described as a good baby, calm, and placid. There may be delays in gross motor milestones. Non-specific hand wringing and decelerating head growth may be present.

Stage II: Rapid Destructive

Age: 1 to 4 years
Duration: weeks to months

This stage can have a rapid onset or it can be more gradual as purposeful hand skills and spoken language are lost. Stereotyped hand movements begin to emerge, and often include hand-to-mouth movements as the first expression. Movements are most often midline hand wringing or hand washing, and persist while the girl is awake but disappear during sleep. Other hand movements include hand clapping or tapping. Hands are sometimes clasped behind the back or held at the sides in a specific pose, with random touching, grasping, and releasing.

Breathing irregularities may be noticed, and may include episodes of breath holding and hyperventilation associated with vacant spells. However, breathing is usually normal during sleep. Some girls appear autistic with loss of social interaction and communication. General irritability and sleep irregularity may be seen.

Periods of tremulousness may be obvious, especially when excited. Gait patterns are unsteady, and initiating motor movements can be difficult. Slowing of head growth is usually noticed from 3 months–4 years, when the girl's head circumference falls on a percentile chart (compared to children at the same age).

Stage III: Plateau

Age: Pre-school to school years
Duration: years

This stage, from 2-10 years, follows the rapid destructive period. Apraxia, motor problems, and seizures are more prominent. However, improvement is seen in behavior with less irritability and crying and less autistic features. She shows more interest in her surroundings, and her alertness, attention span and communication skills improve. Many girls with RS remain in Stage III for most of their lifetime.

Stage IV A (Previously Ambulant) and Stage IV B (Never Ambulant): Late Motor Deterioration

Age: When stage III ceases, 5-15-25-? years
Duration: up to decades

This stage usually begins after age 10, and is characterized by reduced mobility. Some girls stop walking, while others have never walked. However, there is no decline in cognition, communication, or hand skills. Repetitive hand movements may decrease. Scoliosis is a prominent feature. Eye gaze usually improves. Rigidity (stiffness) and dystonia (increased muscle tone with abnormal extremity or trunk positions) are characteristic. Puberty begins at the expected age in most girls.

Revised Diagnostic Criteria for Rett Syndrome

In September 2001, the IRSA convened a panel of international experts in a satellite session of the European Pediatric Neurology Society in Baden Baden, Germany. This meeting was an important first step in the creation of the IRSA RS Clinical Database, which will compare genotypes (gene mutations) and phenotypes (symptoms). The Clinical Database will be linked with the new IRSA MECP2 Variations Database.

The aim of this meeting was to establish as simple a data set as possible to assist physicians in making the clinical diagnosis of RS. The meeting resulted in an updated set of diagnostic/clinical criteria, based on observations and knowledge gained from understanding the natural history of RS, and from new information based on the discovery of the MECP2 gene. While the original nine essential clinical criteria have been retained, the revised criteria clarify ambiguities in language, which could affect their broad application or implementation in phenotype-genotype correlation studies. The panel is also in the process of examining several different models of severity scales in an attempt to create a suitable scale that can be applied universally.

The new diagnostic criteria and severity scale are of significant importance to research, giving a set of rules which all labs and diagnosticians should apply when making the diagnosis and determining severity. Without these, it would be difficult to get a true genotype/ phenotype correlation, or comparison of the location/length of the different mutations and correlating symptoms. In addition, the new criteria includes information on atypical or borderline variants of RS, which is so important for increasing physician awareness and for expanded understanding of RS.

Since the initial criteria were established in 1985, there has been remarkable progress in our understanding of the clinical, neurobiologic, and molecular genetic characteristics of RS. These include greater definition of the timing and pattern of clinical features, recognition of RS as a neurodevelopmental disorder instead of a degenerative disorder, and the identification of mutations in MECP2 as the molecular basis for more than 80% of girls fulfilling criteria for classic RS.

Commentary

It is important to emphasize that at our present level of knowledge, the diagnosis of RS remains a clinical one and is not made solely on the basis of MECP2 mutations. This means that RS can occur with or without mutations in MECP2, and MECP2 mutations can occur without the diagnosis of RS. Therefore, consensus on the diagnostic criteria for classic and variant forms of RS is essential and these criteria must be applied consistently for the accuracy of phenotype-genotype correlation studies.

Rett Syndrome and MECP2 Mutations

- Rett Syndrome is a clinical diagnosis
- Rett Syndrome is not synonymous with MECP2 mutations
- Rett Syndrome may be seen with MECP2 mutations
- Rett Syndrome may be seen without MECP2 mutations
- MECP2 mutations may be seen without Rett Syndrome

Rett Syndrome Phenotypes Noted with MECP2 Mutations

Females

- Rett syndrome
- Preserved speech variant
- Delayed onset variant
- Mild learning disability
- Angelman syndrome
- Normal carriers

Males

- Fatal encephalopathy
- Rett/Klinefelter syndrome
- Angelman syndrome
- X-linked mental retardation/progressive spasticity
- Somatic mosaicism/neurodevelopmental delay

Diagnostic Criteria

Necessary Criteria

1. Apparently normal prenatal and perinatal history
2. Psychomotor development largely normal through the first six months or may be delayed from birth
3. Normal head circumference at birth
4. Postnatal deceleration of head growth in the majority
5. Loss of achieved purposeful hand skill between ages 1/2 – 2-1/2 years

6. Stereotypic hand movements such as hand wringing/squeezing, clapping/tapping, mouthing, and washing/rubbing automatisms

7. Emerging social withdrawal, communication dysfunction, loss of learned words, and cognitive impairment

8. Impaired (dyspraxic) or failing locomotion

Supportive criteria

1. Awake disturbances of breathing (hyperventilation, breath-holding, forced expulsion of air or saliva, air swallowing)

2. Bruxism

3. Impaired sleep pattern from early infancy

4. Abnormal muscle tone successively associated with muscle wasting and dystonia

5. Peripheral vasomotor disturbances

6. Scoliosis/kyphosis progressing through childhood

7. Growth retardation

8. Hypotrophic small and cold feet; small, thin hands

Exclusion Criteria

1. Organomegaly or other signs of storage disease

2. Retinopathy, optic atrophy, or cataract

3. Evidence of perinatal or postnatal brain damage

4. Existence of identifiable metabolic or other progressive neurological disorder

5. Acquired neurological disorder resulting from severe infections or head trauma

Revised Delineation of Variant Phenotypes

Inclusion Criteria

1. Meet at least 3 of 6 main criteria

2. Meet at least 5 of 11 supportive criteria

Six Main Criteria

1. Absence or reduction of hand skills

2. Reduction or loss of babble speech

3. Monotonous pattern to hand stereotypies

4. Reduction or loss of communication skills

5. Deceleration of head growth from first years of life

6. RS disease profile: a regression stage followed by a recovery of interaction contrasting with slow neuromotor regression

Eleven Supportive Criteria

1. breathing irregularities

2. bloating/air swallowing

3. teeth grinding, harsh sounding type

4. abnormal locomotion

5. scoliosis/kyphosis

6. lower limb amyotrophy

7. cold, purplish feet, usually growth impaired

8. sleep disturbances including night screaming outbursts

9. laughing/screaming spells

10. diminished response to pain

11. intense eye contact/eye pointing

Additional Information

International Rett Syndrome Association

9121 Piscataway Road, Suite 2B
Clinton, MD 20735
Toll-Free: 800-818-7388
Tel: 301-856-3334
Fax: 301-856-3336
Website: www.rettsyndrome.org
E-mail: irsa@rettsyndrome.org

Rett Syndrome Research Foundation
4600 Devitt Drive
Cincinnati, OH 45246
Tel: 513-874-3020
Fax: 513-874-2520
Website: www.rsrf.org

Easter Seals
230 W. Monroe Street, Suite 1800
Chicago, IL 60606-4802
Toll-Free: 800-221-6827
Tel: 312-762-6200
Fax: 312-726-1494
TTY: 312-726-4258
Website: www.easter-seals.org

National Institute of Child Health and Human Development
Building 31, Room 2A32
Bethesda, MD 20892-2425
Toll-Free: 800-370-2943
Tel: 301-496-5133
Website: www.nichd.nih.gov
E-mail: nichdclearinghouse@mail.nih.gov

Brain Resources and Information Network (BRAIN)
P.O. Box 5801
Bethesda, MD 20824
Toll-Free: 800-352-9424
Tel: 301-496-5751
TTY: 301-468-5981
Website: www.ninds.nih.gov

Chapter 23

Spina Bifida

Did You Know?

Incidence

- All women capable of becoming pregnant are at risk of having a child born with spina bifida.

- Half of all U.S. pregnancies are unplanned.

- 90–95 percent of babies born with spina bifida are born to parents with no family history of spina bifida.

- Each year in the U.S. about 4,000 pregnancies are affected by spina bifida and anencephaly, an average of 11 pregnancies per day.

- Spina bifida affects approximately 1 out of every 1,000 newborns in the U.S.

- These birth defects occur very early in pregnancy, about 3-4 weeks after conception, before most women know that they are pregnant.

- Spina bifida and anencephaly are the most common preventable birth defects.

This chapter includes "Did You Know?" and "Facts about Spina Bifida." This information is reprinted with permission from the Spina Bifida Association of America. © 2001 Spina Bifida Association of America. All rights reserved. Also included are excerpts from "NINDS Spina Bifida Information Page," National Institute of Neurological Disorders and Stroke (NINDS), reviewed 7/1/2001.

- In the U.S., there are 60 million women in the 15-45 age group, with over 6 million pregnancies (resulting in 4 million births) each year.

Recurrence

- If parents have 1 child with spina bifida, the risk of recurrence increases to between 1 and 5 out of 100.

- If one parent has spina bifida, the chances of having a child with spina bifida are between 1 and 5 percent.

- If both parents have spina bifida, the chances of having a child with spina bifida increases to 15 percent.

Prevention

- The cause of spina bifida is unknown. Recent studies have shown that taking the B-vitamin folic acid before conception and during the first few weeks of pregnancy may help reduce the risk of spina bifida.

- Studies have shown that if all women who could become pregnant were to take a multivitamin with folic acid, the risk of neural tube defects could be reduced by up to 75%.

For women at higher risk for spina bifida or other neural tube defects, an increased level of folic acid is recommended by prescription. Research has shown that 4000 micrograms of folic acid reduces the risk of neural tube defects for these women.

Life Expectancy

- Today's medical advances in the fields of neurosurgery and urology (early treatment is important) are making it possible for a majority of infants born with spina bifida to live into adulthood.

Facts about Spina Bifida

What Are Neural Tube Defects?

Neural tube defects (NTDs) are serious birth defects that involve incomplete development of the brain, spinal cord, and/or protective coverings for these organs. There are 3 types of NTDs: anencephaly, encephalocele, and spina bifida.

Babies born with anencephaly have underdeveloped brains and incomplete skulls. Most infants born with anencephaly do not survive more than a few hours after birth. Encephalocele results in a hole in the skull through which brain tissue protrudes. Although most babies with encephalocele do not live or are severely retarded, early surgery has been able to save a few children.

What Is Spina Bifida?

Spina bifida is the most frequently occurring permanently disabling birth defect. It affects approximately one out of every 1,000 newborns in the United States.

Spina bifida, the most common NTD, is one of the most devastating of all birth defects. It results from the failure of the spine to close properly during the first month of pregnancy. In severe cases, the spinal cord protrudes through the back and may be covered by skin or a thin membrane. Surgery to close a newborn's back is generally performed within 24 hours after birth to minimize the risk of infection and to preserve existing function in the spinal cord.

Because of the paralysis resulting from the damage to the spinal cord, people born with spina bifida may need surgeries and other extensive medical care. The condition can also cause bowel and bladder complications. A large percentage of children born with spina bifida also have hydrocephalus, the accumulation of fluid in the brain. Hydrocephalus is controlled by a surgical procedure called shunting which relieves the fluid build up in the brain by redirecting it into the abdominal area. Most children born with spina bifida live well into adulthood as a result of today's sophisticated medical techniques.

Who Is at Higher Risk?

Women who

- have a child with spina bifida
- have spina bifida themselves
- have already had a pregnancy affected by any neural defect

are at greater risk of having a child affected by spina bifida or another neural tube defect. These women may need to get a prescription for folic acid before trying to become pregnant, so it's important to plan any future pregnancy. Please speak with your health care provider about folic acid.

I've Heard That Children with Spina Bifida Have Learning Problems. Is This True?

Some children with spina bifida do experience learning problems. They may have difficulty with paying attention, expressing or understanding language, organizing, sequencing, and grasping reading and math.

How Can We Help Those with Learning Problems?

Early intervention can help considerably to prepare these children for school. Students should be in the least restrictive environment and their day to day activities should be as normal as possible. It often helps to have a psychological evaluation, which tests the child's intelligence, academic levels (reading, spelling, math, etc.), and basic learning abilities (visual perception, receptive and expressive language skills).

What about the Physical Limitations?

Children with spina bifida need to learn mobility skills, and often with the use of crutches, braces, or wheelchairs can achieve more independence. Also, with new techniques children can become independent in managing their bowel and bladder problems. Physical disabilities like spina bifida can have profound effects on the child's emotional and social development. It is important that health care professionals, teachers, and parents understand the child's physical capabilities and limitations. To promote personal growth, they should encourage children (within the limits of safety and health) to be independent, to participate in activities with their non-disabled peers, and to assume responsibility for their own care.

What Are Secondary Conditions Associated with Spina Bifida?

Special attention is needed to identify and treat secondary disabilities. Due to the wide range of neurological damage and mobility impairment it can be difficult to identify some secondary disabilities. Attention should be focused on the psychological and social development of children and young adults with spina bifida. Many recent studies, including the SBAA's Adult Network Survey, clearly indicate the presence of emotional problems that result from factors such as low self-esteem and lack of social skills training.

Examples of secondary conditions associated with spina bifida are latex allergy, tendinitis, obesity, skin breakdown, gastrointestinal disorders, learning disabilities, attaining and retaining mobility, depression, and social and sexual issues.

What Is Latex Allergy?

Allergic responses to latex (rubber) products. Typical symptoms include watery eyes, wheezing, hives, rash, swelling, and in severe cases, anaphylaxis (a life threatening reaction). These responses can occur when items containing latex touch the skin, the mucous membranes (like the mouth, genitals, bladder, or rectum), open areas, or bloodstream (especially during surgery).

Who Is Allergic to Latex?

While it is not known exactly how this allergy develops, anybody can develop a latex allergy. However, certain groups of individuals have been identified as having a greater risk of becoming latex allergic. Those at higher risk include people who are frequently exposed to latex, such as children and adults with spina bifida and health professionals. Research has shown that spina bifida patients have the potential to become allergic (to some degree) to latex. Anyone with a latex allergy should avoid exposure to all products that contain latex.

What Are Some Common Products That Contain Latex?

Catheters, elastic bandages, baby bottle nipples, pacifiers, and balloons are just a few common products that contain latex. For a more extensive list of items containing latex often found at home, in your community, and in hospitals, contact the SBAA. If you are in doubt about a specific product, check with its distributor or manufacturer.

Can Anything Be Done to Prevent Spina Bifida?

Birth defects can happen in any family. Many things can affect a pregnancy, including family genes and things women may come in contact with during pregnancy. Recent studies have shown that folic acid is one factor that may reduce the risk of having an NTD baby. Taking folic acid cannot guarantee having a healthy baby, but it can help.

Taking folic acid before and during early pregnancy reduces the risk of spina bifida and other neural tube defects. Here's what you can do:

- Take a vitamin with 400 micrograms (mcg) folic acid every day.

  This amount is also written as 0.4 milligrams (mg). All women should take this amount every day while not planning to become pregnant.

- If you have a child with spina bifida, have spina bifida yourself, or have had a history of pregnancy affected by a neural tube defect, and you are thinking about becoming pregnant, you need a higher dose of folic acid. You should take 4000 micrograms (mcg) of folic acid by prescription for 1 to 3 months before becoming pregnant.

  This amount is also written as 4.0 milligrams (mg). Taking this amount of folic acid by prescription may reduce the chance of a neural tube defect like spina bifida in future pregnancies. Please see your doctor. Do not take this extra folic acid by taking more multivitamins because too much of some of the other vitamins could harm you and your future baby.

- Plan your next pregnancy.

  Speak with your health care provider about your personal risk of having a baby with a neural tube defect. You may need to get a prescription for folic acid before you try to become pregnant.

What Is Folic Acid?

Folic acid, a common water-soluble B vitamin, is essential for the functioning of the human body. During periods of rapid growth, such as pregnancy and fetal development, the body's requirement for this vitamin increases. Folic acid can be found in multivitamins, fortified breakfast cereals, dark green leafy vegetables such as broccoli and spinach, egg yolks, and some fruits and fruit juices. However, the average American diet does not supply the recommended level of folic acid.

Additional Information

Disabled Sports USA
451 Hungerford Drive
Suite 100
Rockville, MD 20850
Tel: 301-217-0960 or 301-217-9736
Fax: 301-217-0968

Website: www.dsusa.org
E-mail: dsusa@dsusa.org

Lipomyelomeningocele Family Support Net.
9217 Sayornis Court
Raleigh, NC 27615
Tel: 919-844-2043
Fax: 919-844-2044
Website: www.lfsn.org
E-mail: bborchert@mindspring.com

March of Dimes Birth Defects Foundation
1275 Mamaroneck Avenue
White Plains, NY 10605
Toll-Free: 888-MODIMES (663-4637)
Tel: 914-428-7100
Fax: 914-428-8203
Website: www.modimes.org
E-mail: resourcecenter@modimes.org

National Information Center for Children and Youth with Disabilities
P.O. Box 1492
Washington, DC 20013-1492
Toll-Free: 800-695-0285
Tel: 202-884-8200
Fax: 202-884-8441
Website: www.nichcy.org
E-mail: nichcy@aed.org

Spina Bifida Association of America
4590 MacArthur Blvd. NW
Suite 250
Washington, DC 20007-4266
Toll-Free: 800-621-3141
Tel: 202-944-3285
Fax: 202-944-3295
Website: www.sbaa.org
E-mail: sbaa@sbaa.org

Chapter 24

Spinal Muscular Atrophy (SMA)

Quick Facts about Spinal Muscular Atrophy

The Disease

Spinal muscular atrophy (SMA), the number one genetic killer of children under the age of two, is a group of inherited and often fatal diseases that destroys the nerves controlling voluntary muscle movement, which affects crawling, walking, head and neck control, and even swallowing.

Who Is Affected?

SMA is one of the most prevalent genetic disorders.

- One in every 6,000 babies is born with SMA. Of children diagnosed before age two, 50 percent will die before their second birthday.

- SMA can strike anyone of any age, race, or gender.

- One in every 40 people carries the gene that causes SMA. The child of two carriers has a one in four chance of developing SMA.

Types of SMA

- **Type I**, or Werdnig-Hoffman Disease, is the most severe form of SMA. Children with Type I tend to be weak and lack motor development, rendering movement difficult. Children afflicted with Type I cannot sit unaided and have trouble breathing, sucking, and swallowing. Type I SMA strikes infants between birth and six months.

- **Type II** is slightly less severe. Type II patients may be able to sit unaided or even stand with support and usually do not suffer from feeding and swallowing difficulties. However, they are at increased risk for complications from respiratory infections. Type II SMA affects infants between seven and 18 months old.

- **Type III**, also known as Kugelberg-Welander Disease, is the least deadly form of childhood-onset SMA. Type III patients are able to stand, but weakness is prevalent and tends to eventually sentence its victims to a wheelchair. Type III SMA strikes children after the age of 18 months, but can surface even in adulthood.

- **Type IV** is the adult form of the disease in which symptoms tend to begin after age 35. Symptoms usually begin in the hands, feet, and tongue, and spread to other areas of the body.

- **Adult Onset X-Linked SMA**, also known as Kennedy's Syndrome or Bulbo-Spinal Muscular Atrophy, occurs only in men. Facial and tongue muscles are noticeably affected. In addition, these men also often have breast enlargement known as gynecomastia. Like all forms of SMA, the course of the disease is variable, but in general tends to progress slowly.

SMA does not affect sensation and intellectual activity in patients. It commonly is observed that patients with SMA are unusually bright and sociable.

Testing

Prenatal counseling is available to couples who are carriers of SMA or who have lost a child to SMA.

Understanding Spinal Muscular Atrophy: A Comprehensive Guide

This chapter is to serve as a source of information and support to those involved with children and adults with Spinal Muscular Atrophy

(SMA). Families of SMA was founded by a group of parents of children with SMA Type II. They all continue to be actively involved working to raise money to distribute educational materials, provide patient services, and support research, which will lead to a treatment and cure. These efforts have aided in the 1990 discovery of the chromosome which houses the SMA gene, and of the finding of the gene itself, including testing for SMA.

Whether you have a family member or close friend, your interest in this is probably based on the fact that you or someone you care about is awaiting diagnosis of SMA or has been diagnosed with SMA. The concern that you might have upon hearing the term, Werdnig-Hoffmann, Kugelberg-Welander, Spinal Muscular Atrophy is understood. We've all heard of leukemia, AIDS, and cystic fibrosis but Spinal Muscular Atrophy is an unknown. It is still an unknown despite the fact that 1 in 40 people are carriers, and 1 in every 6,000 live births is affected which is why so much research is being conducted to discover its cause(s) and cure.

What Is Spinal Muscular Atrophy?

Spinal Muscular Atrophy (SMA) is a disease of the anterior horn cells. Anterior horn cells are located in the spinal cord. SMA affects the voluntary muscles for activities such as crawling, walking, head and neck control, and swallowing.

It mainly affects the proximal muscles, or in other words the muscles closest to the point of origin, in this case those closest to the trunk of one's body. Weakness in the legs is generally greater than weakness in the arms. Some abnormal movements of the tongue, called tongue fasciculations may be present in patients with Type I and some patients with Type II. The senses/feelings are normal as is intellectual activity. In fact it is often observed that patients with SMA are unusually bright and sociable.

Type I Acute (Severe)

Type I SMA is also called Werdnig-Hoffmann Disease. The diagnosis of children with this type is usually made before 6 months of age and in the majority of cases before 3 months, there may be lack of fetal movement in the final months of pregnancy.

Usually a child with Type I, (Werdnig-Hoffmann) is never able to lift his/her head or accomplish normal physical milestones. Swallowing and feeding may be difficult and the child may show some difficulties with their own secretions. There is a general weakness in the intercostals and accessory respiratory muscles (the muscles situated between the ribs). The chest may appear concave (sunken in) due to the diaphragmatic (tummy) breathing.

Please note: Although diagnosis may be made before 6 months of age it does not necessarily follow the same course of severity for each patient.

Type II (Chronic)

Diagnosis of Type II is almost always made before 2 years of age with the majority of cases diagnosed by 15 months. Children with this type may sit unsupported although they are usually unable to come to a sitting position without assistance. At some point they may be able to stand. This is most often accomplished with the aid of bracing and/or a parapodium/standing frame.

Feeding and swallowing problems are not usually characteristic of Type II although in some patients this can occur and a feeding tube may become necessary. Tongue fasciculations are less often found in children with Type II but a fine tremor in the outstretched fingers is common. Children with Type II are also diaphragmatic breathers.

Type III (Mild)

Diagnosis of Type III, often referred to as Kugelberg-Welander or Juvenile Spinal Muscular Atrophy, is made sometime after 18 months of age and as late as adolescence. The patient with Type III can stand alone and walk, but may show difficulty with walking and/or getting up from a sitting or bent over position. With Type III, a fine tremor can be seen in the outstretched fingers but tongue fasciculations are seldom seen.

Spinal Muscular Atrophy Types I, II and III are usually nonprogressive.

Type IV (Adult Onset)

Typically in the adult form symptoms begin after age 35. It is very rare for Spinal Muscular Atrophy to begin between the ages of 18 and 30. Adult SMA is characterized by insidious onset and very slow progression. The bulbar muscles, those muscles used for swallowing and respiratory function, are rarely affected in Type IV.

Adult Onset X-Linked SMA

This form also known as Kennedy's Syndrome or Bulbo-Spinal Muscular Atrophy, occurs only in males, although 50% of female offspring are carriers. This form of SMA is associated with a mutation in the gene that codes for part of the androgen receptor and therefore these male patients often have breast enlargement known as gynecomastia. Also noticeably affected are the facial and tongue muscles. Like all forms of SMA the course of the disease is variable, but in general tends to be slowly progressive or nonprogressive.

Diagnosing Spinal Muscular Atrophy

It is important that we all understand the tests that we must endure. This is especially important when it comes to our children. After having gone through this testing we often do not remember to ask for an explanation of all of the tests. If and when we did ask, we weren't clearheaded enough to hear or understand the explanation.

As parents, we have gathered information to answer these initial questions and explain as simply as possible their diagnostic uses. Up until 1995 there were 3 major lab tests used for diagnosis, as well as the clinical exam.

1. Serum Enzymes

This is a normal blood test. The enzyme most commonly studied is CPK (creatine-phosphokinase). In Type I (Werdnig-Hoffmann) this enzyme tends to be normal, but moderate elevation may occur in the milder forms.

2. EMG (Electromyography)

This test measures the electrical activity of muscle. In this procedure small needles are inserted into the patient's muscles, usually the arms and thighs, while an electrical pattern is observed and recorded. The readout is similar to that of an EKG or lie detector.

In addition, a nerve conduction velocity (NVC) may also be performed. In this test the response of a nerve to an electrical stimulus is measured. When performing this test on a child, if at all possible, it should be performed by a doctor experienced in dealing with children. Also be sure to bring lots of things with which to keep your child occupied. Hold your child on your lap during the procedure, as it is a tremendous help in making an unpleasant procedure somewhat bearable. Ask your doctor whether your child/the patient should be given a mild pain killer or sedative prior to the test.

In the fall of 1995, probes were updated that detect deletions in Types I, II, and III SMA were reported. One of these probes called Spinal Motor Neuron (SMN) detects the absence of gene sequences in approximately 90-94% of SMA patients and is not absent in normal individuals. This information makes this SMN gene test very useful for the diagnosis of SMA. However the defect in this gene cannot be used to indicate the severity of the disease. It is believed that with a blood test to screen for SMN deletion together with an EMG and clinical examination it may not be necessary for a muscle biopsy to be performed.

The results may show that there is no deletion of the SMN gene. If this is the case then a muscle biopsy would be necessary to confirm the diagnosis.

3. Muscle Biopsy

This is a surgical procedure where an incision, approximately 3 inches long, is made and a small section of muscle is removed, usually from the thigh. The biopsy is used to check for degeneration. Although many doctors may persuade you of the necessity of a general anesthetic, this procedure can be done with a local anesthetic. It is an especially important point when dealing with children who may be suffering from a neuromuscular disorder and may have weak respiratory function.

Please Note: There is an alternative to the biopsy, it is a procedure known as a needle biopsy. Instead of a 2 to 3 inch incision, only a small nick in the skin is necessary. Ask your doctor about this procedure.

- No matter what, understand that you as a parent or as a patient have rights and that you are not alone.

- Most hospitals have social service departments that can give you a shoulder to lean on.

- Don't be afraid to say no if something doesn't seem right.

- Don't be intimidated or afraid to ask questions.

- If you forget to ask something call your doctor or contact Families of S.M.A. for suggestions.

Prognosis: What Does it Mean? What Are We to Expect?

Type I Acute

In the acute type of this disease the bulbar muscles are often affected, and this may make feeding and swallowing extremely difficult. Breathing is often labored due to reduced strength of the chest muscles, and most breathing can be seen in the abdominal areas, with the chest appearing sunken in. Because of increasing overall weakness or repeated respiratory infections, the prognosis is poor. Death in the majority of children with Type I S.M.A. usually occurs by 2 years of age.

It is important to note the overlap of types I and II.

Type II Chronic

Because of the range of progression seen in patients with Type II it is hard to tell how fast, if at all, the weakness will progress. Some children may learn to walk with the aid of bracing and may survive into adulthood. However, others, due to weakened chest and respiratory muscles may become increasingly weak with probable respiratory infections such as pneumonia. There are many cases in which the initial progressive weakness may remain the same, or there may be periods of worsening followed by long periods of stability. With such variables, age of death can vary greatly. It can take place as early as 3 years as in Type I or not until adulthood.

Although not all children diagnosed with Type II develop respiratory weakness, respiratory failure is usually the cause of death following a bout of pneumonia or other respiratory infection.

Type III Mild

Patients with Type III will again vary greatly. However the prognosis is very good. Often walking will be possible, or the patient will be fully functional for years before assistance is necessary. As with Type I and Type II respiratory infections should be prevented and necessary precautions taken.

Type IV Adult Onset

There is nothing unusual or distinctive about the current management of the adult forms of Spinal Muscular Atrophy. Proper diagnosis, genetic counseling, and appropriate physical therapy remain mainstays.

Taking the Diagnosis Home: What Can We Do?

Our first reaction when the doctors told us we could take our child home was "Home?" How could they expect us to go home with a child whom we had brought in "well," and now they are sending us home with a child who has a life-threatening disease? It is hard to accept that with so many modern medical advances there is so little help. The medical field has yet to find any drug, therapy, or surgery to cure the Spinal Muscular Atrophy diseases.

Type I (and Some Type II)

While most children diagnosed with Type I are still infants there are a myriad of things that can be done to assist in the cognitive and emotional health of your child. Using balloons and feathers as toys makes for wonderful stimulation and allows them that feeling of independence and accomplishment. Reaching games are a form of physical therapy that can be very helpful. Instructions in range of motion and other physical therapy ideas by a licensed physical therapist are important no matter how young the child. Your physical therapist can also suggest ideal seating systems that will be most helpful in the comfort and maximum mobility of your child.

Also getting in touch with a respiratory therapist is very important especially so you can be instructed in CPT (chest physiotherapy). CPT is a means of clearing the lungs of accumulated mucus, by using a series of procedures to assist in coughing.

Saliva can settle in the nasopharynx causing a faint gurgling sound. Often the secretions or mucus cannot be cleared with these noninvasive measures and the use of a suction machine may be necessary. Blowing raspberries, bubbles, anything encourages respiratory strength.

Water therapy can be very helpful as the buoyancy of the water allows movement of the arms and legs that may otherwise not be there. Be sure that the water temperature is at least 90°F and that the child's head does not go under the water or into the water. You must watch so that the child has no possibility of aspirating (getting fluid into their lungs).

Aspirating can also become a problem with children when eating. Sometimes the child may even aspirate his/her own secretions. As this becomes a problem loss of weight may also be noted and assistive feeding may be necessary.

Two possible options are:

1. **Naso Gastric Tube:** which is a tube inserted through the nose which goes directly into the stomach.

2. **Gastric Tube:** is a more permanent option. It is a surgical procedure to insert a tube or button directly into the stomach.

Although many doctors may try to persuade you of the necessity of a general anesthetic, this procedure can be done with a local anesthetic and an intravenous (IV) sedation drip.

It will be necessary to monitor respiratory distress by measuring the level of oxygen and to determine if oxygen from an outside source is necessary. The tool used to measure this is called a Biox-oximeter. This is a small clip which is usually placed on the patient's index finger to determine the oxygen saturation.

To help the child with breathing a ventilator can be used. There are several possibilities when considering ventilation.

1. **Negative Pressure Ventilation** can be achieved by placing the patient in a Port-A-Lung. This is a much smaller version of the old fashioned Iron Lung. It works by using external ventilation to create negative pressure to set the rate of breathing.

2. **Bi-Pap (Biphasic Positive Airway Pressure).** This ventilation unit uses a nasal mask with a cap, which fits over the head to hold it in place over the nose. A small hose is attached that feeds oxygen. This unit allows maximum inspiration and expiration. A small alarm is also attached to detect for leaks.

For long-term ventilation a tracheotomy is usually performed. There may be other options available. Consult your physicians and respiratory therapists or contact Families of S.M.A. for literature.

It is important to understand your rights when it comes to making life-sustaining decisions for your child. Be sure that both parents discuss their feelings about this very delicate topic. It is a decision that cannot be made lightly and all options should be covered. Talking to a counselor in the department of social services at your hospital may be helpful. Once your decision has been reached be sure that you put it in writing, and that all necessary medical personal and family members are aware of your wishes. This is your decision, one you have reached with great care and anguish, and under no circumstances should you allow others to judge you or place their values upon you. You are never alone. Families of SMA is always just a phone call away.

Type II (and some Type III)

Raising a child with SMA should be no different than raising a child who is not affected. Do as many things as possible that are age appropriate. Many times this means making adaptations. It is very important that children with SMA are assisted in reaching their utmost potential. This includes getting the child upright at the earliest possible age.

Standing is important in the development of all children. It allows for better respiratory function, greater bowel function, and encourages greater mobility. Getting your child in an upright position can sometimes take pushing on the part of the parent to encourage the physician to write a prescription for standing aids.

There are several options to consider when choosing the appropriate standing aid. Among them are a standing frame and a parapodium. For added mobility and independence a standing wheelchair is ideal. A child as young as 13 months can use this. Bracing is also an option. Reciprocating Gait Orthosis (RGOs) have been found to work for children with Type II, and these children have been able to take some steps.

The use of a lightweight manual wheelchair can be an exciting addition for the SMA child. It can provide mobility, independence, and a taste of adventure, while still allowing them to use some of their own strength. However, it should be understood that for true independence and mobility, a power wheelchair is necessary.

Scoliosis (curvature of the spine) occurs at some point in all children with SMA Type I and II and some Type III. The degree of the scoliosis will be a factor in deciding how to treat it. Because scoliosis can restrict breathing and pulmonary function, necessary precautions should be taken early. Among these options are custom seating systems, seating aids, and a body jacket. Later spinal fusion may need to be considered.

If your child is having continuous upper respiratory infections you may want to inquire about an IPPB (Intermittent Positive Pressure Breathing) machine. The IPPB may assist with respiratory function and help prevent the lungs from becoming stiff. IPPB is also helpful in eliminating secretions. Using an Incentive Spirometer daily allows you to measure lung capacity. When volumes are low it usually indicates an increase in mucus and/or a cold developing. Diet as with any growing child is very important.

Your child's diet deserves careful consideration. Excessive weight can make mobility more difficult. Good eating habits help contribute to strong minds and strong bodies. Constant contact with your physician and a nutritionist is very important in this aspect of maintenance.

Type III

Because children with Type III walk at some point unassisted, it is important that they be monitored so that any difficulty may be detected at an early stage. The use of a walker and bracing may become necessary. The use of a lightweight manual wheelchair may be considered for distance as well as an electric scooter or other motorized chair. Physical and occupational therapists should be consulted. Diet should also be watched.

Type IV: Adult Onset

As an adult you are aware of your weaknesses and limitations. You should work together with your physician, physical therapist, and occupational therapist to work out the best possible program for you. As with Types I, II, and III diet and nutrition are an important factor in your well-being. It is important to keep your body and mind healthy.

The diagnosis of Spinal Muscular Atrophy can be a frightening prospect, but it can also be looked on as a gift. Unfortunately in life, it seems to take something tragic or earth shattering to make us open our eyes to the joys of today. Having a child with SMA or being an adult with SMA gives life a different perspective. We become more aware of the simple pleasures—the seasons, the smiles, the tears. We become grateful for the simple things, getting a glass of water, taking a step, and breathing. We learn to accept diversity and challenges with a new found enthusiasm and drive and we learn how many people there are who truly care.

What Causes Spinal Muscular Atrophy?

Spinal Muscular Atrophy is an autosomal recessive disease, which means that both parents must be carriers. Both parents must have the gene responsible and these genes must be passed onto their child. When a child has received this gene from each of its parents it will then be affected by SMA. Although both parents are carriers the likelihood of passing this gene along to a child and having an affected child is 25%, or 1 in 4.

Familial Forms (affecting other family members) of Spinal Muscular Atrophy in the older age group can occur as autosomal recessive, mutants, or autosomal dominant. The genetic defects underlying these diseases make it necessary to be precise regarding the inheritance pattern in a particular family.

I Am a Carrier of the SMA Gene, What Can I Do?

If you find you are a carrier of the SMA gene it is necessary that you seek the advice of a genetic counselor. This counselor will assist biological parents to better understand the risks and chances of having another affected child. The genetic counselor will take a complete family history which will include any diseases, deaths, causes of death, stillbirths, and miscarriages of each family member. Using this information helps them to identify persons likely to carry a defective gene. Sometimes laboratory studies will follow.

The information presently available allows for prenatal testing with 98% reliability. The decision to have prenatal testing performed and the options available once the results of the testing are back can be difficult. These are individual decisions and very personal. It is important that both parents have discussed their feelings together and with their genetic counselor who will offer unbiased support in their decision. Often times a family may also wish to consult with their clergyman. Once a decision has been made it is important to be supportive of one another and to allow any necessary time to grieve. This is a difficult decision, one that has taken great anguish and thought.

Under no circumstances should you allow others' values or judgment to affect you. Remember you are not alone. Families of SMA is only a phone call away.

Ongoing Research

Through the Indiana University Roster which is funded by Families of SMA one of the key families in the gene location was found. This roster continues to be a useful tool to researchers in their quest to correct the defective gene(s). Families participation is an important factor to this discovery.

Researchers throughout the country are funded by Families of SMA in efforts to not only alleviate but to cure the Spinal Muscular Atrophy diseases. They are looking at all avenues from nutritional based studies, missing proteins, to neurotrophic based drug studies. It is an exciting thought that we can almost see the pot of gold at the end of the rainbow.

How Families of SMA Can Help

As caring parents and professionals who have experienced the day to day trials and tribulations of raising a child with Spinal Muscular Atrophy or have had to deal with the loss of a child or family member with Spinal Muscular Atrophy, SMA can offer support and understanding when it is most needed. By phone and networking Families of SMA volunteer staff and members are there when you need them. They are willing to listen and share.

The publishing of a quarterly newsletter keeps families and professionals up to date on the latest in research, technology, and day to day coping in regards to Spinal Muscular Atrophy. The sponsoring of Biannual conferences allows families and professionals hands on techniques and family to family support, while also giving the children a great opportunity to make new friends and have a great time.

Because Families of SMA understands the financial hardship living with Spinal Muscular Atrophy can cause, they have a very large equipment pool which is available free of charge to members of Families of SMA.

Most of all Families of SMA can offer friendship and hope. Please contact us so that we can help you with any questions you may have or support you may need. We are all here for each other.

Additional Information

Families of S.M.A. (Spinal Muscular Atrophy)
National Headquarters
P.O. Box 196
Libertyville, IL 60048-0196
Toll-Free: 800-886-1762
Tel: 847-367-7620
Fax: 847-367-7623
E-mail: info@fsma.org

Chapter 25

Tourette Syndrome

What Is Tourette Syndrome?

Tourette Syndrome (TS) is a neurological disorder characterized by tics—involuntary, rapid, sudden movements or vocalizations that occur repeatedly in the same way. The symptoms include:

1. Both multiple motor and one or more vocal tics present at some time during the illness although not necessarily simultaneously;

2. The occurrence of tics many times a day (usually in bouts) nearly every day or intermittently throughout a span of more than one year; and

3. Periodic changes in the number, frequency, type, and location of the tics, and waxing and waning of their severity. Symptoms can sometimes disappear for weeks or months at a time.

4. Onset before the age of 18.

The term, involuntary, used to describe TS tics is sometimes confusing since it is known that most people with TS do have some control over their symptoms. What is not recognized is that the control, which can be exercised anywhere from seconds to hours at a time, may merely postpone more severe outbursts of symptoms. Tics are experienced as irresistible and (as with the urge to sneeze) eventually must be expressed. People with TS often seek a secluded spot to release their symptoms after delaying them in school or at work. Typically, tics increase as a result of tension or stress, and decrease with relaxation or when focusing on an absorbing task.

How Would a Typical Case of TS Be Described?

The term typical cannot be applied to TS. The expression of symptoms covers a spectrum from very mild to quite severe. However, the majority of cases can be categorized as mild.

Is Obscene Language (Coprolalia) a Typical Symptom of TS?

Definitely not. The fact is that cursing, uttering obscenities, and ethnic slurs are manifested by fewer than 15% of people with TS. Too often, however, the media seize upon this symptom for its sensational effect.

What Causes the Symptoms?

The cause has not been established, although current research presents considerable evidence that the disorder stems from the abnormal metabolism of at least one brain chemical (neurotransmitter) called dopamine. Undoubtedly, other neurotransmitters, e.g. serotonin, are involved as well.

How Is TS Diagnosed?

A diagnosis is made by observing symptoms and by evaluating the history of their onset. No blood analysis or other type of neurological testing exists to diagnose TS. However, some physicians may wish to order an EEG, MRI, CAT scan, or certain blood tests to rule out other ailments that might be confused with TS. Rating scales are available for assessment of tic severity.

What Are the First Symptoms?

The most common first symptom is a facial tic such as rapidly blinking eyes or twitches of the mouth. However, involuntary sounds such as throat clearing and sniffing, or tics of the limbs may be initial signs.

For a minority, the disorder begins abruptly with multiple symptoms of movements and sounds.

How Are Tics Classified?

Two categories of tics and several other examples are:

Simple

- Motor—Eye blinking, head jerking, shoulder shrugging, and facial grimacing.

- Vocal—Throat clearing, yelping and other noises, sniffing, and tongue clicking.

Complex

- Motor—Jumping, touching other people or things, smelling, twirling about, and only rarely, self-injurious actions including hitting or biting oneself.

- Vocal—Uttering words or phrases out of context and coprolalia (vocalizing socially unacceptable words).

The range of tics or tic-like symptoms that can be seen in TS is very broad. The complexity of some symptoms is often perplexing to family members, friends, teachers, and employers who may find it hard to believe that the actions or vocal utterances are involuntary.

How Is TS Treated?

The majority of people with TS are not significantly disabled by their tics or behavioral symptoms, and therefore do not require medication. However, there are medications available to help control the symptoms when they interfere with functioning. The drugs include haloperidol (Haldol), clonidine (Catapres), pimozide (Orap), fluphenazine (Prolixin, Permitil), and clonazepam (Klonopin). Stimulants such as Ritalin, Cylert, and Dexedrine that are prescribed for ADHD may increase tics. Their use is controversial. For obsessive compulsive traits that interfere significantly with daily functioning, fluoxetine (Prozac), clomipramine (Anafranil), sertraline (Zoloft), risperidone (Risperdal), and paroxetine (Paxil) are prescribed.

Dosages which achieve maximum control of symptoms vary for each patient and must be gauged carefully by a doctor. The medicine is administered in small doses with gradual increases to the point where there is maximum alleviation of symptoms with minimal side effects. Some of the undesirable reactions to medications are weight gain, muscular rigidity, fatigue, motor restlessness, and social withdrawal, most of which can be reduced with specific medications. Side effects such as depression and cognitive impairment can be alleviated with dosage reduction or a change of medication.

Other types of therapy may also be helpful. Psychotherapy can assist a person with TS and help his/her family cope, and some behavior therapies can teach the substitution of one tic for another that is more acceptable. The use of relaxation techniques and/or biofeedback can serve to alleviate stress reactions that cause tics to increase.

Is It Important to Treat Tourette Syndrome Early?

Yes, especially in those instances when the symptoms are viewed by some people as bizarre, disruptive, and frightening. Sometimes TS symptoms provoke ridicule and rejection by peers, neighbors, teachers, and even casual observers. Parents may be overwhelmed by the strangeness of their child's behavior. The child may be threatened, excluded from activities, and prevented from enjoying normal interpersonal relationships. These difficulties may become greater during adolescence—an especially trying period for young people and even more so for a person coping with a neurological problem. To avoid psychological harm, early diagnosis and treatment are crucial. Moreover, in more serious cases, it is possible to control many of the symptoms with medication.

Do All People with TS Have Associated Behaviors in Addition to Tics?

No, but many do have one or more additional problems which may include:

- **Obsessions** which consist of repetitive, unwanted, or bothersome thoughts.

- **Compulsions and ritualistic behaviors** which occur when a person feels that something must be done over and over and/or in a certain way. Examples include touching an object with one hand after touching it with the other hand to even things up or repeatedly checking to see that the flame on the stove is turned

288

off. Children sometimes beg their parents to repeat a sentence many times until it sounds right.

- **Attention Deficit Disorder with or without hyperactivity (ADD or ADHD)** occurs in many people with TS. Children may show signs of hyperactivity before TS symptoms appear. Indications of ADHD may include: difficulty with concentration; failing to finish what is started; not listening; being easily distracted; often acting before thinking; shifting constantly from one activity to another; needing a great deal of supervision; and general fidgeting. Adults too may exhibit signs of ADHD such as overly impulsive behavior and concentration difficulties and the need to move constantly. ADD without hyperactivity includes all of the above symptoms except for the high level of activity. As children with ADHD mature, the need to move is more likely to be expressed by restless, fidgety behavior. Difficulties with concentration and poor impulse control persist.

- **Learning disabilities** may include reading and writing difficulties, problems with mathematics, and perceptual problems.

- **Difficulties with impulse control** which may result, in rare instances, in overly aggressive behaviors or socially inappropriate acts. Also, defiant and angry behaviors can occur.

- **Sleep disorders** are fairly common among people with TS. These include frequent awakenings or walking or talking in one's sleep.

Do Students with TS Have Special Educational Needs?

While school children with TS as a group have the same IQ range as the population at large, many have special educational needs. Data show that many may have some kind of learning problem. TS children with learning difficulties, combined with attention deficits and the difficulty of coping with frequent tics, often call for special educational assistance. The use of tape recorders, typewriters, or computers for reading and writing problems, untimed exams (in a private room if vocal tics are a problem), and permission to leave the classroom when tics become overwhelming are often helpful. Some children need extra help such as access to tutoring in a resource room.

When difficulties in school cannot be resolved, an educational evaluation may be indicated. A resulting identification as other health impaired under federal law will entitle the student to an Individual

Education Plan (IEP) which addresses specific educational problems in school. Such an approach can significantly reduce the learning difficulties that prevent the young person from performing at his/her potential. The child who cannot be adequately educated in a public school with special services geared to his/her individual needs may be best served by enrollment in a special school.

Is TS Inherited?

Genetic studies indicate that TS is inherited as a dominant gene (or genes) causing different symptoms in different family members. A person with TS has about a 50% chance of passing the gene to one of his/her children with each separate pregnancy. However, that genetic predisposition may express itself as TS, as a milder tic disorder or as obsessive compulsive symptoms with no tics at all. It is known that a higher than normal incidence of milder tic disorders and obsessive compulsive behaviors occur in the families of TS patients.

The sex of the offspring also influences the expression of the gene. The chance that the gene-carrying child of a person with TS will have symptoms is at least three to four times higher for a son than for a daughter. Yet only about 10% of the children who inherit the gene will have symptoms severe enough to ever require medical attention. In some cases TS may not be inherited, and cases such as these are identified as sporadic TS. The cause in these instances is unknown.

Is There a Cure?

Not yet.

Is There Ever a Remission?

Many people experience marked improvement in their late teens or early twenties. Most people with TS get better, not worse, as they mature, and those diagnosed with TS have a normal life span. As many as 1/3 of TS patients experience remission of tic symptoms in adulthood.

How Many People in the U.S. Have TS?

Since many people with TS have yet to be diagnosed, there are no absolute figures. The official estimate by the National Institutes of Health is that 100,000 Americans have full-blown TS. Some genetic studies suggest that the figure may be as high as one in two hundred if those with chronic multiple tics and/or transient childhood tics are included in the count.

What Is the History of TS?

In 1825 the first case of TS was reported in medical literature with a description of the Marquise de Dampierre, a noblewoman whose symptoms included involuntary tics of many parts of her body and various vocalizations including coprolalia and echolalia. Later, Dr. Georges Gilles de la Tourette, the French neurologist for whom the disorder is named, first described nine cases in 1885. Samuel Johnson, the lexicographer, and Andre Malraux, the French author, are among the famous people who are thought to have had TS.

What Is the Current Focus of Research?

Since 1984, the TSA has directly funded important research investigations in a number of scientific areas relevant to TS. Recently, studies have intensified to understand how the disorder is transmitted from one generation to the next, and researchers are working toward locating the gene marker for TS. That focus has been enhanced by the efforts of a TSA supported international group of scientists who have formed a unique network to share what they know about the genetics of TS and to systematically cooperate to unravel the unknown. Additional insights are being obtained from studies of large families (kindreds) with numerous members who have TS. At the same time, investigators continue to study specific groups of brain chemicals to better understand the syndrome and to identify new and improved medications.

What Type of Services for Families Exist?

Local TSA affiliates and support groups allow families to exchange ideas and feelings about their common problems. Often family therapy is helpful. Parents of a child with TS have to walk a fine line between understanding and overprotection. They are constantly faced with deciding whether or not certain actions are the expression of TS or just poor behavior. Parents then must determine the appropriate response. For socially unacceptable behavior, a child should be encouraged to control what he/she can whenever possible, and try to substitute what is more socially acceptable. Parents are urged to give their children with TS the opportunity for as much independence as possible, while gently but firmly limiting attempts by some children to use their symptoms to control those around them.

What Is the Tourette Syndrome Association?

TSA, founded in 1972, is the only national voluntary non-profit membership organization dedicated to:

- Identifying the cause;
- Finding the cure; and
- Controlling the effects of TS.

Members include individuals with the disorder, their relatives, and other interested, concerned people. The Association develops and disseminates educational material to individuals, professionals, and to agencies in the fields of health care, education, and government; coordinates support services to help people and their families cope with the problems that occur with TS; funds research that will ultimately find the cause of and cure for TS and, at the same time, lead to improved medications and treatments.

TSA also:

- Offers direct help to TS families in crisis situations through its Information and Referral Service.
- Organizes workshops and symposiums for scientists, clinicians, and others working in the field of TS.
- Promotes public awareness and understanding.
- Maintains a database of allied professionals.
- Sponsors the Tourette Syndrome Brain Bank Program involving collection of sorely needed tissue for scientific research.
- Serves many thousands of members throughout the USA and abroad.
- Increases the knowledge and sensitivity of health care professionals to TS through exhibits at conferences, the dissemination of literature, and the organization of national meetings.
- Develops and maintains state-by-state lists of doctors who can diagnose and treat TS, as well as medical referrals in other

countries; lists of allied professionals (psychologists, social workers) by state; ABA lists of pro-bono attorneys by state; advocate lists by state; and lists of health insurance resources by state.

- Organizes and assists local chapters and support groups throughout the US and around the world.

- Represents the interests of members to the government on critical policy issues including orphan drugs, health insurance, and employment.

These questions and answers are intended to provide basic information about TS. They are not intended to, nor do they constitute medical advice. Readers are warned against changing medical schedules or life activities based on this information without first consulting a physician.

Part Five

Adult-Onset Neurological-Based Movement Disorders

Chapter 26

Amyotrophic Lateral Sclerosis (Lou Gehrig's Disease)

What Is Amyotrophic Lateral Sclerosis?

Amyotrophic lateral sclerosis (ALS), sometimes called Lou Gehrig's disease, is a rapidly progressive, invariably fatal neurological disease that attacks the nerve cells (neurons) responsible for controlling voluntary muscles. The disease belongs to a group of disorders known as motor neuron diseases, which are characterized by the gradual degeneration and death of motor neurons.

Motor neurons are nerve cells located in the brain, brainstem, and spinal cord that serve as controlling units and vital communication links between the nervous system and the voluntary muscles of the body. Messages from motor neurons in the brain (called upper motor neurons) are transmitted to motor neurons in the spinal cord (called lower motor neurons) and from them to particular muscles. In ALS, both the upper motor neurons and the lower motor neurons degenerate or die, ceasing to send messages to muscles. Unable to function, the muscles gradually weaken, waste away (atrophy), and twitch (fasciculations). Eventually, the ability of the brain to start and control voluntary movement is lost.

ALS causes weakness with a wide range of disabilities (see section titled "What are the symptoms?"). Eventually, all muscles under voluntary control are affected, and patients lose their strength and the ability to move their arms, legs, and body. When muscles in the

"Amyotrophic Lateral Sclerosis," Fact Sheet, National Institute of Neurological Disorders and Stroke (NINDS), reviewed July 1, 2001.

diaphragm and chest wall fail, patients lose the ability to breathe without ventilation support. Most people with ALS die from respiratory failure, usually within 3 to 5 years from the onset of symptoms. However, about 10 percent of ALS patients survive for 10 or more years.

Because ALS affects only motor neurons, the disease does not impair a person's mind, personality, intelligence, or memory. Nor does it affect a person's ability to see, smell, taste, hear, or recognize touch. Patients usually maintain control of eye muscles and bladder and bowel functions.

Who Gets ALS?

As many as 20,000 Americans have ALS, and an estimated 5,000 people in the United States are diagnosed with the disease each year. ALS is one of the most common neuromuscular diseases worldwide, and people of all races and ethnic backgrounds are affected. ALS most commonly strikes people between 40 and 60 years of age, but younger and older people also can develop the disease. Men are affected more often than women.

In 90 to 95 percent of all ALS cases, the disease occurs apparently at random with no clearly associated risk factors. Patients do not have a family history of the disease, and their family members are not considered to be at increased risk for developing ALS.

About 5 to 10 percent of all ALS cases are inherited. The familial form of ALS usually results from a pattern of inheritance that requires only one parent to carry the gene responsible for the disease. About 20 percent of all familial cases result from a specific genetic defect that leads to mutation of the enzyme known as superoxide dismutase 1 (SOD1). Research on this mutation is providing clues about the possible causes of motor neuron death in ALS. Not all familial ALS cases are due to the SOD1 mutation, therefore other unidentified genetic causes clearly exist.

What Are the Symptoms?

The onset of ALS may be so subtle that the symptoms are frequently overlooked. The earliest symptoms may include twitching, cramping, or stiffness of muscles; muscle weakness affecting an arm or a leg; slurred and nasal speech; or difficulty chewing or swallowing. These general complaints then develop into more obvious weakness or atrophy that may cause a physician to suspect ALS.

The parts of the body affected by early symptoms of ALS depend on which muscles in the body are damaged first. In some cases, symptoms initially affect one of the legs, and patients experience awkwardness when walking or running or they notice that they are tripping or stumbling more often. Some patients first see the effects of the disease on a hand or arm as they experience difficulty with simple tasks requiring manual dexterity such as buttoning a shirt, writing, or turning a key in a lock. Other patients notice speech problems.

Regardless of the part of the body first affected by the disease, muscle weakness and atrophy spread to other parts of the body as the disease progresses. Patients have increasing problems with moving, swallowing (dysphagia), and speaking or forming words (dysarthria). Symptoms of upper motor neuron involvement include tight and stiff muscles (spasticity) and exaggerated reflexes (hyperreflexia) including an overactive gag reflex. An abnormal reflex commonly called Babinski's sign (the large toe extends upward as the sole of the foot is stimulated in a certain way) also indicates upper motor neuron damage. Symptoms of lower motor neuron degeneration include muscle weakness and atrophy, muscle cramps, and fleeting twitches of muscles that can be seen under the skin (fasciculations).

To be diagnosed with ALS, patients must have signs and symptoms of both upper and lower motor neuron damage that cannot be attributed to other causes.

Although the sequence of emerging symptoms and the rate of disease progression vary from person to person, eventually patients will not be able to stand or walk, get in or out of bed on their own, or use their hands and arms. Difficulty swallowing and chewing impair the patient's ability to eat normally and increase the risk of choking. Maintaining weight will then become a problem. Because the disease usually does not affect cognitive abilities, patients are aware of their progressive loss of function and may become anxious and depressed. Health care professionals need to explain the course of the disease and describe available treatment options so that patients can make informed decisions in advance. In later stages of the disease, patients have difficulty breathing as the muscles of the respiratory system weaken. Patients eventually lose the ability to breathe on their own and must depend on ventilation support for survival. Patients also face an increased risk of pneumonia during later stages of ALS.

How Is ALS Diagnosed?

No one test can provide a definitive diagnosis of ALS, although the presence of upper and lower motor neuron signs in a single limb is strongly suggestive. Instead, the diagnosis of ALS is primarily based on the symptoms and signs the physician observes in the patient and a series of tests to rule out other diseases. Physicians obtain the patient's full medical history and usually conduct a neurologic examination at regular intervals to assess whether symptoms such as muscle weakness, atrophy of muscles, hyperreflexia, and spasticity are getting progressively worse.

Because symptoms of ALS can be similar to those of a wide variety of other, more treatable diseases or disorders, appropriate tests must be conducted to exclude the possibility of other conditions. One of these tests is electromyography (EMG), a special recording technique that detects electrical activity in muscles. Certain EMG findings can support the diagnosis of ALS. Another common test measures nerve conduction velocity (NCV). Specific abnormalities in the NCV results may suggest, for example, that the patient has a form of peripheral neuropathy (damage to peripheral nerves) or myopathy (muscle disease) rather than ALS. The physician may order magnetic resonance imaging (MRI), a noninvasive procedure that uses a magnetic field and radio waves to take detailed images of the brain and spinal cord. Although these MRI scans are often normal in patients with ALS, they can reveal evidence of other problems that may be causing the symptoms, such as a spinal cord tumor, a herniated disk in the neck, syringomyelia, or cervical spondylosis.

Based on the patient's symptoms and findings from the examination and from these tests, the physician may order tests on blood and urine samples to eliminate the possibility of other diseases as well as routine laboratory tests. In some cases, for example, if a physician suspects that the patient may have a myopathy rather than ALS, a muscle biopsy may be performed.

Infectious diseases such as human immunodeficiency virus (HIV), human T-cell leukemia virus (HTLV), and Lyme disease can in some cases cause ALS-like symptoms. Neurological disorders such as multiple sclerosis, post-polio syndrome, multifocal motor neuropathy, and spinal muscular atrophy also can mimic certain facets of the disease and should be considered by physicians attempting to make a diagnosis. Because of the prognosis carried by this diagnosis and the variety of diseases or disorders that can resemble ALS in the early stages of the disease, patients may wish to obtain a second neurological opinion.

What Causes ALS?

The cause of ALS is not known, and scientists do not yet know why ALS strikes some people and not others. An important step toward answering that question came in 1993 when scientists supported by the National Institute of Neurological Disorders and Stroke (NINDS) discovered that mutations in the gene that produces the SOD1 enzyme were associated with some cases of familial ALS. This enzyme is a powerful antioxidant that protects the body from damage caused by free radicals. Free radicals are highly unstable molecules produced by cells during normal metabolism. If not neutralized, free radicals can accumulate and cause random damage to the DNA and proteins within cells. Although it is not yet clear how the SOD1 gene mutation leads to motor neuron degeneration, researchers have theorized that an accumulation of free radicals may result from the faulty functioning of this gene. In support of this, animal studies have shown that motor neuron degeneration and deficits in motor function accompany the presence of the SOD1 mutation.

Studies also have focused on the role of glutamate in motor neuron degeneration. Glutamate is one of the chemical messengers or neurotransmitters in the brain. Scientists have found that, compared to healthy people, ALS patients have higher levels of glutamate in the serum and spinal fluid. Laboratory studies have demonstrated that neurons begin to die off when they are exposed over long periods to excessive amounts of glutamate. Now, scientists are trying to understand what mechanisms lead to a buildup of unneeded glutamate in the spinal fluid and how this imbalance could contribute to the development of ALS.

Autoimmune responses—which occur when the body's immune system attacks normal cells—have been suggested as one possible cause for motor neuron degeneration in ALS. Some scientists theorize that antibodies may directly or indirectly impair the function of motor neurons, interfering with the transmission of signals between the brain and muscles.

In searching for the cause of ALS, researchers have also studied environmental factors such as exposure to toxic or infectious agents. Other research has examined the possible role of dietary deficiency or trauma. However, as of yet, there is insufficient evidence to implicate these factors as causes of ALS. Future research may show that many factors, including a genetic predisposition, are involved in the development of ALS.

How Is ALS Treated?

No cure has yet been found for ALS. However, the Food and Drug Administration (FDA) has approved the first drug treatment for the disease—riluzole (Rilutek). Riluzole is believed to reduce damage to motor neurons by decreasing the release of glutamate. Clinical trials with ALS patients showed that riluzole prolongs survival by several months, mainly in those with difficulty swallowing. The drug also extends the time before a patient needs ventilation support. Riluzole does not reverse the damage already done to motor neurons, and patients taking the drug must be monitored for liver damage and other possible side effects. However, this first disease-specific therapy offers hope that the progression of ALS may one day be slowed by new medications or combinations of drugs.

Other treatments for ALS are designed to relieve symptoms and improve the quality of life for patients. This supportive care is best provided by multidisciplinary teams of health care professionals such as physicians; pharmacists; physical, occupational and speech therapists; nutritionists; social workers; and home care and hospice nurses. Working with patients and caregivers, these teams can design an individualized plan of medical and physical therapy and provide special equipment aimed at keeping patients as mobile and comfortable as possible.

Physicians can prescribe medications to help reduce fatigue, ease muscle cramps, control spasticity, and reduce excess saliva and phlegm. Drugs also are available to help patients with pain, depression, sleep disturbances, and constipation. Pharmacists can give advice on the proper use of medications and monitor a patient's prescriptions to avoid risks of drug interactions.

Physical therapy and special equipment can enhance patients' independence and safety throughout the course of ALS. Gentle, low-impact aerobic exercise such as walking, swimming, and stationary bicycling can strengthen unaffected muscles, improve cardiovascular health, and help patients fight fatigue and depression. Range of motion and stretching exercises can help prevent painful spasticity and shortening (contracture) of muscles. Physical therapists can recommend exercises that provide these benefits without overworking muscles. Occupational therapists can suggest devices such as ramps, braces, walkers, and wheelchairs that help patients conserve energy and remain mobile.

ALS patients who have difficulty speaking may benefit from working with a speech therapist. These health professionals can teach patients adaptive strategies such as techniques to help them speak louder and more clearly. As ALS progresses, speech therapists can help patients develop ways for responding to yes or no questions with their eyes or by other nonverbal means and can recommend aids such as speech synthesizers and computer-based communication systems. These methods and devices help patients communicate when they can no longer speak or produce vocal sounds.

Patients and caregivers can learn from speech therapists and nutritionists how to plan and prepare numerous small meals throughout the day that provide enough calories, fiber, and fluid along with how to avoid foods that are difficult to swallow. Patients may begin using suction devices to remove excess fluids or saliva and prevent choking. When patients can no longer get enough nourishment from eating, doctors may advise inserting a feeding tube into the stomach. The use of a feeding tube also reduces the risk of choking and pneumonia that can result from inhaling liquids into the lungs. The tube is not painful and does not prevent patients from eating food orally if they wish.

When the muscles that assist in breathing weaken, use of nocturnal ventilation assistance (intermittent positive pressure ventilation [IPPV] or bilevel positive airway pressure [BIPAP]) may be used to aid breathing during sleep. Such devices artificially inflate the patient's lungs from various external sources that are applied directly to the face or body. When muscles are no longer able to maintain oxygen and carbon dioxide levels, these devices may be used full-time.

Patients may eventually consider forms of mechanical ventilation (respirators) in which a machine inflates and deflates the lungs. To be effective, this may require a tube that passes from the nose or mouth to the windpipe (trachea) and for long-term use, an operation such as a tracheostomy, in which a plastic breathing tube is inserted directly in the patient's windpipe through an opening in the neck. Patients and their families should consider several factors when deciding whether and when to use one of these options. Ventilation devices differ in their effect on the patient's quality of life and in cost. Although ventilation support can ease problems with breathing and prolong survival, it does not affect the progression of ALS. Patients need to be fully informed about these considerations and the long-term effects of life without movement before they make decisions about ventilation support.

Social workers and home care and hospice nurses help patients, families, and caregivers with the medical, emotional, and financial challenges of coping with ALS, particularly during the final stages of the disease. Social workers provide support such as assistance in obtaining financial aid, arranging durable power of attorney, preparing a living will, and finding support groups for patients and caregivers. Home care nurses are available not only to provide medical care but also to teach caregivers about tasks such as maintaining respirators, giving tube feedings, and moving patients to avoid painful skin problems and contractures. Home hospice nurses work in consultation with physicians to ensure proper medication, pain control, and other care affecting the quality of life of patients who wish to remain at home. The home hospice team can also counsel patients and caregivers about end-of-life issues.

What Research Is Being Done?

The National Institute of Neurological Disorders and Stroke, part of the National Institutes of Health, is the Federal Government's leading supporter of biomedical research on ALS. The goals of this research are to find the cause or causes of ALS, understand the mechanisms involved in the progression of the disease, and develop effective treatment.

Scientists are seeking to understand the mechanisms that trigger selective motor neurons to degenerate in ALS and to find effective approaches to halt the processes leading to cell death. This work includes studies in animals to identify the means by which SOD1 mutations lead to the destruction of neurons. The excessive accumulation of free radicals, which has been implicated in a number of neurodegenerative diseases including ALS, is also being closely studied. In addition, researchers are examining how the loss of neurotrophic factors may be involved in ALS. Neurotrophic factors are chemicals found in the brain and spinal cord that play a vital role in the development, specification, maintenance, and protection of neurons. Studying how these factors may be lost and how such a loss may contribute to motor neuron degeneration may lead to a greater understanding of ALS and the development of neuroprotective strategies. By exploring these and other possible factors, researchers hope to find the cause or causes of motor neuron degeneration in ALS and develop therapies to slow the progression of the disease.

Researchers are also conducting investigations to increase their understanding of the role of programmed cell death or apoptosis in ALS. In normal physiological processes, apoptosis acts as a means to rid the body of cells that are no longer needed by prompting the cells to commit "cell suicide." The critical balance between necessary cell death and the maintenance of essential cells is thought to be controlled by trophic factors. In addition to ALS, apoptosis is pervasive in other chronic neurodegenerative conditions such as Parkinson's disease and Alzheimer's disease and is thought to be a major cause of the secondary brain damage seen after stroke and trauma. Discovering what triggers apoptosis may eventually lead to therapeutic interventions for ALS and other neurological diseases.

Scientists have not yet identified a reliable biological marker for ALS—a biochemical abnormality shared by all patients with the disease. Once such a biomarker is discovered and tests are developed to detect the marker in patients, allowing early detection and diagnosis of ALS, physicians will have a valuable tool to help them follow the effects of new therapies and monitor disease progression.

NINDS-supported researchers are studying families with ALS who lack the SOD1 mutation to locate additional genes that cause the disease. Identification of additional ALS genes will allow genetic testing useful for diagnostic confirmation of ALS and prenatal screening for the disease. This work with familial ALS could lead to a greater understanding of sporadic ALS as well. Because familial ALS is virtually indistinguishable from sporadic ALS clinically, some researchers believe that familial ALS genes may also be involved in the manifestations of the more common sporadic form of ALS. Scientists also hope to identify genetic risk factors that predispose people to sporadic ALS.

Potential therapies for ALS are being investigated in animal models. Some of this work involves experimental treatments with normal SOD1 and other antioxidants. In addition, neurotrophic factors are being studied for their potential to protect motor neurons from pathological degeneration. Investigators are optimistic that these and other basic research studies will eventually lead to treatments for ALS.

Additional Information

ALS Association of America (ALSA)
27001 Agoura Road, Suite 150
Calabasas Hills, CA 91301-5104
Toll-Free: 800-782-4747
Tel: 818-880-9007
Website: www.alsa.org

Center for Neurologic Study
9850 Genesee Avenue, Suite 320
LaJolla, CA 92037
Tel: 858-455-5463
Fax: 858-455-1713
Website: www.cnsonline.org
E-mail: cns@cts.com

Forbes Norris ALS Research Center
California Pacific Medical Center
2324 Sacramento Street
San Francisco, CA 94115
Tel: 415-923-3604
Fax: 415-673-5184
Website: www.cpmc.org/services/als

Les Turner ALS Foundation
8142 North Lawndale Avenue
Skokie, IL 60076-3322
Toll-Free: 888-ALS-1107
Tel: 847-679-3311
Fax: 847-679-9109
Website: www.lesturnerals.org
E-mail: info@lesturnerals.org

The Muscular Dystrophy Association
3300 East Sunrise Drive
Tucson, AZ 85718-3208
Toll-Free: 800-572-1717
Tel: 520-529-2000
Website: www.mdausa.org
E-mail: mda@mdausa.org

Project ALS
511 Avenue of the Americas, Suite 341
New York, NY 10011
Toll-Free: 800-603-0270
Tel: 212-969-0329
Fax: 212-337-9915
Website: www.projectals.org
E-mail: projectals@aol.com

Chapter 27

Charcot-Marie-Tooth Disease

Charcot-Marie-Tooth (CMT) disease is a common neuromuscular disorder named for the three physicians—Jean Martin Charcot, Pierre Marie, and Howard Henry Tooth—who first identified it more than 100 years ago.

In 1886, Charcot and Marie, in France, and Tooth, in England, reported almost simultaneously on a disease of the peripheral nerves. These nerves have cell bodies in the brain and spinal cord and fibers that run from the brain and spinal cord to the whole body, sending signals that control voluntary muscles. They also have receptors in the periphery of the body that send sensory signals, such as those for pain, pressure, temperature, and position, back to the brain and spinal cord along different fibers. Therefore, CMT largely affects muscular and sensory function in the limbs. The disorder is one of the 40 diseases in the Muscular Dystrophy Association's program.

MDA is committed to helping people with CMT through research aimed at finding causes and treatments for the disease, and through medical services provided at 230 MDA clinics across the United States.

MDA-funded scientists have made significant progress in the 1990s. They've identified three different genes that, when abnormal, can each cause CMT. Each of these genes affects the insulating sheath that surrounds nerves. These findings have led to better diagnostic tests and may also eventually lead to specific treatments, because understanding the genetic causes of CMT and their effects on the nervous system gives doctors important clues about how resulting problems might be corrected.

Questions and Answers

What Is CMT?

CMT is actually a broad term used to describe a group of genetic disorders that affects the peripheral nerves, which carry motor (relating to movement) and sensory (relating to sensation) signals between the brain and spinal cord and the rest of the body.

CMT most frequently affects the lower legs, feet, and hands, resulting in weakness and atrophy, or loss of muscle bulk, as well as causing a mild degree of loss of sensation. However, the motor problems are much more significant than the sensory problems, which are usually minor.

About one in 2,500 people has a form of CMT. Overall, it affects about 100,000 to 125,000 people in the United States alone, making it one of the most common hereditary disorders.

Are There Other Names for CMT?

Yes. CMT disorders are sometimes referred to as hereditary motor and sensory neuropathies (HMSNs). An old name for CMT is peroneal muscular atrophy. The peroneal muscles are in the lower leg and may atrophy in this disorder.

Is There More Than One Variety of the Disease?

CMT is usually divided into types 1 and 2, according to the specific site of the peripheral nerve problem. About two-thirds of people with CMT have type 1, which affects the myelin sheath, the insulating covering that surrounds nerve fibers. Approximately one-third of patients have type 2, which affects the nerve fibers (also called axons) themselves. The peripheral nerves are made of bundles of these fibers.

Some physicians use the term type 3 CMT to describe a disease that is also known as Dejerine-Sottas disease. This is a severe form of CMT.

Nerve fibers are often compared to electrical wires and myelin to insulation, and the comparison holds up fairly well. However, whereas electrical impulses can travel along an uninsulated wire, nerve impulses travel very poorly along an uninsulated fiber.

Doctors can check the function of the myelin sheath by measuring the speed with which nerve impulses travel from one point to another along a nerve. In type 1 CMT, the nerve impulses travel more slowly than is normal. In type 2 CMT, the speed of nerve impulses is normal, but the size or amount of the impulses is smaller than normal, indicating a problem with the axons (nerve fibers).

CMT can be further classified by the location of the genetic defect that underlies the disorder. For example, type 1 CMT, caused by a defect on chromosome 17, is called CMT1A, and type 1 CMT, caused by a defect on chromosome 1, is CMT1B.

When Do Signs of the Disease First Become Apparent?

Due to the slow progression of this disease, its onset is often difficult to determine. Type 1 (the myelin-related type) is usually noticed during late childhood or adolescence. Type 2 (the axonal type) is often diagnosed a little later than type 1.

What Are the Early Symptoms of CMT?

The first symptoms of CMT are usually foot abnormalities, such as a high arch or flexed toes. It can be difficult to hold up the foot, which may result in tripping on curbs, having to take a higher than normal step (picking up the foot by bending the knee), and walking with deliberation.

How Disabling Is CMT?

CMT varies highly in severity, even among members of the same family. Some people are so mildly affected they don't notice any symptoms. For those with symptoms, foot abnormalities and walking difficulties pose the most serious problems.

Although exceptions exist, most people with CMT have trouble participating in sports. Sprained ankles and fractures of the ankles and lower legs are common. The leg and foot problems are rarely disabling enough to require a wheelchair, and many people with CMT pursue active, vigorous lives.

If the muscles of the hands are affected, aids may be required for such daily activities as writing, fastening buttons, and turning door knobs and screw caps.

CMT doesn't affect most physical functions, including the cardiovascular system, and has no effect on intellect. Life expectancy isn't shortened by CMT.

How Is CMT Diagnosed?

A diagnosis is reached after an experienced doctor performs a thorough physical examination, notes a CMT-like pattern of foot, leg, and hand weakness, and obtains a family history. The doctor will often then order tests to confirm the suspected diagnosis of CMT.

An important test is one known as nerve conduction velocity, or NCV, which measures the speed at which nerve impulses travel along the nerves. Nerve impulses are slowed in type 1 CMT and may show other abnormalities in type 2 CMT.

Another useful test is an electromyogram, or EMG, which records the electrical activity of muscle cells. Damage to nerves causes the muscles that would normally receive signals from those nerves to show a characteristic pattern of electrical activity.

These tests may be somewhat uncomfortable, but they're extremely valuable, because they allow nerve function to be directly examined. They serve a function similar to that served by electrocardiograms in diagnosing heart problems. Other testing is sometimes done to exclude the possibility of disorders with signs and symptoms similar to those of CMT.

Genetic testing is available for at least one form of CMT (the type caused by a defect on chromosome 17), but new developments in CMT genetic testing are expected. See your physician or genetic counselor for up-to-date information about genetic testing.

What Causes CMT?

CMT is caused by defects in genes that affect the function of the peripheral nerves. Genes are the instructions, or blueprints, for proteins in the body. When a gene is abnormal, the protein is likewise abnormal, or altered. The genes that, when altered, cause CMT, affect either the nerve fiber itself or the myelin sheath that surrounds it.

MDA-supported researchers have so far identified three genes that, when abnormal, result in type 1 CMT. The genes are on chromosomes 1, 17, and the X chromosome. All of them affect myelin, and the X chromosome type may affect the nerve fiber itself as well.

The most common form of CMT is the kind that involves a gene on chromosome 17 known as PMP22, or peripheral myelin protein 22. The problem is usually a duplication of a small section of chromosome 17 that includes the PMP22 gene. Patients with this type of CMT actually have a total of three copies of the PMP22 gene in each cell, instead of the usual two copies. Having this extra copy leads to the CMT symptoms. In a few cases, a different kind of problem—one that alters the PMP22 gene itself instead of duplicating it—has been found.

Other patients with type 1 CMT have a defect in a gene on chromosome 1 known as the myelin protein zero (P0) gene. Both the chromosome 17 type and the chromosome 1 type are inherited in an autosomal dominant pattern, which means that a child only needs to inherit an abnormal gene from one parent to show symptoms of the disease. Still other patients with type 1 CMT have a defect in a gene located on the X chromosome known as connexin 32 (Cx32).

Females have two X chromosomes and males have an X and a Y chromosome. Because of this difference, females are usually not as severely affected by genetic abnormalities on the X chromosome as are males and often escape symptoms of an X chromosome disease entirely. This is because they have a normal gene on the other X chromosome to serve as a backup. Males, with their single X chromosome, have no such backup and usually show more severe symptoms.

In Cx32-related CMT, girls and women show the disease to varying degrees. This has prompted researchers to call Cx32-related CMT an X-linked dominant condition. In X-linked dominant conditions, males and females need only one abnormal X chromosome gene to show the disease.

Type 2 (axonal) CMT is usually inherited in an autosomal dominant pattern. The genes for type 2 CMT haven't been specifically identified, but two of them have been mapped to small regions of chromosomes 1 and 3. In at least some patients with X-linked CMT, there are features that resemble type 2 CMT.

Note: Although autosomal and X-linked dominant diseases can be inherited when an affected parent passes the gene to his or her child, they aren't necessarily inherited—at least not in this strict sense. Genes are carried from parent to child via sperm and egg cells, and sometimes genetic defects occur only in these cells, not in the rest of the parent's cells. In these cases, parents won't show any disease symptoms and genetic testing of parents won't reveal any defects.

Is Charcot-Marie-Tooth Disease Contagious?

No. Genetic diseases are not contagious.

Is There Any Cure or Treatment for the Disease?

There is no cure for CMT, although MDA-supported research is aimed at understanding exactly how the gene defects lead to the disease, with the ultimate goal of compensating for these defects. For now, treatment may involve physical therapy, lightweight lower leg braces or shoe inserts, and sometimes surgery to correct foot deformities.

Dejerine-Sottas Disease

Dejerine-Sottas disease is closely related to CMT and is, in fact, sometimes referred to as type 3 CMT. However, many clinicians still refer to it by the names of the French doctors who first described it in the late 19th century, Joseph Jules Dejerine and Jules Sottas.

Characteristics of Dejerine-Sottas disease include:

- slow development of early motor skills, including walking, which is sometimes not achieved until the third or fourth year;

- possible loss of the ability to walk during the adult years;

- hearing loss in some cases;

- severe sensory problems;

- an autosomal dominant inheritance pattern when inheritance can be traced.

Dejerine-Sottas disease can be caused by abnormalities in the same genes that can cause two forms of type 1 CMT—the PMP22 gene on chromosome 17 and the P gene on chromosome 1. However, the defects in these genes are not the same defects that cause the type 1 CMT disorders. Researchers are studying mice and rats with defects that cause a Dejerine-Sottas-like condition.

As with CMT, there are likely to be other genes that, when abnormal, can cause this disorder. Dejerine-Sottas disease often occurs without a family history.

Inheritance Patterns

In autosomal dominant disorders, a child need inherit only one abnormal gene to have the disease. The chance of a child inheriting this one abnormal gene is 50 percent with each conception.

X-linked diseases are caused by defects in genes on the X chromosome. Females have two Xs, and males have only one, paired with a Y chromosome.

In X-linked dominant diseases, an abnormal X chromosome gene from either parent can cause the disease. The chances of a child getting the disease is 50 percent if the mother has the defect on one of her Xs. If it's the father who has the defect, only girl children will inherit it, because boys get a Y chromosome from the father, not an X. All female children will inherit the defect, since they all get their father's sole X chromosome.

Chapter 28

Corticobasal Ganglionic Degeneration (CBD)

Corticobasal ganglionic degeneration (which we will call CBD) is a rare progressive neurological disorder characterized by a combination of Parkinsonism and cortical dysfunction. It is a rare sporadic progressive disorder first reported in 1968. CBD appears to be closely related to another, less rare, sporadic extrapyramidal degenerative disorder named Progressive Supranuclear Palsy (PSP). In CBD, cognitive symptoms dominate, while in PSP, eye movement symptoms dominate the picture.

The Parkinsonism is generally an asymmetric akinetic rigid syndrome, unresponsive to levodopa, similar to that of multiple system atrophy and PSP. Eye movement abnormalities are common, as in PSP, and a supranuclear gaze palsy can be seen as in PSP. Given the genetic similarities between CBD and PSP, it seems possible that they are simply two "faces" of the same disease.

Neuroradiological imaging studies in CBD demonstrate cortical atrophy, which may be symmetrical or asymmetrical. Other cortical signs include

- Alien limb phenomenon
- Apraxia
- Dysphasia
- Cortical sensory loss
- Pyramidal signs

The information in this chapter is from "Corticobasal ganglionic degeneration (CBD)," by Timothy C. Hain, MD. Dr. Hain is a Professor of Neurology at Northwestern University in Chicago, IL © 2001. Reprinted with permission.

Proposed diagnostic criteria include at least three of the following:

- bradykinesia and rigidity that does not respond to levodopa
- alien limb phenomena
- cortical sensory signs
- focal limb dystonia
- action tremor
- myoclonus

The alien limb symptom is highly specific but it is not necessary for the diagnosis. Arm levitation resembling alien limb phenomena has been reported in PSP (Barclay et al, 1999), which certainly can also show focal limb dystonia and bradykinesia. Other aspects of this picture could easily be mistaken for other neurodegenerative disease such as Alzheimer's or Picks disease, and in fact, even experienced clinicians are correct 50% of the time or less when judged by pathological criteria. Onset in the sixth or seventh decade is typical. Disease progression is quicker than in Parkinsonism but similar to that of PSP. Recently language disturbance has been documented to be frequent (Frattali et al, 2000).

Pathology

There is neuronal loss and gliosis and swollen achromatic neurons (ballooned neurons) are found in all cortical layers, but especially so in superior frontal and parietal gyri. There is extensive loss of myelinated axons in the white matter. Scattered neuronal inclusions may be seen similar to Pick bodies. Ballooned neurons are strongly reactive for phosphorylated neurofilaments and may include the tau protein. (Dickson et al, 1986). Neuronal loss and gliosis are also observed in the nuclei of the basal ganglia. Lewy bodies and neurofibrillary tangles are absent. The substantia nigra shows neuronal loss with extraneuronal melanin, gliosis and neurofibrillary inclusions, called corticobasal bodies.

Differential Diagnosis

CBD is difficult to diagnose in early stages, and experienced examiners typically diagnose it correctly less than 50% of the time (Litvan et al, 1997). CBD and may also be impossible to differentiate from PSP or a striatonigral type of MSA. As more cortical signs develop in later stages, the disorders below may be possible to separate. As diagnostic sensitivity is poor, neuropathological confirmation remains the gold standard. Even here, one wonders if this disorder can be defined.

- Parkinsonism
- PSP (progressive supranuclear palsy, related by tau)
- MSA (multiple system atrophy)
- Picks disease

While CBD patients have normal saccadic velocity, this may be an artifact of case definition. If PSP and CBD share the same pathologic mechanism, they may simply be two different presentations of the same disease.

The cause of CBD is presently unknown but because the tau protein accumulates in this disorder, it may be related to a mutation in the tau gene. (Higgins et al, 1999). Tau is a microtubule-binding protein that is normally abundant in neurons. Other tauopathies include Alzheimer's disease, Picks disease, frontotemporal dementia and parkinsonism, ALS-Parkinson dementia complex of Guam, and progressive supranuclear palsy (PSP) (Higgins et al, 1999). According to Di Maria et al (2000) and Houlden et al (2001), CBD shares the same tau haplotype as do PSP patients, suggesting that both CBD and PSP share the same genetic background, and possibly the same pathologic mechanism.

Conventional Treatment

CBD patients do not respond to levodopa treatment (the standard treatment for Parkinsonism). Management is based on appropriate use of appliances, prevention of medical complications, and appropriate use of nursing. Patients with CBD and caregivers should establish early on the plan regarding invasive care—intubation, feeding tubes, as these issues are almost certain to come up in the course of the disease.

References

Barclay CL, Bergeron C, Lang AE. Arm levitation in progressive supranuclear palsy. *Neurology* 1999:52:879-882.

Di Maria et al. Corticobasal degeneration shares a common genetic background with progressive supranuclear palsy. *Ann Neurol* 2000:47:374-377.

Dickson DW and others. Ballooned neurons in select neurodegenerative disease contain phosphorylated neurofilament epitopes. *Acta Neuropathol* 71:216-223, 1986).

Frattali CM and others. Language disturbances in corticobasal degeneration. *Neurology* 2000:54:990-992.

Higgins JJ, Litvan I, Nee LE, Loveless BS. A lack of the R406W tau mutation in progressive supranuclear palsy and corticobasal degeneration. *Neurology* 1999:52:404-406.

Houlden H and others. Corticobasal degeneration and progressive supranuclear palsy share a common tau haplotype. *Neurology* 2001: 56:1702-6.

Koller WC, Montgomery EB. Issues in the early diagnosis of Parkinson's disease. *Neurology* 1997:49 (Suppl 1), S10-25.

Litvan I, and others. Accuracy of the clinical diagnosis of corticobasal degeneration: a clinicopathologic study. *Neurology* 1997:48:119-125.

Riley DE, Lange AE, Lewis A, et al. Cortico-basal ganglionic degeneration. *Neurology* 1990;40:1203-1212.

Chapter 29

Friedreich's Ataxia

Questions and Answers

What Is Friedreich's Ataxia?

Friedreich's ataxia is an inherited (genetic), progressive disorder of the nervous system that affects balance, coordination, movement, and sensation. Ataxia means a loss of coordination and is usually the earliest and most prominent characteristic of the disease. Increasing impairment of balance and movement eventually lead to the loss of the ability to walk. Speech and swallowing difficulties may occur as well. FRDA also causes cardiac disease in most people who have it. Friedreich's is the most common inherited type of ataxia.

Who Gets Friedreich's Ataxia?

FRDA affects approximately two out of every 100,000 people, or about 5,000 people in the United States. Males and females are equally affected. FRDA is slightly more common among French Canadians. The first symptoms of FRDA usually occur before age 20, but occasionally, onset can be as late as the 50s.

FRDA is an inherited disease and, therefore, can't be spread from person to person like an infectious disease.

How Is Friedreich's Ataxia Inherited?

FRDA is due to defects in a gene on chromosome 9 that carries the recipe, or code, for a cellular protein known as frataxin. The defects keep the affected cells from making a normal amount of frataxin.

Every person has two copies of the frataxin gene, one inherited from each parent. A person with one defective gene copy will not develop

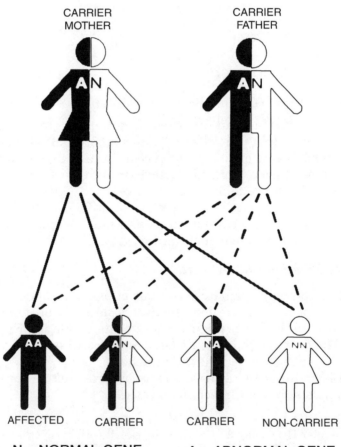

RECESIVE INHERITANCE

Figure 29.1. Inheritance Diagram

FRDA but is instead a carrier of the disease gene, who can then pass it on to his or her children. A person who inherits two defective frataxin genes will develop FRDA. The disorder is said to be recessive because it shows this pattern of inheritance. In a recessive disease, it's necessary for both parents to be carriers in order to have a child who has the disease.

When both parents are FRDA carriers, they have a one-in-four chance in each pregnancy of conceiving a child who will develop the disease, as shown in the inheritance diagram. The chances for each successive pregnancy aren't affected by the results of earlier ones. Boys and girls have equal chances of inheriting FRDA.

How Do Genetic Defects Cause Friedreich's Ataxia?

Recent research has revealed that the probable role of the frataxin protein in cells is to regulate the amount of iron located in the cells' mitochondria, tiny energy-producing units found inside the cells (see Figure 29.2).

Without frataxin, iron builds up in the mitochondria and damages them. The resulting cellular energy shortage can kill the cell.

In FRDA, some of the cells in the nervous system degenerate over time. The cells most affected are those that transmit sensory and

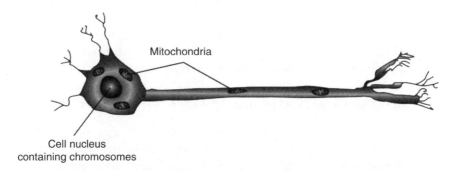

Figure 29.2. *Motor Nerve Cell. Motor nerve cells control muscle movement throughout the body via their long fibers, which transmit signals between the brain and spinal cord and the muscles. These fibers degenerate in Friedreich's ataxia, perhaps because their mitochondria can't regulate iron properly.*

Cells in the body's sensory system (sensory nerve cells) also have fibers, and these too are lost in Friedreich's ataxia.

movement signals via long fibers. The fibers run between the central nervous system (the brain and spinal cord) and the rest of the body.

Cells in the heart and pancreas are also affected in this disorder. Some of these cells probably die because of the direct effects of the loss of frataxin; others may die because of secondary effects. Current MDA-supported research is working on sorting this out, with an eye to treatment possibilities.

What Is Wrong with the Frataxin Gene in a Person with Friedreich's Ataxia?

The most common flaw (mutation) in the frataxin gene that leads to FRDA is known as a triplet repeat. In this type of mutation, a section of DNA is repeated over and over again, from as many as 100 to more than 1,000 times. The presence of this extra bit of genetic material interferes with the normal production of frataxin protein. Research has shown that the number of repeat units varies among people with FRDA, and even among tissues in the same person.

A second type of gene flaw, called a point mutation, is much less common. In this type of mutation, a very small amount of DNA is altered. FRDA occurs when a person inherits two triplet repeats or a point mutation and a triplet repeat. Theoretically, two point mutations could also lead to the disorder, but this combination hasn't been seen in people with the disease.

Recent research indicates that people with smaller numbers of repeats generally have later disease onset, slower progression and less severe heart problems. However, there is too much variability in the course of the disease among people with similar numbers of repeats to allow predictions about disease severity from this factor alone.

What Are the First Symptoms of Friedreich's Ataxia?

The most common early symptoms involve trouble with balance and coordination. A person with FRDA may have difficulty walking and running, may appear clumsy and may have difficulty negotiating doorways or corners. Lack of control may also affect the arms and hands early on and interfere with hand-eye coordination. Skin sensations may be decreased as well.

Most people with FRDA develop speech difficulties, called dysarthria, early in their disease. A person with FRDA may have trouble coordinating precise movements of the lips and tongue, leading to speech that is slower or more difficult to understand. FRDA doesn't affect the thinking and feeling portions of the brain, and speech difficulties don't indicate any loss of mental abilities.

Cardiac (heart) disease and scoliosis (curvature of the spine) may occur early and generally worsen over time.

How Is Friedreich's Ataxia Diagnosed?

Diagnosis of FRDA begins with a careful medical history and physical exam. A neurological exam is performed, in which balance, sensation, reflexes, and strength are tested. People with FRDA usually have decreased reflexes in their lower limbs and, sometimes, in their upper limbs. Strength is usually normal early on. The ability to sense light touch or vibration may be decreased.

Two electrical tests are often used as part of the diagnostic process. In a nerve conduction velocity test, small needles are inserted below the skin to determine the strength and speed of electrical impulses traveling along the nerves (bundles of nerve fibers). In FRDA, the strength of these signals is abnormal.

An electromyogram (EMG) uses a similar procedure to test the electrical responses of muscle at rest and during contraction. Characteristic EMG changes are seen in FRDA.

Since the discovery of the frataxin gene, genetic testing has become the most accurate way to diagnose FRDA. The genetic test examines DNA from a blood sample to look for the triplet repeats or point mutations associated with FRDA.

Is There a Cure for Friedreich's Ataxia?

At this point, there's no cure and no way known to slow the progression of the disease. MDA is currently funding a wide range of investigations to more fully understand the role of frataxin and its effects in cells. It's likely that this research will lead to the development of treatments that can partially make up for the loss of frataxin, and in this way slow down or even halt the degenerative process.

How Is a Person Affected by Friedreich's Ataxia as the Disease Progresses?

FRDA progresses at different rates in different people. This makes predicting the course of the disease in any particular person especially difficult. Even siblings with FRDA may progress at very different rates. For this reason, remember that the information presented here on the usual course of the disease only represents the average. Some people will have a very mild disease course, while others may be more severely affected.

Through your MDA clinic, FRDA can be treated by a coordinated team approach, in which all of the medical and social professionals work together to develop a treatment plan.

Loss of balance and coordination will usually require a person with FRDA to use mobility aids such as braces, a cane, or a walker within a decade of the diagnosis. A wheelchair is often needed for mobility several years afterward. Progressive weakness of the lower limbs can compound the problems caused by loss of coordination.

Some people with FRDA develop extremely high arches (pes cavus) and other foot deformities as a result of uneven muscle weakening. Without regular stretching, the involved muscles may become permanently shortened (a condition called contracture), which can be painful. Muscle stiffness, spasms, and cramps may also cause pain.

These problems are addressed by a physiatrist or physical therapist, who can offer advice on choosing the right mobility aids and develop a physical therapy program to minimize contractures and maintain strength. Regular stretching and exercise are usually an important part of the program. Surgical correction of foot deformities and contractures is possible. Painful muscle tightening can usually be controlled with medication.

Loss of coordination in the upper limbs occurs later in the disease and is more variable in its severity. It may interfere with activities of daily living, such as writing, eating, and dressing. Some people with FRDA experience loss of muscle bulk (wasting), especially in the small muscles of the hands. Arm weakness is usually not a significant problem until late in the disease. An occupational therapist helps determine the appropriate devices and strategies to make the most of remaining abilities and to improve function in the activities of daily living.

Curvature of the spine (scoliosis) occurs in some people with FRDA. Scoliosis can impair the ability to breathe fully, can be painful, and may affect self-image. Mild scoliosis is sometimes treated with a brace fitted around the chest and abdomen. More severe scoliosis can be corrected by surgery.

What about Speech and Swallowing Problems?

Dysarthria affects almost all people with FRDA either early or later on in the disease. Some of the same nerve pathways involved in speech production also control swallowing, and swallowing difficulties (dysphagia) are common later in FRDA. Dysphagia can cause food to enter the airways, increasing the possibility of pneumonia. It can also make it more difficult to obtain adequate nutrition and can lead to choking on food.

A speech-language pathologist or speech therapist can help the person with FRDA learn compensatory techniques for both speech and swallowing. A dietitian or nutritionist advises on meals and preparation techniques that make food easier to swallow and increase nutritional content. Family members should be trained in performing the Heimlich maneuver (a technique for dislodging food from the airways) before dysphagia becomes a problem.

How Does Friedreich's Ataxia Affect the Heart?

Heart disease is one of the most significant complications of FRDA. Ninety percent of people with FRDA develop cardiac disease, either cardiomyopathy (heart muscle disease) or arrhythmia (affecting the electrical pacing system that controls the heart rate and rhythm). These problems may be life-threatening if untreated. For this reason, a cardiologist familiar with FRDA is a critical part of the care team.

The most common type of heart problem is left ventricular hypertrophy, in which the muscular wall of the left ventricle (the main pumping chamber of the heart) becomes thickened. Types of arrhythmias include a slowing of the heart rate (bradycardia) and rapid heart rate (tachycardia). Symptoms of cardiac disease may include shortness of breath, dizziness, fainting, and chest pain. The good news is that effective treatments are available. Treatment depends on the type of problem and may include drug therapy or implantation of a pacemaker.

Are There Other Physical Problems with FRDA?

About 10 percent of people with FRDA develop diabetes mellitus—an inability to control the level of sugar in the blood. Diabetes can usually be successfully controlled through diet and monitoring of blood sugar levels, with insulin administration if needed. Diabetes may cause pain or abnormal sensation in the extremities. Medications are available to help control these symptoms.

Partial deafness and loss of visual acuity occur in a small proportion of people with FRDA. Hearing aids can be used if hearing loss isn't too severe.

FRDA doesn't affect the parts of the brain responsible for thinking and feeling. Reasoning, memory, and emotion are all normal in people with FRDA.

How Does Friedreich's Ataxia Affect Life Span?

As with other aspects of the disease, the effect of FRDA on life span varies from person to person. On average, people with FRDA live for three to four decades after their diagnosis. People with milder disease and later age of onset often live even longer. Heart disease has the most significant impact on life span. In the last two decades, the recognition and treatment of cardiac disease in FRDA has allowed many people to live longer than in the past.

Additional Information

Friedreich's Ataxia Research Alliance (FARA)
2001 Jefferson Davis Hwy.
Suite 209
Arlington, VA 22202
Tel: 703-413-4468
Fax: 703-413-4467
Website: www.frda.org
E-mail: fara@frda.org

Genetic Alliance
4301 Connecticut Avenue, N.W.
Suite 404
Washington, DC 20008-2304
Toll-Free: 800-336-GENE (4363)
Tel: 202-966-5557
Fax: 202-966-8553
Website: www.geneticalliance.org
E-mail: info@geneticalliance.org

Muscular Dystrophy Association
3300 East Sunrise Drive
Tucson, AZ 85718-3208
Toll-Free: 800-572-1717
Tel: 520-529-2000
Fax: 520-529-5300
Website: www.mdausa.org
E-mail: mda@mdausa.org

National Ataxia Foundation (NAF)
2600 Fernbrook Lane
Suite 119
Minneapolis, MN 55447-4752
Tel: 763-553-0020
Fax: 763-553-0167
Website: www.ataxia.org
E-mail: naf@ataxia.org

National Organization for Rare Disorders (NORD)
P.O. Box 1968
Danbury, CT 06813-1968
Toll-Free: 800-999-NORD (6673)
Tel: 203-746-6518
Fax: 203-746-6481
Website: www.rarediseases.org
E-mail: orphan@rarediseases.org

Chapter 30

Huntington's Disease

In 1872, the American physician George Huntington wrote about an illness that he called "an heirloom from generations away back in the dim past." He was not the first to describe the disorder, which has been traced back to the Middle Ages at least. One of its earliest names was chorea, which, as in choreography, is the Greek word for dance. The term chorea describes how people affected with the disorder writhe, twist, and turn in a constant, uncontrollable dance-like motion. Later, other descriptive names evolved. *Hereditary chorea* emphasizes how the disease is passed from parent to child. *Chronic progressive chorea* stresses how symptoms of the disease worsen over time. Today, physicians commonly use the simple term Huntington's disease (HD) to describe this highly complex disorder that causes untold suffering for thousands of families.

In the United States alone, about 30,000 people have HD; estimates of its prevalence are about 1 in every 10,000 persons. At least 150,000 others have a 50 percent risk of developing the disease and thousands more of their relatives live with the possibility that they, too, might develop HD.

Until recently, scientists understood very little about HD and could only watch as the disease continued to pass from generation to generation. Families saw the disease destroy their loved ones' ability to feel, think, and move. In the last several years, scientists working with support from the National Institute of Neurological Disorders and

"Huntington's Disease—Hope Through Research," National Institute of Neurological Disorders and Stroke (NINDS), reviewed July 1, 2001.

327

Stroke (NINDS) have made several breakthroughs in the area of HD research. With these advances, our understanding of the disease continues to improve.

This chapter presents information about HD, and about current research progress, to health professionals, scientists, caregivers, and, most important, to those already too familiar with the disorder—the many families who are affected by HD.

What Causes Huntington's Disease?

HD results from genetically programmed degeneration of nerve cells, called neurons, in certain areas of the brain. This degeneration causes uncontrolled movements, loss of intellectual faculties, and emotional disturbance. Specifically affected are cells of the basal ganglia, structures deep within the brain that have many important functions, including coordinating movement. Within the basal ganglia, HD especially targets neurons of the striatum, particularly those in the caudate nuclei and the pallidum. Also affected is the brain's outer surface, or cortex, which controls thought, perception, and memory.

How Is HD Inherited?

HD is found in every country of the world. It is a familial disease, passed from parent to child through a mutation or misspelling in the normal gene.

A single abnormal gene, the basic biological unit of heredity, produces HD. Genes are composed of deoxyribonucleic acid (DNA), a molecule shaped like a spiral ladder. Each rung of this ladder is composed of two paired chemicals called bases. There are four types of bases—adenine, thymine, cytosine, and guanine—each abbreviated by the first letter of its name: A, T, C, and G. Certain bases always pair together, and different combinations of base pairs join to form coded messages. A gene is a long string of this DNA in various combinations of A, T, C, and G. These unique combinations determine the gene's function, much like letters join together to form words. Each person has about 30,000 genes—a billion base pairs of DNA or bits of information repeated in the nuclei of human cells—which determine individual characteristics or traits.

Genes are arranged in precise locations along 23 rod-like pairs of chromosomes. One chromosome from each pair comes from an individual's mother, the other from the father. Each half of a chromosome pair is similar to the other, except for one pair, which determines the sex of the individual. This pair has two X chromosomes in females and one X and one Y chromosome in males. The gene that produces HD lies on chromosome 4, one of the 22 non-sex-linked, or autosomal, pairs of chromosomes, placing men and women at equal risk of acquiring the disease.

The impact of a gene depends partly on whether it is dominant or recessive. If a gene is dominant, then only one of the paired chromosomes is required to produce its called-for effect. If the gene is recessive, both parents must provide chromosomal copies for the trait to be present. HD is called an autosomal dominant disorder because only one copy of the defective gene, inherited from one parent, is necessary to produce the disease.

The genetic defect responsible for HD is a small sequence of DNA on chromosome 4 in which several base pairs are repeated many, many times. The normal gene has three DNA bases, composed of the sequence CAG. In people with HD, the sequence abnormally repeats itself dozens of times. Over time—and with each successive generation—the number of CAG repeats may expand further.

Each parent has two copies of every chromosome but gives only one copy to each child. Each child of an HD parent has a 50-50 chance of inheriting the HD gene. If a child does not inherit the HD gene, he or she will not develop the disease and cannot pass it to subsequent generations. A person who inherits the HD gene, and survives long enough, will sooner or later develop the disease. In some families, all the children may inherit the HD gene; in others, none do. Whether one child inherits the gene has no bearing on whether others will or will not share the same fate.

A small number of cases of HD are sporadic, that is, they occur even though there is no family history of the disorder. These cases are thought to be caused by a new genetic mutation—an alteration in the gene that occurs during sperm development and that brings the number of CAG repeats into the range that causes disease.

What Are the Major Effects of the Disease?

Early signs of the disease vary greatly from person to person. A common observation is that the earlier the symptoms appear, the faster the disease progresses.

Family members may first notice that the individual experiences mood swings or becomes uncharacteristically irritable, apathetic, passive, depressed, or angry. These symptoms may lessen as the disease progresses or, in some individuals, may continue and include hostile outbursts or deep bouts of depression.

HD may affect the individual's judgment, memory, and other cognitive functions. Early signs might include having trouble driving, learning new things, remembering a fact, answering a question, or making a decision. Some may even display changes in handwriting. As the disease progresses, concentration on intellectual tasks becomes increasingly difficult.

In some individuals, the disease may begin with uncontrolled movements in the fingers, feet, face, or trunk. These movements—which are signs of chorea—often intensify when the person is anxious. HD can also begin with mild clumsiness or problems with balance. Some people develop choreic movements later, after the disease has progressed. They may stumble or appear uncoordinated. Chorea often creates serious problems with walking, increasing the likelihood of falls.

The disease can reach the point where speech is slurred and vital functions, such as swallowing, eating, speaking, and especially walking, continue to decline. Some individuals cannot recognize other family members. Many, however, remain aware of their environment and are able to express emotions.

Some physicians have employed a recently developed Unified HD Rating Scale, or UHDRS, to assess the clinical features, stages, and course of HD. In general, the duration of the illness ranges from 10 to 30 years. The most common causes of death are infection (most often pneumonia), injuries related to a fall, or other complications.

At What Age Does HD Appear?

The rate of disease progression and the age at onset vary from person to person. Adult-onset HD, with its disabling, uncontrolled movements, most often begins in middle age. There are, however, other variations of HD distinguished not just by age at onset but by a distinct array of symptoms. For example, some persons develop the disease as adults, but without chorea. They may appear rigid and move very little, or not at all, a condition called akinesia.

Some individuals develop symptoms of HD when they are very young—before age 20. The terms early-onset or juvenile HD are often used to describe HD that appears in a young person. A common sign of HD in a younger individual is a rapid decline in school performance. Symptoms can also include subtle changes in handwriting and slight problems with movement, such as slowness, rigidity, tremor, and rapid muscular twitching, called myoclonus. Several of these symptoms are similar to those seen in Parkinson's disease, and they differ from the chorea seen in individuals who develop the disease as adults.

These young individuals are said to have akinetic-rigid HD or the Westphal variant of HD. People with juvenile HD may also have seizures and mental disabilities. The earlier the onset, the faster the disease seems to progress. The disease progresses most rapidly in individuals with juvenile or early-onset HD, and death often follows within 10 years.

Individuals with juvenile HD usually inherit the disease from their fathers. These individuals also tend to have the largest number of CAG repeats. The reason for this may be found in the process of sperm production. Unlike eggs, sperm are produced in the millions. Because DNA is copied millions of times during this process, there is an increased possibility for genetic mistakes to occur. To verify the link between the number of CAG repeats in the HD gene and the age at onset of symptoms, scientists studied a boy who developed HD symptoms at the age of two, one of the youngest and most severe cases ever recorded. They found that he had the largest number of CAG repeats of anyone studied so far—nearly 100. The boy's case was central to the identification of the HD gene and at the same time helped confirm that juveniles with HD have the longest segments of CAG repeats, the only proven correlation between repeat length and age at onset.

A few individuals develop HD after age 55. Diagnosis in these people can be very difficult. The symptoms of HD may be masked by other health problems, or the person may not display the severity of symptoms seen in individuals with HD of earlier onset. These individuals may also show symptoms of depression rather than anger or irritability, or they may retain sharp control over their intellectual functions, such as memory, reasoning, and problem-solving.

There is also a related disorder called senile chorea. Some elderly individuals display the symptoms of HD, especially choreic movements, but do not become demented, have a normal gene, and lack a family history of the disorder. Some scientists believe that a different gene mutation may account for this small number of cases, but this has not been proven.

How Is HD Diagnosed?

The great American folk singer and composer Woody Guthrie died on October 3, 1967, after suffering from HD for 13 years. He had been misdiagnosed, considered an alcoholic, and shuttled in and out of mental institutions and hospitals for years before being properly diagnosed. His case, sadly, is not extraordinary, although the diagnosis can be made easily by experienced neurologists.

A neurologist will interview the individual intensively to obtain the medical history and rule out other conditions. A tool used by physicians to diagnose HD is to take the family history, sometimes called a pedigree or genealogy. It is extremely important for family members to be candid and truthful with a doctor who is taking a family history.

The doctor will also ask about recent intellectual or emotional problems, which may be indications of HD, and will test the person's hearing, eye movements, strength, coordination, involuntary movements (chorea), sensation, reflexes, balance, movement, and mental status, and will probably order a number of laboratory tests as well.

People with HD commonly have impairments in the way the eye follows or fixes on a moving target. Abnormalities of eye movements vary from person to person and differ, depending on the stage and duration of the illness.

The discovery of the HD gene in 1993 resulted in a direct genetic test to make or confirm a diagnosis of HD in an individual who is exhibiting HD-like symptoms. Using a blood sample, the genetic test analyzes DNA for the HD mutation by counting the number of repeats in the HD gene region. Individuals who do not have HD usually have 28 or fewer CAG repeats. Individuals with HD usually have 40 or more repeats. A small percentage of individuals, however, have a number of repeats that fall within a borderline region (see Table 30.1).

The physician may ask the individual to undergo a brain imaging test. Computed tomography (CT) and magnetic resonance imaging (MRI) provide excellent images of brain structures with little if any discomfort. Those with HD may show shrinkage of some parts of the brain—particularly two areas known as the caudate nuclei and putamen—and enlargement of fluid-filled cavities within the brain called ventricles. These changes do not definitely indicate HD, however, because they

Table 30.1. Outcome of CAG Repeats

No. of CAG repeats	Outcome
< or equal to 28	Normal range; individual will not develop HD
29-34	Individual will not develop HD but the next generation is at risk
35-39	Some, but not all, individuals in this range will develop HD; next generation is also at risk
or equal to 40	Individual will develop HD

can also occur in other disorders. In addition, a person can have early symptoms of HD and still have a normal CT scan. When used in conjunction with a family history and record of clinical symptoms, however, CT can be an important diagnostic tool.

Another technology for brain imaging includes positron emission tomography (PET,) which is important in HD research efforts but is not often needed for diagnosis.

What Is Presymptomatic Testing?

Presymptomatic testing is used for people who have a family history of HD but have no symptoms themselves. If either parent had HD, the person's chance would be 50-50. In the past, no laboratory test could positively identify people carrying the HD gene—or those fated to develop HD—before the onset of symptoms. That situation changed in 1983, when a team of scientists supported by the NINDS located the first genetic marker for HD—the initial step in developing a laboratory test for the disease.

A marker is a piece of DNA that lies near a gene and is usually inherited with it. Discovery of the first HD marker allowed scientists to locate the HD gene on chromosome 4. The marker discovery quickly led to the development of a presymptomatic test for some individuals, but this test required blood or tissue samples from both affected and unaffected family members in order to identify markers unique to that particular family. For this reason, adopted individuals, orphans, and people who had few living family members were unable to use the test.

Discovery of the HD gene has led to a less expensive, scientifically simpler, and far more accurate presymptomatic test that is applicable to the majority of at-risk people. The new test uses CAG repeat length to detect the presence of the HD mutation in blood. This is discussed further in the next section.

There are many complicating factors that reflect the complexity of diagnosing HD. In a small number of individuals with HD—1 to 3 percent—no family history of HD can be found. Some individuals may not be aware of their genetic legacy, or a family member may conceal a genetic disorder from fear of social stigma. A parent may not want to worry children, scare them, or deter them from marrying. In other cases, a family member may die of another cause before he or she begins to show signs of HD. Sometimes, the cause of death for a relative may not be known, or the family is not aware of a relative's death. Adopted children may not know their genetic heritage, or early symptoms in an individual may be too slight to attract attention.

How Is the Presymptomatic Test Conducted?

An individual who wishes to be tested should contact the nearest testing center. (A list of such centers can be obtained from the Huntington Disease Society of America at 1-800-345-HDSA.) The testing process should include several components. Most testing programs include a neurological examination, pretest counseling, and follow-up. The purpose of the neurological examination is to determine whether or not the person requesting testing is showing any clinical symptoms of HD. It is important to remember that if an individual is showing even slight symptoms of HD, he or she risks being diagnosed with the disease during the neurological examination, even before the genetic test. During pretest counseling, the individual will learn about HD, and about his or her own level of risk, about the testing procedure. The person will be told about the test's limitations, the accuracy of the test, and possible outcomes. He or she can then weigh the risks and benefits of testing and may even decide at that time against pursuing further testing.

If a person decides to be tested, a team of highly trained specialists will be involved, which may include neurologists, genetic counselors, social workers, psychiatrists, and psychologists. This team of professionals helps the at-risk person decide if testing is the right thing to do and carefully prepares the person for a negative, positive, or inconclusive test result.

Individuals who decide to continue the testing process should be accompanied to counseling sessions by a spouse, a friend, or a relative who is not at risk. Other interested family members may participate in the counseling sessions if the individual being tested so desires.

The genetic testing itself involves donating a small sample of blood that is screened in the laboratory for the presence or absence of the HD mutation. Testing may require a sample of DNA from a closely related affected relative, preferably a parent, for the purpose of confirming the diagnosis of HD in the family. This is especially important if the family history for HD is unclear or unusual in some way.

Results of the test should be given only in person and only to the individual being tested. Test results are confidential. Regardless of test results, follow-up is recommended. In order to protect the interests of minors, including confidentiality, testing is not recommended for those under the age of 18 unless there is a compelling medical reason (for example, the child is exhibiting symptoms).

Testing of a fetus (prenatal testing) presents special challenges and risks; in fact some centers do not perform genetic testing on fetuses.

Because a positive test result using direct genetic testing means the at-risk parent is also a gene carrier, at-risk individuals who are considering a pregnancy are advised to seek genetic counseling prior to conception.

Some at-risk parents may wish to know the risk to their fetus but not their own. In this situation, parents may opt for prenatal testing using linked DNA markers rather than direct gene testing. In this case, testing does not look for the HD gene itself but instead indicates whether or not the fetus has inherited a chromosome 4 from the affected grandparent or from the unaffected grandparent on the side of the family with HD. If the test shows that the fetus has inherited a chromosome 4 from the affected grandparent, the parents then learn that the fetus's risk is the same as the parent (50-50), but they learn nothing new about the parent's risk. If the test shows that the fetus has inherited a chromosome 4 from the unaffected grandparent, the risk to the fetus is very low (less than 1%) in most cases.

Another option open to parents is in vitro fertilization with pre-implantation screening. In this procedure, embryos are screened to determine which ones carry the HD mutation. Embryos determined not to have the HD gene mutation are then implanted in the woman's uterus.

In terms of emotional and practical consequences, not only for the individual taking the test, but for his or her entire family, testing is enormously complex and has been surrounded by considerable controversy. For example, people with a positive test result may risk losing health and life insurance, suffer loss of employment, and other liabilities. People undergoing testing may wish to cover the cost themselves, since coverage by an insurer may lead to loss of health insurance in the event of a positive result, although this may change in the future.

With the participation of health professionals and people from families with HD, scientists have developed testing guidelines. All individuals seeking a genetic test should obtain a copy of these guidelines. Use only organizations that perform testing using the established procedures and avoid testing that does not adhere to these guidelines.

How Does a Person Decide Whether to Be Tested?

The anxiety that comes from living with a 50 percent risk for HD can be overwhelming. How does a young person make important choices about long-term education, marriage, and children? How do older parents of adult children cope with their fears about children and grandchildren? How do people come to terms with the ambiguity and uncertainty of living at risk?

Some individuals choose to undergo the test out of a desire for greater certainty about their genetic status. They believe the test will enable them to make more informed decisions about the future. Others choose not to take the test. They are able to make peace with the uncertainty of being at risk, preferring to forego the emotional consequences of a positive result, as well as possible losses of insurance and employment. There is no right or wrong decision, as each choice is highly individual. The guidelines for genetic testing for HD, discussed in the previous section, were developed to help people with this life-changing choice.

Whatever the results of genetic testing, the at-risk individual and family members can expect powerful and complex emotional responses. The health and happiness of spouses, brothers and sisters, children, parents, and grandparents are affected by a positive test result, as are an individual's friends, work associates, neighbors, and others. Because receiving test results may prove to be devastating, testing guidelines call for continued counseling even after the test is complete and the results are known.

Is There a Treatment for HD?

Physicians may prescribe a number of medications to help control emotional and movement problems associated with HD. It is important to remember however, that while medicines may help keep these clinical symptoms under control, there is no treatment to stop or reverse the course of the disease.

Antipsychotic drugs, such as haloperidol, or other drugs, such as clonazepam, may help to alleviate choreic movements and may also be used to help control hallucinations, delusions, and violent outbursts. Antipsychotic drugs, however, are not prescribed for another form of muscle contraction associated with HD, called dystonia, and may in fact worsen the condition, causing stiffness and rigidity. These medications may also have severe side effects, including sedation, and for that reason should be used in the lowest possible doses.

For depression, physicians may prescribe fluoxetine, sertraline, nortriptyline, or other compounds. Tranquilizers can help control anxiety and lithium may be prescribed to combat pathological excitement and severe mood swings. Medications may also be needed to treat the severe obsessive-compulsive rituals of some individuals with HD.

Most drugs used to treat the symptoms of HD have side effects such as fatigue, restlessness, or hyperexcitability. Sometimes it may be difficult to tell if a particular symptom, such as apathy or incontinence, is a sign of the disease or a reaction to medication.

What Kind of Care Does the Individual with HD Need?

Although a psychologist or psychiatrist, a genetic counselor, and other specialists may be needed at different stages of the illness, usually the first step in diagnosis and in finding treatment is to see a neurologist. While the family doctor may be able to diagnose HD, and may continue to monitor the individual's status, it is better to consult with a neurologist about management of the varied symptoms.

Problems may arise when individuals try to express complex thoughts in words they can no longer pronounce intelligibly. It can be helpful to repeat words back to the person with HD so that he or she knows that some thoughts are understood. Sometimes people mistakenly assume that if individuals do not talk, they also do not understand. Never isolate individuals by not talking, and try to keep their environment as normal as possible. Speech therapy may improve the individual's ability to communicate.

It is extremely important for the person with HD to maintain physical fitness as much as his or her condition and the course of the disease allows. Individuals who exercise and keep active tend to do better than those who do not. A daily regimen of exercise can help the person feel better physically and mentally. Although their coordination may be poor, individuals should continue walking, with assistance if necessary. Those who want to walk independently should be allowed to do so as long as possible, and careful attention should be given to keeping their environment free of hard, sharp objects. This will help ensure maximal independence while minimizing the risk of injury from a fall. Individuals can also wear special padding during walks to help protect against injury from falls. Some people have found that small weights around the ankles can help stability. Wearing sturdy shoes that fit well can help too, especially shoes without laces that can be slipped on or off easily.

Impaired coordination may make it difficult for people with HD to feed themselves and to swallow. As the disease progresses, persons with HD may even choke. In helping individuals to eat, caregivers should allow plenty of time for meals. Food can be cut into small pieces, softened, or pureed to ease swallowing and prevent choking. While some foods may require the addition of thickeners, other foods may need to be thinned. Dairy products, in particular, tend to increase the secretion of mucus, which in turn increases the risk of choking. Some individuals may benefit from swallowing therapy, which is especially helpful if started before serious problems arise. Suction cups for plates, special tableware designed for people with disabilities, and plastic cups with tops can help prevent spilling. The individual's physician can offer additional advice about diet and about how to handle swallowing difficulties or gastrointestinal problems that might arise, such as incontinence or constipation.

Caregivers should pay attention to proper nutrition so that the individual with HD takes in enough calories to maintain his or her body weight. Sometimes people with HD, who may burn as many as 5,000 calories a day without gaining weight, require five meals a day to take in the necessary number of calories. Physicians may recommend vitamins or other nutritional supplements. In a long-term care institution, staff will need to assist with meals in order to ensure that the individual's special caloric and nutritional requirements are met. Some individuals and their families choose to use a feeding tube; others choose not to.

Individuals with HD are at special risk for dehydration and therefore require large quantities of fluids, especially during hot weather. Bendable straws can make drinking easier for the person. In some cases, water may have to be thickened with commercial additives to give it the consistency of syrup or honey.

What Community Resources Are Available?

Individuals and families affected by HD can take steps to ensure that they receive the best advice and care possible. Physicians and state and local health service agencies can provide information on community resources and family support groups that may exist. Possible types of help include:

- **Legal and social aid.** HD affects a person's capacity to reason, make judgments, and handle responsibilities. Individuals may need help with legal affairs. Wills and other important documents should be drawn up early to avoid legal problems when the person with HD may no longer be able to represent his or her own interests. Family members should also seek out assistance if they face discrimination regarding insurance, employment, or other matters.

- **Home care services.** Caring for a person with HD at home can be exhausting, but part-time assistance with household chores or physical care of the individual can ease this burden. Domestic help, meal programs, nursing assistance, occupational therapy, or other home services may be available from federal, state, or local health service agencies.

- **Recreation and work centers.** Many people with HD are eager and able to participate in activities outside the home. Therapeutic work and recreation centers give individuals an opportunity to pursue hobbies and interests and to meet new people. Participation in these programs, including occupational, music, and recreational therapy, can reduce the person's dependence on family members and provides home caregivers with a temporary, much needed break.

- **Group housing.** A few communities have group housing facilities that are supervised by a resident attendant and that provide meals, housekeeping services, social activities, and local transportation services for residents. These living arrangements are particularly suited to the needs of individuals who are alone and who, although still independent and capable, risk injury when they undertake routine chores like cooking and cleaning.

- **Institutional care.** The individual's physical and emotional demands on the family may eventually become overwhelming. While many families may prefer to keep relatives with HD at home whenever possible, a long-term care facility may prove to be best. To hospitalize or place a family member in a care facility is a difficult decision; professional counseling can help families with this.

Finding the proper facility can itself prove difficult. Organizations such as the Huntington's Disease Society of America (contact information is available in the "Additional Information" section at the end of the chapter) may be able to refer the family to facilities that have met standards set for the care of individuals with HD. Very few of these exist however, and even fewer have experience with individuals with juvenile or early-onset HD who require special care because of their age and symptoms.

What Research Is Being Done?

Although HD attracted considerable attention from scientists in the early 20th century, there was little sustained research on the disease until the late 1960s when the Committee to Combat Huntington's disease and the Huntington's Chorea Foundation, later called the Hereditary Disease Foundation, first began to fund research and to campaign for federal funding. In 1977, Congress established the *Commission for the Control of Huntington's Disease and Its Consequences*, which made a series of important recommendations. Since then, Congress has provided consistent support for federal research, primarily through the National Institute of Neurological Disorders and Stroke, the government's lead agency for biomedical research on disorders of the brain and nervous system. The effort to combat HD proceeds along the following lines of inquiry, each providing important information about the disease:

- **Basic neurobiology**. Now that the HD gene has been located, investigators in the field of neurobiology—which encompasses the anatomy, physiology, and biochemistry of the nervous system—are continuing to study the HD gene with an eye toward understanding how it causes disease in the human body.

- **Clinical research**. Neurologists, psychologists, psychiatrists, and other investigators are improving our understanding of the symptoms and progression of the disease in patients while attempting to develop new therapeutics.

- **Imaging**. Scientific investigations using PET and other technologies are enabling scientists to see what the defective gene does to various structures in the brain and how it affects the body's chemistry and metabolism.

- **Animal models**. Laboratory animals, such as mice, are being bred in the hope of duplicating the clinical features of HD and can soon be expected to help scientists learn more about the symptoms and progression of the disease.

- **Fetal tissue research**. Investigators are implanting fetal tissue in rodents and nonhuman primates with the hope that success in this area will lead to understanding, restoring, or replacing functions typically lost by neuronal degeneration in individuals with HD.

These areas of research are slowly converging and, in the process, are yielding important clues about the gene's relentless destruction of mind and body. The NINDS supports much of this exciting work.

Molecular Genetics

For 10 years, scientists focused on a segment of chromosome 4 and, in 1993, finally isolated the HD gene. The process of isolating the responsible gene—motivated by the desire to find a cure—was more difficult than anticipated. Scientists now believe that identifying the location of the HD gene is the first step on the road to a cure.

Finding the HD gene involved an intense molecular genetics research effort with cooperating investigators from around the globe. In early 1993, the collaborating scientists announced they had isolated the unstable triplet repeat DNA sequence that has the HD gene. Investigators relied on the NINDS-supported Research Roster for Huntington's Disease, based at Indiana University in Indianapolis, to accomplish this work. First started in 1979, the roster contains data on many American families with HD, provides statistical and demographic data to scientists, and serves as a liaison between investigators and specific families. It provided the DNA from many families affected by HD to investigators involved in the search for the gene and was an important component in the identification of HD markers.

For several years, NINDS-supported investigators involved in the search for the HD gene made yearly visits to the largest known kindred with HD—14,000 individuals—who live on Lake Maracaibo in Venezuela. The continuing trips enable scientists to study inheritance patterns of several interrelated families.

The HD Gene and Its Product

Although scientists know that certain brain cells die in HD, the cause of their death is still unknown. Recessive diseases are usually thought to result from a gene that fails to produce adequate amounts of a substance essential to normal function. This is known as a loss-of-function gene. Some dominantly inherited disorders, such as HD, are thought to involve a gene that actively interferes with the normal function of the cell. This is known as a gain-of-function gene.

How does the defective HD gene cause harm? The HD gene encodes a protein—which has been named huntingtin—the function of which is as yet unknown. The repeated CAG sequence in the gene causes an abnormal form of huntingtin to be made, in which the amino acid glutamine is repeated. It is the presence of this abnormal form, and not the absence of the normal form, that causes harm in HD. This explains why the disease is dominant and why two copies of the defective gene—one from both the mother and the father—do not cause a more serious case than inheritance from only one parent. With the HD gene isolated, NINDS-supported investigators are now turning their attention toward discovering the normal function of huntingtin and how the altered form causes harm. Scientists hope to reproduce, study, and correct these changes in animal models of the disease.

Huntingtin is found everywhere in the body but only outside the cell's nucleus. Mice called knockout mice are bred in the laboratory to produce no huntingtin; they fail to develop past a very early embryo stage and quickly die. Huntingtin, scientists now know, is necessary for life. Investigators hope to learn why the abnormal version of the protein damages only certain parts of the brain. One theory is that cells in these parts of the brain may be supersensitive to this abnormal protein.

Cell Death in HD

Although the precise cause of cell death in HD is not yet known, scientists are paying close attention to the process of genetically programmed cell death that occurs deep within the brains of individuals with HD. This process involves a complex series of interlinked events leading to cellular suicide. Related areas of investigation include:

- **Excitotoxicity.** Overstimulation of cells by natural chemicals found in the brain.

- **Defective energy metabolism.** A defect in the power plant of the cell, called mitochondria, where energy is produced.

- **Oxidative stress.** Normal metabolic activity in the brain that produces toxic compounds called free radicals.

- **Trophic factors.** Natural chemical substances found in the human body that may protect against cell death.

Several HD studies are aimed at understanding losses of nerve cells and receptors in HD. Neurons in the striatum are classified both by their size (large, medium, or small) and appearance (spiny or aspiny). Each type of neuron contains combinations of neurotransmitters. Scientists know that the destructive process of HD affects different subsets of neurons to varying degrees. The hallmark of HD, they are learning, is selective degeneration of medium-sized spiny neurons in the striatum. NINDS-supported studies also suggest that losses of certain types of neurons and receptors are responsible for different symptoms and stages of HD.

What do these changes look like? In spiny neurons, investigators have observed two types of changes, each affecting the nerve cells' dendrites. Dendrites, found on every nerve cell, extend out from the cell body and are responsible for receiving messages from other nerve cells. In the intermediate stages of HD, dendrites grow out of control. New, incomplete branches form and other branches become contorted. In advanced, severe stages of HD, degenerative changes cause sections of dendrites to swell, break off, or disappear altogether. Investigators believe that these alterations may be an attempt by the cell to rebuild nerve cell contacts lost early in the disease. As the new dendrites establish connections, however, they may in fact contribute to nerve cell death. Such studies give compelling, visible evidence of the progressive nature of HD and suggest that new experimental therapies must consider the state of cellular degeneration. Scientists do not yet know exactly how these changes affect subsets of nerve cells outside the striatum.

Animal Models of HD

As more is learned about cellular degeneration in HD, investigators hope to reproduce these changes in animal models and to find a way to correct or halt the process of nerve cell death. Such models serve the scientific community in general by providing a means to test the safety of new classes of drugs in nonhuman primates. NINDS-supported scientists are currently working to develop both nonhuman primate and mouse models to investigate nerve degeneration in HD and to study the effects of excitotoxicity on nerve cells in the brain.

Investigators are working to build genetic models of HD using transgenic mice. To do this, scientists transfer the altered human HD gene into mouse embryos so that the animals will develop the anatomical and biological characteristics of HD. This genetic model of mouse HD will enable in-depth study of the disease and testing of new therapeutic compounds.

Another idea is to insert into mice a section of DNA containing CAG repeats in the abnormal, disease gene range. This mouse equivalent of HD could allow scientists to explore the basis of CAG instability and its role in the disease process.

Fetal Tissue Research

A relatively new field in biomedical research involves the use of brain tissue grafts to study, and potentially treat, neurodegenerative disorders. In this technique, tissue that has degenerated is replaced with implants of fresh, fetal tissue, taken at the very early stages of development. Investigators are interested in applying brain tissue implants to HD research. Extensive animal studies will be required to learn if this technique could be of value in patients with HD.

Clinical Studies

Scientists are pursuing clinical studies that may one day lead to the development of new drugs or other treatments to halt the disease's progression. Examples of NINDS-supported investigations, using both asymptomatic and symptomatic individuals, include:

- **Genetic studies on age of onset, inheritance patterns**, and markers found within families. These studies may shed additional light on how HD is passed from generation to generation.

- **Studies of cognition, intelligence, and movement**. Studies of abnormal eye movements, both horizontal and vertical, and tests of patients' skills in a number of learning, memory, neuropsychological, and motor tasks may serve to identify when the various symptoms of HD appear and to characterize their range and severity.

- **Clinical trials of drugs**. Testing of various drugs may lead to new treatments and at the same time improve our understanding of the disease process in HD. Classes of drugs being tested include those that control symptoms, slow the rate of progression of HD, and block effects of excitotoxins, and those that might correct or replace other metabolic defects contributing to the development and progression of HD.

Imaging

NINDS-supported scientists are using positron emission tomography (PET) to learn how the gene affects the chemical systems of the body. PET visualizes metabolic or chemical abnormalities in the body, and investigators hope to ascertain if PET scans can reveal any abnormalities that signal HD. Investigators conducting HD research are also using PET to characterize neurons that have died and chemicals that are depleted in parts of the brain affected by HD.

Like PET, a form of magnetic resonance imaging (MRI) called functional MRI can measure increases or decreases in certain brain chemicals thought to play a key role in HD. Functional MRI studies are also helping investigators understand how HD kills neurons in different regions of the brain.

Imaging technologies allow investigators to view changes in the volume and structures of the brain and to pinpoint when these changes occur in HD. Scientists know that in brains affected by HD, the basal ganglia, cortex, and ventricles all show atrophy or other alterations.

How Can I Help?

In order to conduct HD research, investigators require samples of tissue or blood from families with HD. Access to individuals with HD and their families may be difficult however, because families with HD are often scattered across the country or around the world. A research project may need individuals of a particular age or gender or from a certain geographic area. Some scientists need only statistical data while others may require a sample of blood, urine, or skin from family members. All of these factors complicate the task of finding volunteers. The following NINDS-supported efforts bring together families with HD, voluntary health agencies, and scientists in an effort to advance science and speed a cure.

The NINDS-sponsored HD Research Roster at the Indiana University Medical Center in Indianapolis, which was discussed earlier, makes research possible by matching scientists with patient and family volunteers. The first DNA bank was established through the roster. Although the gene has already been located, DNA from individuals who have HD is still of great interest to investigators. Of continuing interest are twins, unaffected individuals who have affected offspring, and individuals with two defective HD genes, one from each parent—a very rare occurrence. Participation in the roster and in specific research projects is voluntary and confidential. For more information about the roster and DNA bank, contact:

Indiana University Medical Center
Department of Medical and Molecular Genetics
Medical Research and Library Building
975 W. Walnut Street
Indianapolis, IN 46202-5251
Tel: 317-274-5744 (call collect)
Website: www.biochemistry.iu.edu

Brain tissue is also critical to the HD research effort, and many individuals are willing to donate their brains and other organs to research after they die. The NINDS supports two national human brain specimen banks, one at the Greater Los Angeles Health Care System, and the other at McLean Hospital near Boston. These banks supply investigators around the world with tissue not only from individuals with HD but also from those with other neurological or psychiatric diseases. Both banks need brain tissue to enable scientists to study these disorders more intensely. Prospective donors should contact:

National Neurological Research Specimen Bank
VMAC (W127A)-West Los Angeles
11301 Wilshire Boulevard
Los Angeles, CA 90073
Tel: 310-268-3536

Harvard Brain Tissue Resource Center
McLean Hospital
115 Mill Street
Belmont, MA 02178
Toll-Free: 800-BRAIN-BANK (800-272-4622)
Tel: 617-855-2400
Fax: 617-855-3479
Website: www.brainbank.mclean.org
E-mail: btrc@mclean.Harvard.edu

Glossary

Akinesia: decreased body movements.

At-risk: a description of a person whose mother or father has HD or has inherited the HD gene and who therefore has a 50-50 chance of inheriting the disorder.

Autosomal dominant disorder: a non-sex-linked disorder that can be inherited even if only one parent passes on the defective gene.

Basal ganglia: a region located at the base of the brain composed of four clusters of neurons, or nerve cells. This area is responsible for body movement and coordination. The neuron groups most prominently and consistently affected by HD—the pallidum and striatum— are located here. See neuron, pallidum, striatum.

Caudate nuclei: part of the striatum in the basal ganglia. See basal ganglia, striatum.

Chorea: uncontrolled body movements. Chorea is derived from the Greek word for dance.

Chromosomes: the structures in cells that contain genes. They are composed of deoxyribonucleic acid (DNA) and proteins and, under a microscope, appear as rod-like structures. See deoxyribonucleic acid (DNA), gene.

Computed tomography (CT): a technique used for diagnosing brain disorders. CT uses a computer to produce a high-quality image of brain structures. These images are called CT scans.

Cortex: part of the brain responsible for thought, perception, and memory. HD affects the basal ganglia and cortex. See basal ganglia.

Deoxyribonucleic acid (DNA): the substance of heredity containing the genetic information necessary for cells to divide and produce proteins. DNA carries the code for every inherited characteristic of an organism. See gene.

Dominant: a trait that is apparent even when the gene for that disorder is inherited from only one parent. See autosomal dominant disorder, recessive, gene.

Gene: the basic unit of heredity, composed of a segment of DNA containing the code for a specific trait. See deoxyribonucleic acid (DNA).

Huntingtin: the protein encoded by the gene that carries the HD defect. The repeated CAG sequence in the gene causes an abnormal form of huntingtin to be formed. The function of the normal form of huntingtin is not yet known.

Kindred: a group of related persons, such as a family or clan.

Magnetic resonance imaging (MRI): an imaging technique that uses radiowaves, magnetic fields, and computer analysis to create a picture of body tissues and structures.

Marker: a piece of DNA that lies on the chromosome so close to a gene that the two are inherited together. Like a signpost, markers are used during genetic testing and research to locate the nearby presence of a gene. See chromosome, deoxyribonucleic acid (DNA).

Mitochondria: microscopic, energy-producing bodies within cells that are the cells' power plants.

Mutation: in genetics, any defect in a gene. See gene.

Myoclonus: a condition in which muscles or portions of muscles contract involuntarily in a jerky fashion.

Neuron: Greek word for a nerve cell, the basic impulse-conducting unit of the nervous system. Nerve cells communicate with other cells through an electrochemical process called neurotransmission.

Neurotransmitters: special chemicals that transmit nerve impulses from one cell to another.

Pallidum: part of the basal ganglia of the brain. The pallidum is composed of the globus pallidus and the ventral pallidum. See basal ganglia.

Positron emission tomography (PET): a tool used to diagnose brain functions and disorders. PET produces three-dimensional, colored images of chemicals or substances functioning within the body. These images are called PET scans. PET shows brain function, in contrast to CT or MRI, which show brain structure.

Prevalence: the number of cases of a disease that are present in a particular population at a given time.

Putamen: an area of the brain that decreases in size as a result of the damage produced by HD.

Receptor: proteins that serve as recognition sites on cells and cause a response in the body when stimulated by chemicals called neurotransmitters. They act as on-and-off switches for the next nerve cell. See neuron, neurotransmitters.

Recessive: a trait that is apparent only when the gene or genes for it are inherited from both parents. See dominant, gene.

Senile chorea: a relatively mild and rare disorder found in elderly adults and characterized by choreic movements. It is believed by some scientists to be caused by a different gene mutation than that causing HD.

Striatum: art of the basal ganglia of the brain. The striatum is composed of the caudate nucleus, putamen, and ventral striatum. See basal ganglia, caudate nuclei.

Trait: any genetically determined characteristic. See dominant, gene, recessive.

Transgenic mice: mice that receive injections of foreign genes during the embryonic stage of development. Their cells then follow the instructions of the foreign genes, resulting in the development of a certain trait or characteristic. Transgenic mice can serve as an animal model of a certain disease, telling researchers how genes work in specific cells.

Ventricles: cavities within the brain that are filled with cerebrospinal fluid. In HD, tissue loss causes enlargement of the ventricles.

Additional Information

Brain Resources and Information Network (BRAIN)
P.O. Box 5801
Bethesda, MD 20824
Toll-Free: 800-352-9424
TTY: 301-468-5981
Website: www.ninds.nih.gov

Huntington's Disease Society of America (HDSA)
158 West 29th Street
7th Floor
New York, NY 10001-5300
Toll-Free: 800-345-HDSA (800-345-4372)
Tel: 212-242-1968
Fax: 212-239-3430
Website: www.hdsa.org
E-mail: hdsainfo@hdsa.org

The HDSA supports research, assists families, trains professionals, monitors testing guidelines, and educates the public and professionals about Huntington's disease. The Society publishes brochures, books, a newsletter, reprints, and maintains a list of testing centers. It also sponsors conferences, training programs, and nationwide chapters and support groups.

Hereditary Disease Foundation
11400 W. Olympic Blvd., Suite 855
Los Angeles, CA 90064-1560
Tel: 310-575-9656
Fax: 310-575-9156
Website: www.hdfoundation.org
E-mail: cures@hdfoundation.org

This foundation promotes research on genetic disorders and sponsors workshops and fellowship programs. The group provides additional support to two brain banks.

Chapter 31

Machado-Joseph Disease

What Is Machado-Joseph Disease?

Machado-Joseph disease (MJD)—also called spinocerebellar ataxia type 3—is a rare hereditary ataxia. (Ataxia is a general term meaning lack of muscle control.) The disease is characterized by clumsiness and weakness in the arms and legs, spasticity, a staggering lurching gait easily mistaken for drunkenness, difficulty with speech and swallowing, involuntary eye movements, double vision, and frequent urination. Some patients have dystonia (sustained muscle contractions that cause twisting of the body and limbs, repetitive movements, abnormal postures, and/or rigidity) or symptoms similar to those of Parkinson's disease. Others have twitching of the face or tongue, or peculiar bulging eyes.

The severity of the disease is related to the age of onset, with earlier onset associated with a more severe form of the disease. Symptoms can begin any time between early adolescence and about 70 years of age. MJD is also a progressive disease, meaning that symptoms get worse with time. Life expectancy ranges from the mid-thirties for those with severe forms of MJD to a normal life expectancy for those with mild forms. For those who die early from the disease, the cause of death is often aspiration pneumonia.

The name, Machado-Joseph, comes from two families of Portuguese/Azorean descent who were among the first families described

"Machado-Joseph Disease," Fact Sheet, National Institute of Neurological Disease and Stroke (NINDS), reviewed November 28, 2001.

351

with the unique symptoms of the disease in the 1970s. The prevalence of the disease is still highest among people of Portuguese/Azorean descent. For immigrants of Portuguese ancestry in New England, the prevalence is around one in 4,000. The highest prevalence in the world, about one in 140, occurs on the small Azorean island of Flores. Recently, researchers have identified MJD in several family groups not of obvious Portuguese descent, including an African-American family from North Carolina, an Italian-American family, and several Japanese families. On a worldwide basis, MJD is the most prevalent autosomal dominant inherited form of ataxia, based on DNA studies.

What Are the Different Types of Machado-Joseph Disease?

The types of MJD are distinguished by the age of onset and range of symptoms. Type I is characterized by onset between 10 and 30 years of age, fast progression, and severe dystonia and rigidity. Type II MJD generally begins between the ages of 20 and 50 years, has an intermediate progression, and causes symptoms that include spasticity (continuous, uncontrollable muscle contractions), spastic gait, and exaggerated reflex responses. Type III MJD patients have an onset between 40 and 70 years of age, a relatively slow progression, and some muscle twitching, muscle atrophy, and unpleasant sensations such as numbness, tingling, cramps, and pain in the hands, feet, and limbs. Almost all MJD patients experience vision problems, including double vision (diplopia) or blurred vision, loss of ability to distinguish color and/or contrast, and inability to control eye movements. Some MJD patients also experience Parkinson's-like symptoms, such as slowness of movement, rigidity or stiffness of the limbs and trunk, tremor or trembling in the hands, and impaired balance and coordination.

What Causes Machado-Joseph Disease?

MJD is classified as a disorder of movement, specifically a spinocerebellar ataxia. In these disorders, degeneration of cells in an area of the brain called the hindbrain leads to deficits in movement. The hindbrain includes the cerebellum (a bundle of tissue about the size of an apricot located at the back of the head), the brainstem, and the upper part of the spinal cord. MJD is an inherited, autosomal dominant disease, meaning that if a child inherits one copy of the defective gene from either parent, the child will develop symptoms of the disease. People with a defective gene have a 50 percent chance of passing the mutation on to their children.

MJD belongs to a class of genetic disorders called triplet repeat diseases. The genetic mutation in triplet repeat diseases involves the extensive abnormal repetition of three letters of the DNA genetic code. In the case of MJD the code CAG is repeated within a gene located on chromosome 14q. The MJD gene produces a mutated protein called ataxin-3. This protein accumulates in affected cells and forms intranuclear inclusion bodies, which are insoluble spheres located in the nucleus of the cell. These spheres interfere with the normal operation of the nucleus and cause the cell to degenerate and die.

One trait of MJD and other triplet repeat diseases is a phenomenon called anticipation, in which the children of affected parents tend to develop symptoms of the disease much earlier in life, have a faster progression of the disease, and experience more severe symptoms. This is due to the tendency of the triplet repeat mutation to expand with the passing of genetic material to offspring. A longer expansion is associated with an earlier age of onset and a more severe form of the disease. It is impossible to predict precisely the course of the disease for an individual based solely on the repeat length.

How Is Machado-Joseph Disease Diagnosed?

Physicians diagnose MJD by recognizing the symptoms of the disease and by taking a family history. They ask detailed questions about family members who show, or showed, symptoms of the disease, the kinds of symptoms these relatives had, the ages of disease onset, and the progression and severity of symptoms. A definitive diagnosis of MJD can only be made with a genetic test. Unfortunately, many legal and ethical considerations, such as loss of health insurance and employment discrimination, may discourage some individuals with symptoms from getting tested. For the same reasons, many physicians recommend against genetic testing for those individuals who have a family history of the disease but do not show symptoms.

How Is Machado-Joseph Disease Treated?

MJD is incurable, but some symptoms of the disease can be treated. For those patients who show parkinsonian features, levodopa therapy can help for many years. Treatment with antispasmodic drugs, such as baclofen, can help reduce spasticity. Botulinum toxin can also treat severe spasticity as well as some symptoms of dystonia. However, botulinum toxin should be used as a last resort due to the possibility of side effects, such as swallowing problems (dysphagia). Speech problems (dysarthria) and dysphagia can be treated with medication and speech therapy. Wearing prism glasses can reduce blurred or double vision, but eye surgery has only short-term benefits due to the progressive degeneration of eye muscles. Physiotherapy can help patients cope with disability associated with gait problems, and physical aids, such as walkers and wheelchairs, can assist the patient with everyday activities. Other problems, such as sleep disturbances, cramps, and urinary dysfunction, can be treated with medications and medical care.

What Research Is Being Done?

The National Institute of Neurological Disorders and Stroke (NINDS) supports research on MJD and other neurodegenerative diseases in an effort to learn how to better treat, prevent, and even cure these diseases. Ongoing research includes efforts to better understand the genetic, molecular, and cellular mechanisms that underlie triplet repeat diseases. Other research areas include the development of novel therapies to treat the symptoms of MJD, efforts to identify diagnostic markers and to improve current diagnostic procedures for the disease, and population studies to identify affected families.

Additional Information

Brain Resources and Information Network (BRAIN)
P.O. Box 5801
Bethesda, MD 20824
Toll-Free: 800-352-9424
TTY: 301-468-5981
Website: www.ninds.nih.gov

International Joseph Disease Foundation, Inc.
P.O. Box 2550
Livermore, CA 94531-2550
Tel: 925-371-1288
Website: www.ijdf.net

National Ataxia Foundation (NAF)
2600 Fernbrook Lane, Suite 119
Minneapolis, MN 55447-4752
Tel: 763-553-0020

Fax: 763-553-0167
Website: www.ataxia.org
E-mail: naf@ataxia.org

National Organization for Rare Disorders (NORD)
P.O. Box 1968
Danbury, CT 06813-1968
Toll-Free: 800-999-NORD (6673)
Tel: 203-746-6518
Website: www.rarediseases.org

Dystonia Medical Research Foundation
1 East Wacker Drive, Suite 2430
Chicago, IL 60601-1905
Toll-Free in Canada: 800-361-8061
Tel: 312-755-0198
Website: www.dystonia-foundation.org

Worldwide Education & Awareness for Movement Disorders (WE MOVE)
204 West 84th Street
New York, NY 10024
Toll-Free: 800-437-MOV2 (6682)
Fax: 212-875-8389
Website: www.wemove.org
E-mail: wemove@wemove.org

National Aphasia Association
29 John St., Suite 1103
New York, NY 10038
Toll-Free: 800-922-4NAA (4622)
Tel: 212-255-4329
Website: www.aphasia.org
E-mail: naa@aphasia.org

American Speech-Language-Hearing Association (ASHA)
10801 Rockville Pike
Rockville, MD 20852-3279
Toll-Free: 800-638-8255
Tel: 301-897-5700
Website: www.asha.org
Email: actioncenter@asha.org

Family Caregiver Alliance
690 Market Street, Suite 600
San Francisco, CA 94104
Tel: 415-434-3388
Fax: 415-434-3508
Website: www.caregiver.org
E-mail: info@caregiver.org

National Family Caregivers Association
10400 Connecticut Avenue, Suite 500
Kensington, MD 20895-3944
Toll-Free: 800-896-3650
Tel: 301-942-6430
Fax: 301-942-2302
Website: www.nfcacares.org
E-mail: info@nfccares.org

Organizations That Provide Information on Genetic Testing and Counseling:

National Society of Genetic Counselors, Inc.
233 Canterbury Drive
Wallingford, PA 19086-6617
Tel: 610-872-7608
Website: www.nsgc.org
E-mail: nsgc@nsgc.org

Alliance of Genetic Support Groups
4301 Connecticut Avenue, NW, Suite 404
Washington, DC 20008-2304
Toll-Free: 800-336-GENE (4363)
Tel: 202-966-5557
Fax: 202-966-8553
Website: www.geneticalliance.org
E-mail: info@geneticalliance.org

Chapter 32

Multiple Sclerosis

Definition

Multiple sclerosis (MS) is a chronic autoimmune disorder affecting movement, sensation, and bodily functions. It is caused by destruction of the myelin insulation covering nerve fibers (neurons) in the central nervous system (brain and spinal cord).

Description

MS is a nerve disorder caused by destruction of the insulating layer surrounding neurons in the brain and spinal cord. This insulation, called myelin, helps electrical signals pass quickly and smoothly between the brain and the rest of the body. When the myelin is destroyed, nerve messages are sent more slowly and less efficiently. Patches of scar tissue, called plaques, form over the affected areas, further disrupting nerve communication. The symptoms of MS occur when the brain and spinal cord nerves no longer communicate properly with other parts of the body. MS causes a wide variety of symptoms and can affect vision, balance, strength, sensation, coordination, and bodily functions.

Multiple sclerosis affects more than a quarter of a million people in the United States. Most people have their first symptoms between the ages of 20 and 40; symptoms rarely begin before 15 or after 60. Women are almost twice as likely to get MS as men, especially in their early years. People of northern European heritage are more likely to be affected than people of other racial backgrounds, and MS rates are higher in the United States, Canada, and Northern Europe than in other parts of the world. MS is very rare among Asians, North and South American Indians, and Eskimos.

Causes and Symptoms

Causes

Multiple sclerosis is an autoimmune disease, meaning its cause is an attack by the body's own immune system. For unknown reasons, immune cells attack and destroy the myelin sheath that insulates neurons in the brain and spinal cord. This myelin sheath, created by other brain cells called glia, speeds transmission and prevents electrical activity in one cell from short-circuiting to another cell. Disruption of communication between the brain and other parts of the body prevent normal passage of sensations and control messages, leading to the symptoms of MS. The demyelinated areas appear as plaques, small round areas of gray neuron without the white myelin covering. The progression of symptoms in MS is correlated with development of new plaques in the portion of the brain or spinal cord controlling the affected areas. Because there appears to be no pattern in the appearance of new plaques, the progression of MS can be unpredictable.

Despite considerable research, the trigger for this autoimmune destruction is still unknown. At various times, evidence has pointed to genes, environmental factors, viruses, or a combination of these.

The risk of developing MS is higher if another family member is affected, suggesting the influence of genetic factors. In addition, the higher prevalence of MS among people of northern European background suggests some genetic susceptibility.

The role of an environmental factor is suggested by studies of the effect of migration on the risk of developing MS. Age plays an important role in determining this change in risk—young people in low-risk groups who move into countries with higher MS rates display the risk rates of their new surroundings, while older migrants retain the risk of their original home country. One interpretation of these studies is that an environmental factor, either protective or harmful, is acquired in early life; the risk of disease later in life reflects the effects of the early environment.

These same data can be used to support the involvement of a slow-acting virus, one that is acquired early on but begins its destructive effects much later. Slow viruses are known to cause other diseases, including AIDS. In addition, viruses have been implicated in other autoimmune diseases. Many claims have been made for the role of viruses, slow or otherwise, as the trigger for MS, but as of 1997, no strong candidate has emerged.

How a virus could trigger the autoimmune reaction is also unclear. There are two main models of virally-induced autoimmunity. The first suggests the immune system is actually attacking a virus (one too well-hidden for detection in the laboratory), and the myelin damage is an unintentional consequence of fighting the infection. The second model suggests the immune system mistakes myelin for a viral protein, one it encountered during a prior infection. Primed for the attack, it destroys myelin because it resembles the previously-recognized viral invader.

Either of these models allows a role for genetic factors, since certain genes can increase the likelihood of autoimmunity. Environmental factors as well might change the sensitivity of the immune system or interact with myelin to provide the trigger for the secondary immune response. Possible environmental triggers that have been invoked in MS include viral infection, trauma, electrical injury, and chemical exposure, although controlled studies do not support a causative role.

Symptoms

The symptoms of multiple sclerosis may occur in one of three patterns:

- The most common pattern is the *relapsing-remitting pattern*, in which there are clearly defined symptomatic attacks lasting 24 hours or more, followed by complete or almost complete improvement. The period between attacks may be a year or more at the beginning of the disease, but may shrink to several months later on. This pattern is especially common in younger people who develop MS.

- In the *primary progressive pattern*, the disease progresses without remission or with occasional plateaus or slight improvements. This pattern is more common in older people.

- In the *secondary progressive pattern*, the person with MS begins with relapses and remissions, followed by more steady progression of symptoms.

Between 10-20% of people have a benign type of MS, meaning their symptoms progress very little over the course of their lives.

359

Because plaques may form in any part of the central nervous system, the symptoms of MS vary widely from person-to-person and from stage-to-stage of the disease. Initial symptoms often include:

- Muscle weakness, causing difficulty walking
- Loss of coordination or balance
- Numbness, pins and needles, or other abnormal sensations
- Visual disturbances, including blurred or double vision.

Later symptoms may include:

- Fatigue
- Muscle spasticity and stiffness
- Tremors
- Paralysis
- Pain
- Vertigo
- Speech or swallowing difficulty
- Loss of bowel and bladder control
- Incontinence, constipation
- Sexual dysfunction
- Cognitive changes.

Weakness in one or both legs is common, and may be the first symptom noticed by a person with MS. Muscle spasticity, or excessive tightness, is also common and may be more disabling than weakness.

Double vision or eye tremor (nystagmus) may result from involvement of the nerve pathways controlling movement of the eye muscles. Visual disturbances result from involvement of the optic nerves (optic neutrettos) and may include development of blind spots in one or both eyes, changes in color vision, or blindness. Optic neuritis usually involves only one eye at a time and is often associated with movement of the effected eye.

More than half of all people affected by MS have pain during the course of their disease, and many experience chronic pain, including pain from spasticity. Acute pain occurs in about 10% of cases. This pain may be a sharp, stabbing pain especially in the face, neck, or down the back. Facial numbness and weakness are also common.

Cognitive changes, including memory disturbances, depression, and personality changes, are found in people affected by MS, though it is not entirely clear whether these changes are due primarily to the disease or to the psychological reaction to it. Depression may be severe enough to require treatment in up to 25% of those with MS. A smaller number of people experience disease-related euphoria, or abnormally elevated mood, usually after a long disease duration and in combination with other psychological changes.

Symptoms of MS may be worsened by heat or increased body temperature, including fever, intense physical activity, or exposure to sun, hot baths, or showers.

Diagnosis

There is no single test that confirms the diagnosis of multiple sclerosis, and there are a number of other diseases with similar symptoms. While one person's diagnosis may be immediately suggested by her symptoms and history, another's may not be confirmed without multiple tests and prolonged observation. The distribution of symptoms is important: MS affects multiple areas of the body over time. The pattern of symptoms is also critical, especially evidence of the relapsing-remitting pattern, so a detailed medical history is one of the most important parts of the diagnostic process. A thorough search to exclude other causes of a patient's symptoms is especially important if the following features are present:

1. family history of neurologic disease,

2. symptoms and findings attributable to a single anatomic location,

3. persistent back pain,

4. age of onset over 60 or under 15 years of age, or

5. progressively worsening disease.

In addition to the medical history and a standard neurological exam, several lab tests are used to help confirm or rule out a diagnosis of MS:

* Magnetic resonance imaging (MRI) can reveal plaques on the brain and spinal cord. Gadolinium enhancement can distinguish between old and new plaques, allowing a correlation of new plaques with new symptoms. Plaques may be seen in several other diseases as well, including encephalomyelitis, neurosarcoidosis,

361

and cerebral lupus. Plaques on MRI may be difficult to distinguish from small strokes, areas of decreased blood flow, or changes seen with trauma or normal aging.

- A lumbar puncture, or spinal tap, is done to measure levels of immune proteins, which are usually elevated in the cerebrospinal fluid of a person with MS. This test may not be necessary if other tests are diagnostic.

- Evoked potential tests, electrical tests of conduction speed in the nerves, can reveal reduced speeds consistent with the damage caused by plaques. These tests may be done with small electrical charges applied to the skin (somatosensory evoked potential), with light patterns flashed on the eyes (visual evoked potential), or with sounds presented to the ears (auditory evoked potential).

The clinician making the diagnosis, usually a neurologist, may classify the disease as *definite MS*, meaning the symptoms and test results all point toward MS as the cause. *Probable MS* and *possible MS* reflect less certainty and may require more time to pass to observe the progression of the disease and the distribution of symptoms.

Treatment

As of 1997, there are three drugs approved for the treatment of multiple sclerosis which have been shown to affect the course of the disease. None of these drugs is a cure, but they can slow disease progression in many patients.

Avonex and Betaseron are forms of the immune system protein beta interferon, while Copaxone is glatiramer acetate (formerly called copolymer-1). All three have been shown to reduce the rate of relapses in the relapsing-remitting form of MS. Different measurements from tests of each have demonstrated other benefits as well: Avonex may slow the progress of physical impairment, Betaseron may reduce the severity of symptoms, and Copaxone may decrease disability. All three drugs are administered by injection—Copaxone daily, Betaseron every other day, and Avonex weekly. Betaseron, at least, has led to the development of neutralizing antibodies, which reduce the effectiveness of treatment.

Immunosuppressant drugs have been used for many years to treat acute exacerbations (relapses). Drugs used include corticosteroids such as prednisone and methylprednisolone; the hormone adrenocorticotropic hormone (ACTH); and azathioprine. Recent studies indicate that several days of intravenous methylprednisolone may be more effective than other immunosuppressant treatments for acute symptoms. This treatment may require hospitalization.

MS causes a large variety of symptoms, and the treatments for these are equally diverse. Most symptoms can be treated and complications avoided with good care and attention from medical professionals. Good health and nutrition remain important preventive measures. Vaccination against influenza can prevent respiratory complications, and contrary to earlier concerns, is not associated with worsening of symptoms. Preventing complications such as pneumonia, bed sores, injuries from falls, or urinary infection requires attention to the primary problems which may cause them. Shortened life spans with MS are almost always due to complications rather than primary symptoms themselves.

Physical therapy helps the person with MS to strengthen and retrain affected muscles; to maintain range of motion to prevent muscle stiffening; to learn to use assistive devices such as canes and walkers; and to learn safer and more energy-efficient ways of moving, sitting, and transferring. Exercise and stretching programs are usually designed by the physical therapist and taught to the patient and caregivers for use at home. Exercise is an important part of maintaining function for the person with MS. Swimming is often recommended, not only for its low-impact workout, but also because it allows strenuous activity without overheating.

Occupational therapy helps the person with MS adapt to her environment and adapt the environment to her. The occupational therapist suggests alternate strategies and assistive devices for activities of daily living, such as dressing, feeding, and washing, and evaluates the home and work environment for safety and efficiency improvements that may be made.

Training in bowel and bladder care may be needed to prevent or compensate for incontinence. If the urge to urinate becomes great before the bladder is full, some drugs may be helpful, including propantheline bromide (Pro-Banthine), oxybutynin chloride (Ditropan), or imipramine (Tofranil). Baclofen (Lioresal) may relax the sphincter muscle, allowing full emptying. Intermittent catheterization is effective in controlling bladder dysfunction. In this technique, a catheter is used to periodically empty the bladder.

Spasticity can be treated with oral medications, including baclofen and diazepam (Valium), or by injection with botulinum toxin (Botox). Spasticity relief may also bring relief from chronic pain. Other more acute types of pain may respond to carbamazepine (Tegretol) or diphenylhydantoin (Dilantin). Low back pain is common from increased use of the back muscles to compensate for weakened legs. Physical therapy and over-the-counter pain relievers may help.

Fatigue may be partially avoidable with changes in the daily routine to allow more frequent rests. Amantadine (Symmetrel) and pemoline (Cylert) may improve alertness and lessen fatigue. Visual disturbances often respond to corticosteroids. Other symptoms that may be treated with drugs include seizures, vertigo, and tremor.

Myloral, an oral preparation of bovine myelin, has recently been tested in clinical trials for its effectiveness in reducing the frequency and severity of relapses. Preliminary data indicate no difference between it and placebo.

Alternative Treatment

Bee venom has been suggested as a treatment for MS, but no studies or objective reports support this claim.

In British studies, marijuana has been shown to have variable effects on the symptoms of MS. Improvements have been documented for tremor, pain, and spasticity, and worsening for posture and balance. Side effects have included weakness, dizziness, relaxation, and incoordination, as well as euphoria. As a result, marijuana is not recommended as an alternative treatment.

Some studies support the value of high doses of vitamins, minerals, and other dietary supplements for controlling disease progression or improving symptoms. Alpha-linoleic and linoleic acids, as well as selenium and vitamin E, have shown effectiveness in the treatment of MS. The selenium and vitamin E act as antioxidants. In addition, the Swank diet (low in saturated fats), maintained over a long period of time, may retard the disease process.

Removal of mercury fillings has been touted as a possible cure, but is of no proven benefit.

Prognosis

It is difficult to predict how multiple sclerosis will progress in any one person. Most people with MS will be able to continue to walk and function at their work for many years after their diagnosis. The factors associated with the mildest course of MS are being female, having the relapsing-remitting form, having the first symptoms at a younger age, having longer periods of remission between relapses, and initial symptoms of decreased sensation or vision rather than of weakness or incoordination.

Less than 5% of people with MS have a severe progressive form, leading to death from complications within five years. At the other extreme, 10-20% have a benign form, with a very slow or no progression of their symptoms. The most recent studies show that about seven out of 10 people with MS are still alive 25 years after their diagnosis, compared to about nine out of 10 people of similar age without disease. On average, MS shortens the lives of affected women by about six years, and men by 11 years. Suicide is a significant cause of death in MS, especially in younger patients.

The degree of disability a person experiences five years after onset is, on average, about three-quarters of the expected disability at 10-15 years. A benign course for the first five years usually indicates the disease will not cause marked disability.

Prevention

There is no known way to prevent multiple sclerosis. Until the cause of the disease is discovered, this is unlikely to change. Good nutrition; adequate rest; avoidance of stress, heat, and extreme physical exertion; and good bladder hygiene may improve quality of life and reduce symptoms.

Key Terms

Evoked potentials: Tests that measure the brain's electrical response to stimulation of sensory organs (eyes or ears) or peripheral nerves (skin). These tests may help confirm the diagnosis of multiple sclerosis.

Myelin: A layer of insulation that surrounds the nerve fibers in the brain and spinal cord.

Plaque: Patches of scar tissue that form where the layer of myelin covering the nerve fibers is destroyed by the multiple sclerosis disease process.

Primary progressive: A pattern of symptoms of multiple sclerosis in which the disease progresses without remission, or with occasional plateaus or slight improvements.

Relapsing-remitting: A pattern of symptoms of multiple sclerosis in which symptomatic attacks occur that last 24 hours or more, followed by complete or almost complete improvement.

Secondary progressive: A pattern of symptoms of multiple sclerosis in which there are relapses and remissions, followed by more steady progression of symptoms.

Further Reading

Books

Holland, Nancy, T. Jock Murray, and Stephen Reingold. *Multiple Sclerosis: A Guide for the Newly Diagnosed*. Demos Vermande, 1996.

Matthews, Bryan. *Multiple Sclerosis: The Facts*. New York: Oxford University Press, 1993.

Sibley, William. *Therapeutic Claims in Multiple Sclerosis: A Guide to Treatments*. 4th ed. Demos Vermande, 1996.

Swank, R.L., and M.H. Pullen. *The Multiple Sclerosis Diet Book*. Garden City, NY: Doubleday, 1977.

Organizations

ABLEDATA Adaptive Equipment Center
8630 Fenton Street, Suite 930
Silver Spring, MD 20910
Toll-Free: 800-227-0216
Tel: 301-608-8912 (TTY)
Fax: 301-608-8958
Website: www.abledata.com
E-mail: abledate@macroint.com

The National Multiple Sclerosis Society
733 Third Avenue
New York, NY 10017
Toll-Free: 800-FIGHT-MS (800-344-4867)
Website: www.nmss.org.

Chapter 33

Multiple System Atrophy (Shy-Drager Syndrome)

What Is Shy-Drager Syndrome?

Multiple system atrophy (MSA) with postural hypotension, also called Shy-Drager syndrome, is a progressive disorder of the central and sympathetic nervous systems. The disorder is characterized by postural (or orthostatic) hypotension—an excessive drop in blood pressure when the patient stands up, which causes dizziness or momentary blackouts. MSA has been classified clinically into three types, olivopontocerebellar atrophy (OPCA), which primarily affects balance, coordination, and speech; a parkinsonian form (striatonigral degeneration), which can resemble Parkinson's disease because of slow movement and stiff muscles; and a mixed cerebellar and parkinsonian form. In all three forms of MSA, the patient can have orthostatic hypotension. Orthostatic hypotension and symptoms of autonomic failure such as constipation, impotence in men, and urinary incontinence usually predominate early in the course of the disease. Constipation may be unrelenting and hard to manage. Shy-Drager syndrome may be difficult to diagnose in the early stages. For the majority of patients, blood pressure is low when the patients stand up and high when the patients lie down. Other symptoms that may develop include impaired speech, difficulties with breathing and swallowing, and inability to sweat.

"Shy-Drager Syndrome Information Page," National Institute of Neurological Disorders and Stroke (NINDS), reviewed 7/01/2001.

Is There Any Treatment?

Orthostatic hypotension in Shy-Drager syndrome is treatable, but effective treatment for the progression central nervous system degeneration is not known The general treatment course is aimed at controlling symptoms. Antiparkinsonian medication, such as L-dopa, may be helpful. To relieve low blood pressure while standing, dietary increases of salt and fluid may be beneficial. Medications to elevate blood pressure, such as salt-retaining steroids, are often necessary, but they can cause side effects and should be carefully monitored by a physician. Alpha-adrenergic medications, non-steroidal anti-inflammatory drugs, and sympathomimetic amines are sometimes used. Sleeping in a head-up position at night reduces morning orthostatic hypotension. An artificial feeding tube or breathing tube may be surgically inserted for management of swallowing and breathing difficulties.

What Is the Prognosis?

Shy-Drager syndrome usually ends in the patient's death by 7 to 10 years after diagnosis. Breathing problems such as aspiration, stridor (high-pitched breathing sounds due to airway obstruction), or cardiopulmonary arrest are common causes of death.

What Research Is Being Done?

The NINDS carries out and funds research about disorders of the autonomic nervous system, including Shy-Drager syndrome. This research is aimed at discovering ways to diagnose and treat disorders of the autonomic nervous system and ultimately to cure or prevent them.

Additional Information

National Dysautonomia Research Foundation
421 West 4th Street
Red Wing, MN 55066-2555
Tel: 651-267-0525
Fax: 651-267-0524
Website: www.ndrf.org
E-mail: ndrf@ndrf.org

Shy-Drager/Multiple System Atrophy Support Group, Inc.
2004 Howard Lane
Austin, TX 78728

Toll-Free: 800-288-5582
Tel: 866-SDS-4999 (737-4999)
Fax: 512-251-3315
Website: www.shy-drager.com
E-mail: Don.Summers@shy-drager.com

Worldwide Education & Awareness for Movement Disorders (WE MOVE)

204 West 84th Street
New York, NY 10024
Toll-Free: 800-437-MOV2 (6682)
Fax: 212-875-8389
Website: www.wemove.org
E-mail: wemove@wemove.org

Chapter 34

Myasthenia Gravis (MG)

In 1890, German medical professor Wilhelm Erb and two of his colleagues gave the name myasthenia gravis to a neuromuscular disease which had previously been reported by more than one physician. All three physicians noted that the "grave muscular weakness"— whether it affected the eye muscles first, or created difficulty in talking, chewing and swallowing, or in using the arms and legs—was neither hereditary nor contagious.

Myasthenia gravis and the less common Lambert-Eaton (myasthenic) syndrome are diseases affecting how nerve impulses are transmitted to muscle at the neuromuscular junction. Both are autoimmune diseases in which the body generates an immune system attack against its own skeletal muscles. Although people with myasthenia virtually always do very well when treated properly, myasthenia gravis (MG) and Lambert-Eaton syndrome (LEMS) can be life-threatening when muscle weakness interferes with respiration.

A milestone in myasthenia gravis research occurred in the early 1970s when Muscular Dystrophy Association-supported researchers discovered that the disease affected acetylcholine receptors of the skeletal muscles. Using snake venom that binds to acetylcholine receptors, they discovered that myasthenic patients had decreased numbers of these receptors. Acetylcholine receptors are protein molecules on the muscles cell's surface that contain channels which allow electrically charged sodium atoms, or ions, to flow into the cell. When sodium ions enter the muscle cells, they trigger a chain of events leading to muscle contraction. Simultaneously, another MDA-supported group found that, in rabbits, an immune attack against the acetylcholine receptors resulted in muscle membrane damage that is similar to that seen in human myasthenia gravis. Further studies of this rabbit model are responsible for a large portion of what scientists now know about myasthenia gravis.

In addition to advances in understanding myasthenia gravis and Lambert-Eaton syndrome, MDA has fostered great progress in the treatment of these disorders. These diseases are highly treatable, and for many people, the first year of muscle weakness is by far the most severe. While some other neuromuscular disorders get progressively worse over time, with proper and timely treatment, people with MG and LEMS can usually maintain good muscle function.

Questions and Answers

What Is Myasthenia Gravis?

Myasthenia gravis is a neuromuscular disease that causes weakness and fatigue, most commonly in the muscles of the eyes, face, throat and limbs. It's an autoimmune disease, meaning it's caused by an attack of the body's own immune system. MG is an acquired disease, meaning it isn't inherited as a genetic disease is inherited. MG is not contagious, and can't be passed from person to person. The word myasthenia means muscle weakness.

Who Gets Myasthenia Gravis?

MG affects people of both sexes and all ages, races, and nationalities. Women most often develop MG in their late teens and 20s, while for men onset is usually after age 60. Estimates suggest that MG currently affects about 25,000 people in the United States.

What Is an Autoimmune Disease?

An autoimmune disease occurs when the immune system, normally responsible for fighting infection, attacks the body's own tissues. Other examples of autoimmune diseases are rheumatoid arthritis, systemic lupus erythematosus, and multiple sclerosis. In MG, the immune system attack interferes with normal electrical signaling at the muscle surface.

How Does the Immune System Cause MG?

MG occurs when proteins produced by the immune system called antibodies attack the muscles' acetylcholine receptors, which normally receive messages from nerve cells. When this nerve-muscle communication is disrupted, the muscle can't contract as forcefully as it usually does. The result is muscle weakness.

What Are the Symptoms of MG?

Myasthenia gravis causes muscle weakness and rapid fatigue. The first muscles affected are usually those controlling the eyes, and the first symptoms are most often double vision or drooping eyelids. Less commonly, a person with MG first experiences weakness in the muscles of the jaw and throat, called the oropharyngeal muscles. This causes difficulty chewing, swallowing, or talking. Weakness in a limb is also a possible, but uncommon, first symptom.

For about 15 percent of people with MG, weakness remains localized in the eye muscles. For the rest, symptoms may progress over a period of one to several years, leading to limb, throat, and eye muscle weakness unless treated.

Other muscles in the face, neck, and hips may also be involved. The weakness of MG fluctuates, and is usually better in the morning or after rest, and worse at the end of the day or after exertion. Symptoms may be worsened by heat or cold, thyroid conditions, menstruation, illness, or stress.

MG doesn't affect the brain or sensory systems. The muscles of the heart and gastrointestinal tract aren't affected.

How Is MG Diagnosed?

If your doctor thinks you may have myasthenia gravis, you may want to contact your local MDA office to arrange an examination at an MDA clinic.

Diagnosis of MG begins with a careful medical history and a physical exam. A neurological exam is used to test reflexes, strength, and the distribution of weakness.

Several specialized tests are used to confirm a suspected case of MG. In one type of test, called an electromyogram, surface electrodes are used to measure the electrical activity of the muscle as it contracts in response to repeated stimulation of the nerves. In MG, the contraction response lessens as the muscle is repeatedly stimulated, illustrating how the muscle fatigues.

In the Tensilon test, a small quantity of Tensilon (edrophonium chloride) is injected. Tensilon rapidly inhibits the action of cholinesterase, the enzyme that normally breaks down acetylcholine. This temporarily restores muscle strength. A person whose strength increases after injection of Tensilon is very likely to have MG, but a negative response doesn't rule out the diagnosis.

Antibodies to the acetylcholine receptor can be detected with a blood test. About 80 percent to 90 percent of people with MG will test positive for the presence of these antibodies. Those with mild disease or only eye weakness are less likely to have detectable levels of antibodies. People with Lambert-Eaton syndrome have different antibodies that can also be found with a blood test.

Chest x-rays, CT scans, or MRI scans are used to examine the thymus and determine the presence of thymoma.

How Is MG Treated?

Up to 20 percent of all people with MG have complete remission without any treatment at all, and another 20 percent experience some improvement. For this reason, the first question in treatment is whether to treat at all. Decisions about whether, when, and how to treat MG are best made through careful discussions between the person with MG and the doctor. Available treatments include drugs, surgery, and plasma exchange.

What Drugs Are Used to Treat MG?

The usual first treatment for MG is with cholinesterase inhibitors, drugs that increase strength by preventing the normal breakdown of acetylcholine. The most commonly prescribed drug is Mestinon (pyridostigmine bromide). This is an oral drug taken four to six times per day. People with weakness of the mouth and throat muscles may be directed to take their doses shortly before eating, to improve chewing and swallowing strength.

Side effects of Mestinon may include diarrhea, increased production of saliva and mucus, and a slowing of the heart rate. This drug is helpful to most people with MG, but the benefits tend to decrease over time. Some people are unable to tolerate the side effects at an effective dose level.

Immunosuppressant drugs are another effective treatment for MG, and may be combined with cholinesterase inhibitors. The most commonly used drugs are prednisone and azathioprine.

Prednisone usually brings about rapid improvement. Once maximum improvement is achieved, the prednisone dose is reduced very gradually to the minimum effective dose, but it rarely can be eliminated entirely. This is important, since prednisone's side effects can be significant. These may include weight gain, cataracts, gastrointestinal ulcers, mood changes, hypertension, and osteoporosis.

Azathioprine (Imuran) may be used alone or together with prednisone. Azathioprine is a very slow-acting drug, and maximum improvement may take several months to a year or more to achieve. Side effects can include decreased activity of the bone marrow, liver toxicity, and flu-like symptoms. Like prednisone therapy, use of azathioprine requires close monitoring. Other immunosuppressants prescribed include cyclosporine and cyclophosphamide.

A less frequently prescribed treatment for MG is intravenous immunoglobulin (IVIg), a mixture of human blood proteins injected in large quantity into the bloodstream over two to five days. Improvement usually follows within a week, and may last for weeks to months. Side effects are usually minor, and include headache, fever, and nausea. IVIg therapy is very expensive, and is usually used for short-term benefit, to get patients over a difficult period of weakness or to improve a person's strength before surgery. It's also used as an emergency treatment for myasthenic crisis.

What about Plasmapheresis?

Plasmapheresis (also called plasma exchange) is a blood filtering treatment that removes antibodies from the blood. A course of plasmapheresis requires a hospital stay, during which a large intravenous line is placed in a chest or leg vein. Five sessions of plasmapheresis are usually performed, spaced over seven to 10 days. During each, 3 to 4 liters of blood are removed and purified before being returned to the body.

Improvement in strength usually follows within a week and lasts four to eight weeks. The major side effect is low blood pressure. Like IVIg, plasmapheresis is quite expensive, and is usually done only to treat myasthenic crisis, to boost strength before surgery, or if drugs can't provide symptom relief.

The Effect of MG on Muscle Function

Nerve cells link up with muscles at special sites called neuromuscular junctions. (See Figure 34.1) Here, in order to stimulate movement, nerve cells release small packets of a chemical called acetylcholine from their endings. Acetylcholine stimulates a protein on the muscle surface, called the acetylcholine receptor. This triggers a set of reactions in the muscle cell, causing it to contract. To prevent prolonged muscle response to a single nerve signal, acetylcholine is then broken down by an enzyme known as cholinesterase. (Cholinesterase is an important target for drugs used to treat MG.)

In MG, antibodies bind (attach themselves) to the acetylcholine receptors, triggering damage or loss of the receptors, and preventing them from responding to acetylcholine. Although acetylcholine stimulates the remaining receptors, they are reduced in number and the result is weakness in muscle contraction. The weakness increases on repeated effort, a phenomenon known as fatigue. Drugs that block the enzyme cholinesterase allow acetylcholine to remain intact for a

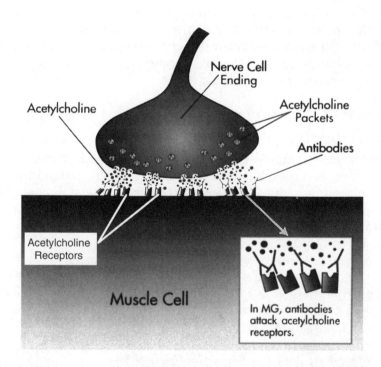

Figure 34.1. Neuromuscular Junction. Normally, acetylcholine flows from nerve to muscle to cause muscle contraction. In MG, antibodies attack the receptors (docking sites) for acetylcholine, leading to muscle weakness.

longer time, and to stimulate the remaining receptors repeatedly. This results in partial improvement of muscle function.

What Is the Thymus, and How Is It Involved in MG?

The thymus is a small gland in the upper chest and lower neck that is part of the immune system. Abnormalities of the thymus occur in 75 percent of people with MG. Eighty-five percent of these abnormalities involve an excess number of cells in the thymus. The other 15 percent are actual thymus tumors, called thymomas. These tumors are benign (not cancer). While the exact connection is still unclear, it's likely that these thymus abnormalities are somehow related to development of MG. Thymectomy—removal of the thymus gland—is an important option in MG therapy, even when no thymoma is found.

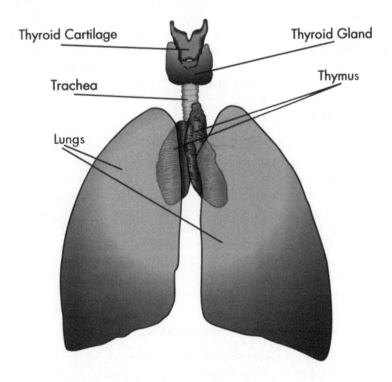

Figure 34.2. *Thymus Gland. The thymus, a small gland in the upper chest, seems to play a role in myasthenia gravis.*

Is Thymectomy Recommended for MG?

Thymectomy (removal of the thymus gland) is recommended for virtually all people with thymomas. It's also increasingly seen as an appropriate initial treatment in a person without thymoma who is younger than age 60 with generalized weakness from MG. Thymectomy is sometimes recommended for those over 60 as well.

About 30 percent of all MG patients who undergo thymectomy may experience clinical remission, and another 50 percent have some improvement. The improvement takes place over a long period of time from many months to years. This surgery requires a stay in the hospital of several days, and a recovery period of several weeks.

What Is the Role of Physical Therapy and other Nonmedical Treatments?

Until medical treatment restores function, swallowing and speech problems may be addressed by a speech therapist, and a nutritionist can help design appetizing meals that are easy to swallow. A physical therapist can design stretching and exercise programs to maintain strength and range of motion, while an occupational therapist suggests adaptive equipment and modifications for the home or workplace to accommodate changes in abilities.

What Is Myasthenic Crisis?

Myasthenic crisis is a potentially life-threatening complication of MG in which the respiratory muscles become too weak to support adequate breathing or the ability to swallow is lost. This is most commonly brought on by a respiratory infection or a change in medication.

Myasthenic crisis is most likely to occur in a person who already has weak oropharyngeal muscles, and may be preceded by increased difficulty swallowing, speaking, or coughing. The onset of a crisis is marked by shortness of breath and difficulty breathing or coughing. If patients are adequately treated during the course of MG, myasthenic crisis is rare.

How Is Myasthenic Crisis Treated?

Myasthenic crisis requires emergency medical attention. Most people in myasthenic crisis require intubation—the placement of a tube into the airway—and the use of a mechanical ventilator to compensate for the weakened respiratory muscles. Intubation may be needed for one to two weeks or more. Drug treatment is used to rapidly improve weakness, and often includes either plasmapheresis or IVIg treatment.

What Is the Usual Course of Myasthenia Gravis?

Most people with MG who receive good medical care are able to lead full, productive lives. The maximum degree of weakness occurs in the first year for about two-thirds of patients. Most people are able to effectively control their symptoms, although some residual weakness may occur in the most severely involved muscles. Weakness serious enough to require a wheelchair is almost unheard of.

Changes in medication may be necessary as time goes on. As noted, improvement or remission is possible for many people with MG, although relapse may occur if the dosage of immunosuppressive medication is reduced below the minimum effective level. The best outlook is for younger people and those without thymoma.

What about Pregnancy and MG?

Symptoms of MG may first appear during pregnancy. For reasons researchers don't understand, pregnancy improves MG symptoms in about one-third of women who already have MG, worsens them in another third, and has no effect in the rest. The effects of one pregnancy can't be used to predict the effects during later ones.

Cholinesterase inhibitors and prednisone are safe to use during pregnancy, but azathioprine is not recommended. Although the uterus isn't affected by MG, delivery can be complicated by weakness of voluntary muscles. Weakness may be worse after delivery.

About 20 percent of infants born to women with MG have temporary weakness because they have absorbed some antibodies from the mother. This can be treated, and isn't associated with development of MG later in the child's life. This temporary form of infant MG isn't the same as a congenital myasthenic syndrome, which is due to an inherited gene defect.

Can Some Drugs Worsen Symptoms of MG?

Yes. A number of drugs increase muscle weakness and should be avoided or used with caution. These include certain antibiotics, cardiovascular drugs, muscle relaxants, and antiseizure medications. Doctors or dentists prescribing any drug for a person with MG should be familiar with its potential for worsening MG symptoms.

A Medic Alert bracelet or card can be used to inform emergency personnel that a person has MG and explain the danger of drug complications. A card can list not only the diagnosis, but also current medications, allergies, the phone number of the treating neurologist, and other critical information.

What Is Lambert-Eaton Syndrome?

Lambert-Eaton syndrome (LEMS), also known as myasthenic syndrome, is a rare autoimmune disease whose symptoms are somewhat similar to those of MG. In LEMS, antibodies attack a protein on the surface of the nerve endings that regulates levels of calcium. Inactivation of this calcium channel protein prevents the nerve cells from releasing normal amounts of acetylcholine.

The muscle weakness caused by LEMS most often appears in the thighs and hips, and rarely affects the eye muscles early in the disease. Weakness spreads as the disease progresses, but eye, jaw, and throat weakness is not as severe as in MG. The weakness usually improves temporarily after a brief exertion, unlike in MG. LEMS also usually affects several involuntary body functions, causing dry mouth, low blood pressure upon standing (postural hypotension), and impotence in men.

LEMS affects men and women about equally often, and usually begins in middle age. Cancer is found in about 40 percent of people with LEMS, either at the time of diagnosis or within several years afterward. Most of these cancers are small-cell lung cancers, although other types of cancer may occur. Since cancer is so often associated with LEMS, people with LEMS should have frequent checkups to monitor for the presence of malignancies. Successful treatment of a malignancy often leads to improvement in the symptoms of LEMS.

Treatments for LEMS may include cholinesterase inhibitors, although these are less likely to lead to improvement than in MG. Guanidine hydrochloride and 3,4-diaminopyridine both increase acetylcholine release, and may be effective. Prednisone and azathioprine may be useful, as may other immunosuppressive drugs. Plasmapheresis and IVIg have also shown temporary effectiveness.

What Are Congenital Myasthenic Syndromes?

The congenital myasthenic syndromes are a group of disorders resulting from inherited gene defects. The symptoms of congenital myasthenic syndromes are similar to those of MG, but begin during infancy or early childhood.

The congenital myasthenic syndromes include a wide variety of inherited disorders involving the acetylcholine receptor of the enzyme cholinesterase. In general, these disorders are inherited in an autosomal recessive pattern, meaning that the affected child must inherit two defective gene copies, one from each parent, neither of whom will show signs of the disease. Diagnosis of the specific nature of the gene defect is important, since the treatments depend on the exact nature of the defect. In fact, treatments that are effective for some forms of congenital myasthenic syndromes are actually harmful in other forms.

The Immune System in Myasthenia Gravis

The immune system is a group of organs and cells located throughout the body, including the thymus, spleen, bone marrow, lymph glands, and circulating white blood cells. Normally the immune system detects and attacks foreign substances, such as viruses and bacteria. In MG, the immune system's antibodies mistakenly attack the part of the muscle that receives messages from nerves, called the acetylcholine receptor.

While scientists know that antibodies are the problem in MG, it's still not clear how the immune system is stimulated to make these antibodies in the first place. Most researchers think that development of MG probably involves several factors. While MG isn't an inherited disease, it's possible that having certain immune system genes increases a person's likelihood of developing MG, given other triggers.

Many researchers believe that a further risk for MG arises in the thymus, a gland located in the chest. Normally, the thymus screens out and destroys cells that can react against the body's own tissues. If this screening process misses those cells that can make antibodies to the muscle receptor, the stage is set for a later autoimmune reaction. The thymus plays an active role in this part of immune system development, and researchers suspect that thymus abnormalities play a major role in the development of MG.

Genetic susceptibility and thymus abnormalities probably combine with other, still unidentified factors to trigger MG. MDA has funded pioneering studies into the causes of MG, and continues to lead in the quest for further understanding of its complex details.

Chapter 35

Post-Polio Syndrome

What Is Post-Polio Syndrome?

Post-polio syndrome (PPS) is a condition that affects polio survivors anywhere from 10 to 40 years after recovery from an initial paralytic attack of the poliomyelitis virus. PPS is characterized by a further weakening of muscles that were previously affected by the polio infection. Symptoms include fatigue, slowly progressive muscle weakness, and, at times, muscular atrophy. Joint pain and increasing skeletal deformities such as scoliosis are common. Some patients experience only minor symptoms, while others develop spinal muscular atrophy, and very rarely, what appears to be, but is not, a form of amyotrophic lateral sclerosis (ALS), also called Lou Gehrig's disease. PPS is rarely life threatening.

The extent to which polio survivors will suffer from PPS depends on how seriously they were affected by the original polio attack. Patients who had only minimal symptoms from the original attack and subsequently develop PPS will most likely experience only mild PPS symptoms. People originally hit hard by the polio virus, who were left with severe residual weakness, may develop a more severe case of PPS with a greater loss of muscle function, difficulty in swallowing, and more periods of fatigue.

"Post-Polio Syndrome," Fact Sheet, National Institute of Neurological Disorders and Stroke (NINDS), NIH Publication No. 96-4030, updated June 2000, reviewed July 1, 2001.

More than 300,000 polio survivors in the United States may be at risk for PPS. Doctors are unable to establish a firm incidence rate, but they estimate that the condition affects 25 percent to 50 percent of these survivors, or possibly more depending on how the disorder is defined.

What Causes PPS?

PPS is caused by the death of individual nerve terminals in the motor units that remain after the initial attack of polio. This deterioration of individual nerve terminals might be an outcome of the recovery process from the acute polio attack. During this recovery process, in an effort to compensate for the loss of nerve cells (neurons), surviving motor neurons sprout new endings to restore function to muscles. This results in large motor units that may add stress to the neuronal cell body. As a result of this rejuvenation, the individual may have normal functioning muscles for some time. But after a number of years, the motor neurons with excessive sprouting may not be able to maintain the metabolic demands of all their new sprouts, and a slow deterioration of the individual terminals may result.

Restoration of nerve function may occur in some fibers a second time, but eventually nerve terminals are destroyed and permanent weakness occurs. This hypothesis is consistent with PPS's slow, stepwise, unpredictable course. Through years of studies, scientists at the National Institute of Neurological Disorders and Stroke have shown that PPS is a very slowly progressing condition marked by long periods of stability.

How Is PPS Diagnosed?

Doctors arrive at a diagnosis of PPS by observing the patient and asking about symptoms, and by excluding other disorders. PPS may be difficult to diagnose in some because it is hard to determine what component of a neuromuscular deficit is old and what is new. Health professionals say that the only way to be sure a person has PPS is through a neurological examination aided by other laboratory studies that exclude all other possible diagnoses. Patients must visit the doctor periodically to establish that their muscle weakness is progressive.

Objective assessment of muscle strength in PPS patients may not be easy. A change in muscle strength is determined in specific muscle groups, or limbs, using various muscle scales, such as the Medical

Research Council (MRC) scale or scales that quantify muscle force. Doctors use magnetic resonance imaging (MRI), neuroimaging, and electrophysiological studies, muscle biopsies, or spinal fluid analysis as tools to investigate the course of decline in muscle strength and exclude other conditions.

Once PPS is diagnosed, some patients worry that they have polio again, or even ALS. In fact, they have neither of these disorders. In general, PPS is not life-threatening. The only exception is in patients left with severe residual respiratory difficulties, who may experience new severe respiratory impairment. Studies have proven that, compared to control populations, PPS patients lack any elevation of antibodies against the polio virus, and since PPS affects only certain muscle groups, it is not considered a recurrence of the original polio. Further, there is no evidence that the polio virus can cause a persistent infection in humans. Other studies have demonstrated that ALS, which progressively weakens muscles, does not occur more frequently in PPS patients, and PPS is not a form of ALS.

How Is PPS Treated?

Scientists are working on a wide variety of treatment possibilities for patients with PPS, including drug treatments, some of which show promise. Doctors at the National Institutes of Health (NIH) have tried treating PPS patients with alpha 2 recombinant interferon, but the treatment proved ineffective. A study in which PPS patients received high doses of prednisone demonstrated a mild improvement in their condition, but the results were not statistically significant. This, in addition to the drug's side effects, led researchers to recommend that prednisone not be used to treat PPS.

In an effort to reduce fatigue in PPS patients, scientists conducted a study using low doses of the drug pyridostigmine (Mestinon). A large, controlled study that has been recently completed showed that pyridostigmine is not helpful for PPS patients. In a controlled study conducted by NIH scientists, the drug amantadine also was not helpful in reducing fatigue.

The future in PPS treatment may center around nerve growth factors. One small study that NINDS scientists participated in showed that insulin-like growth factor (IGF-1), which can enhance the ability of motor neurons to sprout new branches and maintain existing branches, was not helpful. Since PPS results from the degeneration of nerve sprouts, other growth factors may target the heart of the problem and help to regenerate new nerve sprouts.

385

What Is the Role of Exercise in the Treatment of PPS?

There has been much debate about whether to encourage or discourage exercise for polio survivors or individuals who already have PPS. Some doctors believe that too much exercise can worsen the patient's condition, and that rest will preserve energy. These doctors think patients will wear out their muscles by overusing them in exercise activities. However, others consider this notion unfounded and not scientifically documented.

Researchers at the NIH recently conducted a study of exercise in PPS, not only to determine if exercise is helpful, harmful, or ineffective, but also to define the most effective type—isotonic, isometric, isokinetic, or repetitive. Their study showed that exercise is safe and effective, and other investigators have had similar findings. A commonsense approach, in which patients use individual tolerance as their limit, is currently recommended. Tolerance is the level at which one starts having discomfort or fatigue.

Can PPS Be Prevented?

People who are polio survivors often ask if there is a way to prevent PPS. Presently, no prevention has been found. But doctors recommend that polio survivors follow standard healthy lifestyle practices: consuming a well-balanced diet, exercising in moderation, and visiting a doctor regularly.

What Research Is Being Conducted?

Scientists are working on a variety of investigations that may someday help individuals with PPS. Some basic researchers are studying the behavior of motor neurons many years after a polio attack. Others are looking at the mechanism of fatigue, and trying to tease out information from the brain, muscles, and neuromuscular junction (the site where a nerve cell meets the muscle cell it helps activate). Trying to determine if there is an immunological link in PPS is also an area of intense interest. Researchers who discovered inflammation around motor neurons in the muscle are trying to find out if this is due to an immunological response.

Other investigators are searching for the polio virus, or mutated versions of it, fragments of which have been amplified from the spinal fluid. The significance of this finding is not known however, and more research is being done.

Additional Information

Brain Resources and Information Network (BRAIN)
P.O. Box 5801
Bethesda, MD 20824
Toll-Free: 800-352-9424
TTY: 301-468-5981
Website: www.ninds.nih.gov

International Polio Network/Gazette International
4207 Lindell Boulevard, #110
St. Louis, MO 63108-2915
Tel: 314-534-0475
Fax: 314-534-5070
Website: www.post-polio.org
E-mail: gini_intl@msn.com

Polio Connection of America
P.O. Box 182
Howard Beach, NY 11414
Tel: 718-835-5536
Website: www.geocities.com/w1066w
E-mail: w1066polio@hotmail.com

Chapter 36

Progressive Supranuclear Palsy (PSP)

What Is PSP?

PSP is a rare, degenerative brain disorder related to Parkinson's disease. It strikes middle-aged adults and the elderly, slightly more men than women and affects 6.4 in 100,000. Its cause remains a mystery and although there is no cure, symptoms can often be helped. There are estimated to be 20,000 people with PSP in the United States, but only 3,000-4,000 have been diagnosed. In 1963, Dr. John C. Steele, Dr. J.C. Richardson, and Dr. J. Olszewski identified PSP as a distinct neurological disorder. Dudley Moore, famous actor and musician, was diagnosed with PSP in 1999. He passed away in 2002 from pneumonia, a complication of PSP.

What Are the Symptoms?

Early symptoms include falling, difficulty walking, imbalance, and slow movement, similar to Parkinson's disease. People with PSP experience vision problems such as double and blurred vision, as well as difficulty with speech and swallowing. There may also be changes in mood and behavior. In its advanced stages, persons with PSP are bedridden or in wheelchairs and require full-time care.

"Facts about Progressive Supranuclear Palsy (PSP)," and "Progressive Supranuclear Palsy: Some Answers," by Lawrence I. Golbe, MD, © 2000 Society for Progressive Supranuclear Palsy, reprinted with permission. Both documents are available online at the Society for Progressive Supranuclear Palsy's website at www.psp.org.

How Is PSP Diagnosed?

PSP is usually diagnosed by a neurologist. There is no diagnostic test other than the clinical evaluation. Typical findings include features of Parkinson's with limb stiffness, slowness, imbalance, and trouble walking with limitation of upward and downward eye movements.

What Does Progressive Supranuclear Palsy Mean?

Progressive—the symptoms get slowly worse over time, from diagnosis to late stages, typically three to ten years.

Supranuclear—the area of the brainstem that controls up and down eye movements.

Palsy—a weakness, referring to the palsy of moving the eyes.

Can People Die from PSP?

Yes. People with PSP die from complications of immobility and the inability to swallow, including pneumonia and aspiration.

What Is the Treatment?

At present, there is no treatment that can reverse the effects of this disease, yet, a variety of medications and other forms of therapy can help the symptoms.

What Problems Are Unique to Persons with PSP and Their Families?

Because PSP is a rare disease, there is often a delay before the diagnosis is made. Without an early diagnosis and adequate information, families cannot anticipate the future course of the disease and therefore, are unable to plan. Furthermore, people with PSP may live hundreds of miles from each other and knowledgeable health care professionals causing feelings of loneliness and isolation.

How Can the Society for Progressive Supranuclear Palsy Help?

As a worldwide organization, the Society sponsors medical research and provides information, education, support, and advocacy to persons with PSP, their families, and caregivers. The Society educates physicians and allied health professionals on PSP and how to improve care.

Some Answers

It is unlikely that any of the approximately 20,000 people in the United States who have been diagnosed as having progressive supranuclear palsy had ever heard of that disease before. In fact, most patients with PSP report that their family doctors knew nothing about PSP until a neurologist made the diagnosis. Moreover, the neurologist probably thought the diagnosis was Parkinson's disease until several years into the illness. Recently, more and more has appeared in medical journals to help doctors remedy their unfamiliarity with PSP. This chapter was written to help patients and their families do the same.

Why Has No One Heard of PSP?

PSP is poorly known because it is rare—only about 4-5 percent as common as Parkinson's disease—and because even when it does occur, it is often misdiagnosed. This is gradually changing. As more doctors become familiar with PSP, it will be diagnosed more readily. No one even realized it existed until 1964, when several patients were first described at a national neurology research convention and the disease received its name. In retrospect, at least 12 cases of PSP had appeared in the medical literature since 1909, but because of its resemblance to Parkinson's disease, no one had recognized it as a distinct disease until the 1960s.

What Are the Common Early Symptoms of PSP?

The most common first symptom, occurring, on average, in the 60s, is loss of balance while walking. This may take the form of unexplained falls or of a stiffness and awkwardness in the walk that can resemble Parkinson's disease. Sometimes the falls are described by the person experiencing them as attacks of dizziness. This often prompts the doctor to suspect an inner ear problem or hardening of the arteries supplying the brain.

Other common early symptoms are forgetfulness and changes in personality. The latter can take the form of a loss of interest in ordinary pleasurable activities or increased irritability and cantankerousness. These mental changes are misinterpreted as depression or even as senility. Less common early symptoms are trouble with eyesight, slurring of speech, and mild shaking of the hands. Difficulty driving a car, with several accidents or near misses, is common early in the course of PSP. The exact reason for this problem is not clear.

What Happens Next?

The term progressive was included in the name of the disease because, unfortunately, the early symptoms get worse and new symptoms develop sooner or later. After 7 to 9 years, on average, the imbalance and stiffness worsen to make walking very difficult or impossible. If trouble with eyesight was not present early on, it eventually develops in almost all cases and can sometimes be as disabling as the movement difficulty. Difficulty with speech and swallowing are additional important features of PSP that occur eventually in most patients.

What Does the Name Supranuclear Palsy Mean?

In general, a palsy is a weakness or paralysis of a part of the body. The term supranuclear refers to the nature of the eye problem in PSP. Although some patients with PSP describe their symptom as blurring, the actual problem is an inability to aim the eyes properly because of weakness or paralysis (palsy) of the muscles that move the eyeballs. These muscles are controlled by nerve cells residing in clusters or nuclei (NUKE-lee-eye) near the base of the brain, in the brainstem. Most other brain problems that affect the eye movements originate in those nuclei, but in PSP the problem lies in parts of the brain that control those eye-movement nuclei themselves. These higher control areas are what the prefix supra in supranuclear refers to.

Sometimes complicated disease names are avoided by the use of the name of the physician who discovered the disease. However, for PSP, there were three such physicians and the string of names— Steele, Richardson, and Olszewski (ol-SHEF-skee)—is even less convenient than the descriptive name. It is only rarely used in the U.S., but in Great Britain it is the more commonly used term. Continental Europe and the rest of the world seem to use PSP and SRO equally frequently.

Incidentally, although Drs. Richardson and Olszewski are deceased, Dr. John C. Steele, who was a neurology resident (i.e., a trainee) when he collaborated in the original description of PSP, still does neurological research and serves as Honorary Chairman of the Society for PSP.

Is the Visual Problem the Most Important Part of PSP?

In most cases the visual problem is at least as important as the walking difficulty, though it does not appear, on average, until 3 to 5 years after the walking problem. Because the main difficulty with the eyes is in aiming them properly, reading often becomes difficult. The patient finds it hard to shift down to the beginning of the next line automatically after reaching the end of the first line. This is very different from just needing reading glasses. An eye doctor unfamiliar with PSP may be baffled by the patient's complaint of being unable to read a newspaper despite normal ability to read the individual letters on an eye chart. Some patients have their mild cataracts extracted in a vain effort to relieve such a visual problem.

Another common visual problem is an inability to maintain eye contact during conversation. This can give the mistaken impression that the patient is senile, hostile, or uninterested. The same eye movement problem can create the symptom of tunnel vision and can interfere with driving a car.

The most common eye movement problem in PSP is an impaired ability to move the eyes up or down. This can interfere with eating or with descending a flight of stairs, among other things. This problem is not usually as vexing for the patient and family as the inability to maintain eye contact or to coordinate eye movements while reading, but is much easier for the doctor to detect. This reduction in vertical eye movement is usually the first clue to the doctor that the diagnosis is PSP. Other conditions, particularly Parkinson's disease and normal aging, can sometimes cause difficulty moving the eyes up. However, PSP is nearly unique in also causing problems moving the eyes down.

Yet another eye problem in PSP can be abnormal eyelid movement either too much or too little. A few patients experience forceful involuntary closing of the eyes for a few seconds or minutes at a time, called blepharospasm. Others have difficulty opening the eyes, even though the lids seem to be relaxed, and will try to use the muscles of the forehead, or even the fingers, in an effort to open the eyelids (apraxia of lid opening). About 20 percent of patients with PSP eventually develop one of these problems. Others, on the contrary, have trouble closing the eyes and blink very little. While about 15 to 25 blinks per minute is normal, people with PSP blink, on average, only about 3 or 4 times per minute. This can allow the eyes to become irritated. They often react by producing extra tears, which can itself become annoying.

393

What about the Speech Problems?

The same general area of the brain that controls eye movement also controls movements of the mouth, tongue, and throat, and these movements also weaken in PSP. Speech becomes slurred in most patients after 3 or 4 years, on average, although it is the first symptom in a few patients. In Parkinson's disease, the speech problem is characterized by soft volume and rapid succession of words. In PSP, however, the speech may have an irregular, explosive quality (called spastic speech) or a drunken quality (ataxic speech) or may have the features of speech in Parkinson's disease. Most commonly, there is a combination of at least two of these three features in the speech of PSP.

An erroneous impression of senility in PSP can be created by the combination of the speech difficulty, the slight forgetfulness, the slow (albeit accurate) mental responses, the personality change, and the poor eye contact during conversation.

What about the Swallowing Problems?

Swallowing tough foods or thin liquids can become difficult because of throat muscle weakness or incoordination. This tends to occur later than the walking, visual, and speech problems, but can become very troublesome if the patient tends to choke on food. Unlike the other difficulties in PSP, this one can sometimes pose a danger for the patient—the danger of food going down the wrong pipe into the breathing passages, termed aspiration. Usually, difficulty managing thin liquids precedes difficulty with solid food. This is because in PSP, the swallowing muscles have difficulty creating a watertight seal separating the path to the stomach from the path to the lungs. The same is true for the swallowing difficulty of many neurological diseases. For non-neurologic conditions such as stricture of the esophagus, however, difficulties start with solid foods.

Repeated, minor, often unnoticed episodes of small amounts of food and drink dripping into the lungs can cause pneumonia. Often, it is not apparent to the physician or family that the PSP patient's pneumonia is in fact the result of subtle aspiration. But aspiration pneumonia, in fact, is the most common cause of death in PSP.

Does PSP Lead to Dementia as in Alzheimer's Disease?

Although mental confusion in patients with PSP is more apparent than real, most patients do eventually develop a mild or moderate degree of mental impairment. Some are mislabeled as having Alzheimer's disease. This is not very different from the situation in Parkinson's disease.

In PSP, the dementia, if it does occur, does not feature the memory problem that is so apparent in Alzheimer's disease. Rather, the dementia of PSP is characterized by slowed thought and difficulty synthesizing several different ideas into a new idea or plan. These mental functions are performed mostly by the front part of the brain (the frontal lobes). In Alzheimer's, on the other hand, the problem is mostly in the part of the brain just above the ears (the temporal lobes), where memory functions are concentrated.

Alzheimer's disease also includes either difficulty with language (such as trouble recalling correct names of common objects) or difficulty finding one's way around a previous familiar environment. Fortunately, these symptoms almost never occur in PSP.

Slowing of thought can cause major problems for people with PSP by making it difficult to partake in conversation. A question may be answered with great accuracy and detail, but with a delay of several minutes.

How Is PSP Different from Parkinson's Disease?

Early on, PSP may be difficult to distinguish from Parkinson's disease and indeed, PSP is an important cause of parkinsonism. Both PSP and Parkinson's disease cause stiffness, slowness, and clumsiness. However, shaking (tremor), while prominent in most people with Parkinson's disease, is rare in PSP. When tremor does occur in PSP, it is usually quite irregular, mild, and present only when the hand is in use, not at rest as in Parkinson's disease. Patients with PSP usually stand up straight or occasionally even tilt the head backwards and tend to fall backwards, while those with Parkinson's usually are bent forwards. The problems with vision, speech, and swallowing are much more common and severe in PSP than in Parkinson's. Parkinson's causes more difficulty using the hands and more stiffness in the limbs than does PSP. Finally, the main treatment for Parkinson's disease, Sinemet (and a few other drugs) is of much less benefit in PSP.

Parkinson's disease responds better to Sinemet than does PSP because in PD, deficiency of dopamine is by far the most important abnormality, and Sinemet is an excellent way to replace brain dopamine. In PSP, however, deficiencies of several other brain chemicals are at least as severe as the dopamine deficiency, and no good way exists to replace those. Also, in PSP, the brain cells that receive the dopamine-encoded messages are damaged, while these remain intact in Parkinson's.

What about Treatment with Medication?

Several medications, all available only by prescription, can help PSP in some cases.

Sinemet. This is the brand name for a combination of levodopa and carbidopa. Levodopa is the component that helps the disease symptoms. Carbidopa simply helps prevent the nausea that levodopa alone can cause. When levodopa came along in the late 1960s, it was a revolutionary advance for Parkinson's, but unfortunately it is of only modest benefit in PSP. It can help the slowness, stiffness, and balance problems of PSP to a degree, but usually not the mental, speech, visual, or swallowing difficulties. It usually loses its benefit after two or three years, but a few patients with PSP never fully lose their responsiveness to Sinemet.

Some patients with PSP require large dosages, up to 1,500 mg. of levodopa as Sinemet per day, to see an improvement, so the dosage should be pushed to at least that level, under the close supervision of a physician, unless a benefit or intolerable side effects occur sooner. The most common side effects of Sinemet in patients with PSP are confusion, hallucinations, and dizziness. These generally disappear after the drug is stopped. The most common side effect in patients with Parkinson's disease, involuntary writhing movements (chorea or dyskinesias) occur very rarely in PSP, even at high Sinemet dosages.

Patients with PSP should generally receive the standard Sinemet (levodopa/carbidopa) preparation rather than the controlled-release (Sinemet CR) form. The CR form is absorbed from the intestine into the blood slowly and can be useful for people with Parkinson's disease who respond well to Sinemet but need to prolong the number of hours of benefit from each dose. In PSP, however, such response fluctuations almost never occur. Because CR is sometimes absorbed very little or erratically, a poor Sinemet CR response in a patient with PSP might be incorrectly blamed on the fact that the disease is usually unresponsive to the drug. Such a patient might actually respond to the standard form, which reaches the brain in a more predictable pattern.

Dopamine receptor agonists. There are four such drugs on the market—Parlodel (generic name, bromocriptine), Permax (pergolide), Mirapex (pramipexole), and Requip (ropinirole). These are helpful in most people with Parkinson's disease, but in PSP they rarely give any benefit beyond that provided by Sinemet. However, a large trial of Mirapex in PSP has been completed at a number of North American medical centers. The results are pending and will be reported in the newsletter of the Society for PSP.

The main possible side effects of Mirapex and the other dopamine receptor agonists are hallucinations and confusion, which can be more troublesome for PSP than for Parkinson's, excessive involuntary movements, dizziness, and nausea.

Antidepressants. Another group of drugs that has been of some modest success in PSP are the antidepressant drugs. The anti-PSP benefit of these drugs is not related to their ability to relieve depression. The best antidepressant drug for the movement problems of PSP is probably Elavil (generic name, amitriptyline). It has been used against depression since the early 1960s. The dosage should start at 10 mg once daily, preferably at bedtime. It can be increased slowly and taken divided into at least two doses per day. Past 80 mg per day, the likelihood of side effects increases to an unacceptable level for most patients. Elavil is also a good sleep medication for elderly people and may provide this benefit in PSP if taken at bedtime. One important side effect in some people is constipation. Others are dry mouth, confusion and difficulty urinating (in men).

Symmetrel. This drug (generic name, amantadine) has been used for Parkinson's since the 1960s. Because it affects more than just the dopamine system, it can be effective in PSP even if Sinemet is not. It seems to help the gait disorder more than anything else. However, its benefit generally lasts only a few months. Its principal potential side effects are dry mouth, constipation, confusion, and swelling of the ankles.

Ambien. This sleeping pill (genetic name, zolpidem) was found in one double-blind trial to help some aspects of PSP. It is worth a try, starting with a bedtime dose of 5 mg and moving that dose to the morning if there is not intolerable sleepiness.

Nicotine patch. This drug, sold as a smoking cessation aid, can help increase the alertness of a few patients with PSP, but can cause intolerable jitteriness.

Experimental drugs. In the past ten years, research trials have been completed with the drugs physostigmine, idazoxan, and methysergide.

While each showed initial promise and prompted an optimistic article or two in a prestigious neurological journal, none has proven effective enough to justify use in patients. The most recent trial was of efaroxan, a drug similar to idazoxan, but it, too, proven ineffective. Cognex and Aricept, each modestly useful against the dementia of Alzheimer's disease, have been found not to help the mental difficulties of PSP.

Botox. A different sort of drug that can be useful for people whose PSP is complicated by blepharospasm is Botox (botulinum toxin). This substance is produced by certain bacteria that can contaminate food. Its poisonous action occurs because it weakens muscles. A very dilute solution of the toxin can be carefully injected by a neurologist into the eyelid muscles as a temporary remedy for abnormal involuntary eyelid closure.

Botox can also be used for involuntary fuming or bending of the head that occurs in PSP, but injection of Botox into the neck muscles can sometimes cause slight weakness of the swallowing muscles, which are nearby. In PSP, where swallowing is already impaired in many patients, caution should be used when considering use of Botox in neck muscles.

Is Tube Feeding Advisable for Advanced Patients?

An operation that may be advised for extreme cases of poor swallowing where choking is a definite risk is the placement of a tube through the skin of the abdomen into the stomach [gastrostomy or percutaneous endoscopic gastrostomy (PEG)] for feeding purposes. PEG feeding may allow patients to regain lost weight, avoid hunger, and receive the nourishment they need to fight off other potential complications of PSP. A patient who is receiving the necessary nutrients and fluids is much happier and stronger overall and will probably find general movement, speech, and thinking easier.

PEG placement may be considered when any of the following occur: aspiration pneumonia; small amounts of aspiration with each swallow; significant weight loss from insufficient feeding; or when a meal requires so much time that the functioning of the household is disrupted.

The PEG tube can be inserted with the patient awake but sedated, often as an outpatient procedure. The tube is clamped shut and hidden under the clothes when not in use. The feeding can easily be managed at home by pureeing the family's regular food in a blender and injecting it into the tube with what looks like a basting syringe. The skin site where the tube enters requires only a little care that can easily be provided by a family member or even by the patient. If the need for tube feeding disappears (as through a new medication, for example), normal oral feeding can be resumed and the tube can be kept as a backup or removed.

The potential downside of tube feedings for some patients is a loss of the feeling of wholeness or humanity. The issue of how much additional quality will be introduced into the patient's life is one that must be considered carefully. The family, physician, and if possible the patient must all voice their opinions. It may be useful to note that some nursing homes will advise PEG placement because it reduces the personnel time needed to feed the patients and because third-party payors often will pay an additional fee for tube feeding but not for the time-consuming task of hand feeding a patient by mouth.

What about Other Non-Drug Treatment?

Probably the most important part of dealing with PSP is for the patient's family to understand that the problems with visual inattention and personality changes are part of the illness. The patient is not lacking willpower nor faking. Furthermore, many of the problems in PSP are intermittent and can be aggravated by the patient's mental or emotional state. For example, walking, writing, and eating may be poor one hour and better the next. The family should understand that these fluctuations are not under the patient's conscious control and that nagging and shouting usually just make matters worse. A wise policy is to be prepared to take advantage of the good periods to have an outing, a relaxing shower, or some other activity that would be more difficult during the bad times.

Walking aids are often important for patients with PSP. Because of the tendency to fall backwards, if a walker is required it should be weighted in front with sandbags over the lower rung. A better but more expensive solution is a large, heavy walker resembling a small shopping cart with three or four fat, soft rubber wheels and a hand brake. The tendency to fall backwards can also be countered by the use of built-up heels. Leg braces are not helpful because the problem in PSP is coordination and balance rather than actual muscle weakness.

Shoes with smooth soles are often better than rubber soled athletic shoes. In many people with PSP, the gait disorder includes some element of freezing, a phenomenon that makes it difficult to lift a foot from the ground to initiate gait. Such people can fall if they move their body forward before the foot moves. In these cases, a smooth sole could make it easier to slide the first foot forward.

Handrails installed in the home, especially in the bathroom, may also be helpful. The difficulty in looking down dictates that low objects such as throw rugs and low coffee tables be removed from the patient's living space.

To remedy the difficulty of looking down, bifocals or special glasses called prisms are sometimes prescribed for people with PSP. These are sometimes worth trying, but are usually of limited value because there is not only a problem moving the eyes in PSP, but also a problem directing the person's attention (the mind's eye) to objects located below the eyes. If this additional problem exists, special glasses would not help.

Formal physical therapy is of no proven benefit in PSP, but certain exercises done in the home by oneself on a regular schedule can keep the joints limber. Exercise also has a clear psychological benefit that improves the sense of well-being of anyone with a chronic illness. For specific exercises, consult one of the books for patients with Parkinson's disease or the pamphlets distributed by the national Parkinson organizations.

Do Any of the New Brain Operations for Parkinson's Work for PSP?

Not so far, unfortunately. The fetal brain tissue transplant operation for Parkinson's disease has been tried in a few patients with PSP without success. The reason is undoubtedly that in PSP there is other, equally important, damage in the brain cells that would receive the signals from the area where the transplant goes.

Pallidotomy is an operation that heats part of the globus pallidus, a structure (a nucleus) deep in the brain that is overactive in Parkinson's disease. It has been tried in PSP without success. The reason is probably that the globus pallidus is not damaged in Parkinson's and is actually overactive because of insufficient inhibition by the damaged area. In PSP, on the other hand, the globus pallidus is itself damaged and already partly paralyzed. Therefore, paralyzing it further with a pallidotomy would, if anything, worsen things.

Another operation that can help Parkinson's disease is thalamotomy, destruction of part of the thalamus, an important nucleus that serves as a relay station in the brain. However, thalamotomy helps little besides the tremor of Parkinson's, and tremor is never an important symptom in PSP. Also, the thalamus is overactive in Parkinson's because of stimulation by the overactive globus pallidus. In PSP, where the globus pallidus is damaged and underactive, the thalamus would be underactive as a result. Damaging it surgically would therefore, as with pallidotomy, only worsen things.

Two newer procedures for Parkinson's are pallidal stimulation and subthalamic stimulation. In these, the same effect as pallidotomy is achieved by delivering a constant string of tiny electrical shocks to the globus pallidus or subthalamic area via wires implanted deep in the brain and attached to a battery powered device under the skin of the chest. The advantage over pallidotomy is that the wires can be removed or repositioned without leaving much permanent injury. Because the electrical shocks merely temporarily paralyze the area of brain, they would be no more likely to help PSP than would permanent destruction of those areas, for reasons described in the preceding paragraph.

What Is the Cause of PSP?

The symptoms of PSP are caused by a gradual deterioration of brain cells in a few tiny but important places in the base of the brain. The most important such place, the substantia nigra (sub-STAN-cha NYE-gray), is also affected in Parkinson's disease and damage to it accounts for the symptoms that PSP and Parkinson's have in common. However, several important areas are affected in PSP that are normal in Parkinson's (and vice versa). Moreover, under the microscope, the appearance of the damaged brain cells in PSP is quite different from those in Parkinson's and resembles, rather, the degeneration in Alzheimer's disease. However, the location of the damaged cells is quite different in PSP and Alzheimer's. Furthermore, in PSP there are no amyloid plaques, deposits of waxy protein that are a hallmark of brain cells in Alzheimer's.

What Causes the Brain Cells to Degenerate in the First Place?

No one knows yet. The various national organizations that sponsor research in Parkinson's disease sometimes sponsor deserving PSP research. Their support of research in Parkinson's disease adds to our knowledge of PSP, too.

Another way to help research and yourself is to participate in studies of PSP if so requested by a researcher. This may take the form of answering questionnaires, having medical examinations, having medical tests, and/or taking experimental medication. There are so few people with PSP in any one geographical area that each can make a very important contribution in this way. Joining the Society for PSP will allow PSP researchers to contact you regarding participating in new research studies.

Should I Make Arrangements to Donate my Brain after Death?

Another very important way to help PSP research is to make arrangements to donate your brain after death. The Society for PSP sponsors the Eloise H. Troxel Memorial Brain Bank located at the Mayo Clinic in Jacksonville, FL. Brains donated there are stored and used only for research in PSP by legitimate researchers after their proposals are examined and approved by the Society's Medical Advisory Board. Donating to a brain bank does not interfere with funeral arrangements and costs the family a few hundred dollars for expenses of brain removal and transportation. The family will receive at no charge a full diagnostic report from the Mayo Clinic pathologist, Dennis W. Dickson, MD, who is an authority on PSP. Further information is available from the Society for PSP. There are many other brain banks throughout the country, generally located at major university hospitals.

Should I Join Some Sort of Support Group?

The value of membership in a group of other people with the same problem is tremendous. You can exchange helpful tips on ways to cope physically and psychologically with the limitations of the illness and can learn more about the problem and its treatment from guest speakers. Many large medical centers have a Parkinson support group that welcomes members with PSP. While there are far fewer people with PSP than PD in one geographical area, several successful PSP support groups have been organized in the U.S. in more densely populated areas. All it takes is one organizer with some time and energy. Contact the Society for PSP for help.

A major goal of the Society for PSP is to increase awareness of PSP among the public and the medical profession in order allow its correct diagnosis. If, as we suspect, PSP proves to be much more common than has been assumed, improved diagnosis may allow local support groups to flourish, will foster the growth of the Society for

PSP, and will draw the attention of more researchers to finding the cause and cure of this unique and puzzling illness.

Additional Information

Society for Supranuclear Palsy
1838 Greene Tree Road, Suite 515
Baltimore, MD 21208
Toll-Free: 800-457-4777
Website: www.psp.org
E-mail: spsp@psp.org

Chapter 37

Restless Legs Syndrome

Do You Have Restless Legs Syndrome?

1. When sitting or lying down, do you have unpleasant or creepy-crawly sensations in your legs (and sometimes in other parts of your body), tied to a strong feeling or urge to move?

2. Do the sensations and urge to move come on during periods of rest or inactivity and are they relieved by movement?

3. Do the sensations and urge to move bother you more in the evening and at night rather than during the day?

4. Do you often have trouble falling asleep or staying asleep?

5. Does your bed partner tell you that you jerk your legs (or your arms) when you are asleep; do you sometimes, have involuntary leg jerks when you are awake?

6. Are you frequently tired or fatigued during the day?

7. Do you have family members who experience these same sensations and urge to move?

Reprinted with permission from *Living with Restless Legs*, a booklet produced and published by the Restless Legs Syndrome Foundation, © 2001 RLS Foundation; and excerpts from "Restless Legs," Fact Sheet, National Institute of Neurological Disorders and Stroke (NINDS), NIH Publication No. 01-4847, April 2001, reviewed July 1, 2001.

8. Have medical tests not revealed a cause for your sensations and urge to move?

If you do have restless legs syndrome (RLS), you are not alone. Up to 8% of the U.S. population may have this neurologic condition. Many people have a mild form of the disorder, but RLS severely affects the lives of millions of individuals.

Primary Features of RLS

Adults with RLS will typically have all four of these primary features.

- The bothersome, but usually not painful, sensations deep in the legs produce an irresistible urge to move. Some words used to describe these sensations include creeping, itching, pulling, creepy-crawly, or tugging. (These sensations may only involve a strong urge to move the legs. They may also occasionally occur in the arms.)

- Symptoms are worse or exclusively present when the afflicted individual is at rest, and the sensations are typically lessened by voluntary movement of the affected extremity.

- Symptoms are worse in the evening and at night, especially when the individual lies down.

- Movements of the toes, feet, or legs (known as restlessness) are typically seen when the afflicted individual is sitting or lying down in the evening. This restlessness may be seen as fidgetiness or nervousness.

Associated Features of RLS

- RLS symptoms can cause difficulty in falling and staying asleep. Approximately 80% of people with RLS will also have periodic limb movements of sleep, which are jerks that typically occur every 20 to 30 seconds on and off throughout the night, often causing partial arousals that disrupt sleep.

- Because you may experience difficulties with falling and staying asleep at night, you may be abnormally tired or even sleepy during waking hours. Chronic sleep deprivation and its resultant daytime sleepiness can affect your ability to work, participate in social activities, partake in recreational pastimes, and can cause mood swings which can affect your personal relationships.

Cause

Research into the cause of RLS is ongoing and answers are limited, but we do think that RLS may have different but perhaps overlapping causes.

RLS often runs in families. Researchers are currently looking for the gene or genes that may be responsible for this form of RLS, known as primary or familial RLS.

RLS may be the result of another condition, which, when present, worsens the underlying RLS. This is called secondary RLS. During pregnancy, particularly during the last few months, up to 15% of women develop RLS. After delivery, their symptoms often vanish. Anemia and low levels of iron in the blood are associated with symptoms of RLS, as are chronic conditions such as peripheral neuropathy (damage to the nerves in the hands and feet) and kidney failure. Recent literature also points toward an association between RLS and symptoms of attention-deficit hyperactivity disorder. If you have no family history of RLS and no underlying or associated conditions causing the disorder, your RLS is said to be idiopathic, meaning without a known cause.

Age of Onset

Though RLS is diagnosed most often in people in their middle years, many individuals with RLS, particularly those with primary RLS, can trace their symptoms back to childhood. These symptoms may have been called growing pains or the children may have been thought to be hyperactive because they had difficulty sitting quietly.

Diagnosis

With its classic symptoms, RLS is diagnosed by reviewing your medical history. After ruling out other medical conditions as the cause of your symptoms, your healthcare provider can make the diagnosis of RLS by listening to your description of the sensations. No laboratory test exists that can confirm your diagnosis of RLS. However, a thorough physical examination, including the results of necessary laboratory tests, can reveal temporary disorders, such as iron deficiency, that may be associated with RLS. Some people (including those with periodic limb movements of sleep and without the abnormal sensations of RLS) will require an overnight testing of sleep to determine other causes of their sleep disturbance.

Treatment

The goal of any medical treatment, including the treatment of RLS, is to achieve the greatest benefit while incurring the fewest risks. Sound treatment strategy, therefore, involves weighing these risks and benefits and beginning with the least risky treatments. Low-risk therapies involve treating symptoms that are caused by underlying disorders and making lifestyle changes.

If an underlying iron or vitamin deficiency is found to be the cause of your restless legs, supplementing with iron, vitamin B12, or folate (as indicated) may be sufficient to relieve your symptoms. Because the use of even moderate amounts of some minerals (such as iron, magnesium, potassium, and calcium) can impair your body's ability to use other minerals or can cause toxicity, you should use mineral supplements only on the advice of your health care provider. Current recommendations include checking a serum ferritin level (to evaluate iron-storage status) and supplementing with iron if your ferritin level is less than 50 mcg/L.

The use of some medications seems to worsen the symptoms of RLS. These drugs include calcium-channel blockers (used to treat high blood pressure and heart conditions), most anti-nausea medications, some cold and allergy medications, major tranquilizers, phenytoin, and most medications used to treat depression.

Lifestyle changes involve determining, on an individual basis, which habits and activities worsen or improve your symptoms of RLS. A healthy balanced diet is important in reducing the severity of your RLS. Though caffeine consumption may initially appear to relieve your symptoms, the use of caffeine most likely only delays, and often intensifies, your symptoms to a time later in the day. The best solution is to avoid all caffeine containing products, including chocolate and caffeinated beverages such as coffee, tea, and soft drinks. The consumption of alcohol increases the span or intensity of symptoms for most individuals; again, refraining from the use of alcohol is the best solution.

Because fatigue and drowsiness tend to worsen the symptoms of RLS, implementing a program of good sleep hygiene should be a first step toward resolving your symptoms.

Sleep Hygiene

Ideally, sleep hygiene involves having a cool, quiet, and comfortable sleeping environment, going to bed at the same time every night, arising at the same time every morning; and obtaining a sufficient number of hours of sleep to feel well rested. Some people with RLS find that going to bed later and arising later in the day helps them to obtain an adequate amount of sleep. Good sleep hygiene also involves a program of regular, moderate exercise. Typically, sleep experts recommend that exercise should take place at least six hours before bedtime to avoid an adverse impact on your sleep, however, many people with RLS find that exercising, such as using a stationary bike or a treadmill, immediately before bedtime is useful.

You may find that you achieve your best sleep later in the 24-hour cycle—for example, sleeping from 2 a.m. until 10 a.m. may work best for you. Some people find that performing isometric exercises for a few minutes before bed is helpful.

Self-directed activities that counteract your symptoms of RLS appear to be very effective, although temporary, solutions to managing the disorder. You may find that walking, stretching, taking a hot or cold bath, massaging your affected limb, applying hot or cold packs, using vibration, performing acupressure, and practicing relaxation techniques (such as biofeedback, meditation, or yoga) may help reduce or relieve your symptoms. You may also find that keeping your mind actively engaged through activities such as a participating in a stimulating discussion or argument, performing intricate needlework, or playing video games helps during times that you must stay seated, such as when you are traveling.

Unfortunately, in many cases, the symptoms of RLS either initially do not resolve with the treatment of underlying disorders and the implementation of lifestyle changes, or over time progress so that relief is insufficient with these methods. In either case, the use of medications (pharmacologic therapy) may become necessary.

Drug Therapy

No drugs have been approved by the U.S. Food and Drug Administration for the treatment of RLS, but several drugs have undergone clinical studies in RLS and have been approved for other conditions. These medications fall into four main classes—dopaminergic agents, sedatives, pain relievers, and anticonvulsants. Each drug or class of drugs has its own benefits, limitations, and side effect profile. The choice of medication is dependent upon the timing and severity of your symptoms.

Dopaminergic Agents

The primary and first-line treatment for RLS is with dopaminergic agents: primarily dopamine-receptor agonists like Mirapex (pramipexole),

Permax (pergolide), and Requip (ropinirole), but also drugs like Sinemet (carbidopa/levodopa) that add dopamine to the system. Although dopaminergic agents are used to treat Parkinson's disease, RLS is not a form of Parkinson's disease. All of these drugs should be started at low doses and increased very slowly to decrease potential side effects.

Of the dopaminergic agents, Sinemet has been used the longest, but it has recently been found to cause a serious problem, known as augmentation, in the vast majority of patients who take it for the treatment of RLS. If you are taking Sinemet, you need to be aware of this problem and should discuss it with your physician. Also, you should not take Sinemet within two hours after eating a high-protein meal.

Sedatives

Sedative agents are most effective for relieving the nighttime symptoms of RLS. They are used either at bedtime in addition to a dopaminergic agent or for individuals who have primarily nighttime symptoms. The most commonly used sedative is clonazepam (Klonopin).

Pain Relievers

Pain-relieving drugs are used most often for people with severe relentless symptoms of RLS. Some examples of medications in this category include codeine, Darvon or Darvocet (propoxyphene), Dolophine (methadone), Percocet (oxycodone), Ultram (tramadol), and Vicodin (hydrocodone).

Anticonvulsants

These drugs are particularly effective for some, but not all, patients with marked daytime symptoms, particularly people who have pain syndromes associated with their RLS. Gabapentin (Neurontin) is the anticonvulsant that has shown the most promise in treating the symptoms of RLS.

Augmentation

When augmentation occurs, your usual dose of a dopaminergic agent (most often seen with Sinemet) will allow you to obtain relief from your symptoms so that you will be able to sleep at night, but the sensations, the need to move, and the restlessness will develop (frequently with an increased intensity) earlier in the day (during the afternoon or even during the morning). The RLS may also spread to other parts of the body such as your arms.

If augmentation does develop, increasing your dosage of medication will probably worsen rather than improve your symptoms. Most people who develop augmentation must switch to another medication; however, do not stop taking your current medication abruptly. Instead, consult your healthcare provider.

Summary

By arming yourself with information, you have taken the first step toward defeating RLS. Your optimum treatment plan requires a close interaction between you and your healthcare provider. Choosing a healthy lifestyle, eliminating symptom producing substances, taking vitamin and mineral supplements as necessary, and engaging in self directed activities will all work toward reducing or eliminating the need for pharmacologic intervention.

If you do need medications, careful trials are typically necessary to find the best medication and the best dosage for you. Many patients report that a combination of medications works best, and some find that a medication that has worked for an extended period of time suddenly becomes ineffective and another medication must be substituted. Quite clearly, you must be cautious when combining a variety of medications and should only do so under the supervision of your healthcare provider.

Because no single treatment for RLS is entirely effective for everyone, continued research is of vital importance. Until we find the cause of RLS and a cure, working closely with your healthcare provider, interacting with a local support group, and exploring non-drug treatments as well as pharmacologic therapy will help you find the answer to living a happy productive life in spite of having RLS.

Living with RLS

Living with RLS involves developing coping strategies that work for you.

- **Talk about RLS**. Sharing information about RLS will help your family members, friends, and coworkers understand when they see you pacing the halls at night, standing at the back of

411

the theater, or walking to the water cooler many times through-out the day.

- **Don't fight it**. If you attempt to suppress the urge to move, you may find that your symptoms only get worse. Get out of bed. Find an activity that takes your mind off of your legs. Stop frequently when traveling.

- **Keep a sleep diary**. If you can't sit to write, dictate into a small tape recorder. Keep track of the medications and strategies that help or hinder your battle with RLS, and share this information with your healthcare provider.

- **Occupy your mind**. Keeping your mind actively engaged may lessen your symptoms of RLS. Find an activity that you enjoy to help you through those times when your symptoms are particularly troublesome.

- **Rise to new levels**. You may be more comfortable if you elevate your desktop or bookstand to a height that will allow you to stand while you work or read.

- **Stretch out your day**. Begin and end your day with stretching exercises or gentle massage.

- **Help others**. Support groups bring together family members and people with RLS. By participating in a group, you can help yourself and your insights may help someone else.

Note: RLS can be a serious disorder and is treatable. Persons suspecting that they may have RLS should consult a qualified healthcare provider. Literature concerning RLS that is distributed by the Restless Legs Syndrome Foundation, Inc., is offered for information purposes only and should not be considered a substitute for the advice of a healthcare provider. The Restless Legs Syndrome Foundation does not advertise, endorse, or sponsor any products or services.

Additional Information

RLS Foundation, Inc.
819 Second Street, S.W.
Rochester, MN 55902
Tel: 507-287-6465
Website: www.ris.org
E-mail: RLSFoundation@rls.org

National Sleep Foundation
1522 K Street, NW, Suite 500
Washington, DC 20005
Tel: 202-347-3471
Fax: 202-347-3472
Website: www.sleepfoundation.org
E-mail: nsf@sleepfoundation.org

Worldwide Education and Awareness for Movement Disorders (WE MOVE)
204 W. 84th Street
New York, NY 10024
Toll-Free: 800-437-6682
Fax: 212-875-8389
Website: www.wemove.org
E-mail: wemove@wemove.org

National Heart, Lung, and Blood Institute
National Center on Sleep Disorders Research
Two Rockledge Center, Suite 10038
6701 Rockledge Drive, MSC 7920
Bethesda, MD 20892-7920
Tel: 301-435-0199
Fax: 301-480-3451
Website: www.nhlbi.nih.gov/about/ncsdr
E-mail: ncsdr@prospectassoc.com

Chapter 38

Spastic Paraplegia

General Information about Hereditary Spastic Paraplegia (HSP)

What Is HSP?

HSP (Hereditary Spastic Paraparesis—or Paraplegia) is a name used to represent a group of inherited degenerative spinal cord disorders whose primary symptom is progressive spasticity (stiffness) and weakness of the leg and hip muscles. This causes increasing difficulty in walking. Canes or walkers often become needed, and sometimes wheelchairs. Most people have symptom onset between the second and fourth decade of life, but it can start at any age from early childhood through late adulthood. It is estimated to affect 10,000 to 20,000 people in the U.S.

There are many other names used for this disorder group. Hereditary Spastic Paraparesis (or Paraplegia), Familial Spastic Paraparesis (or Paraplegia) and Strümpell-Lorrain Disease are the most common. Others are Spastic Paraplegia, Strümpell Disease, Hereditary

---

The information in this chapter, "General Information about HSP," "General Information about PLS," "What is Happening in HSP and PLS?" and "A Look at Primary Upper Motor Neuron Diseases," is reprinted with permission by the Spastic Paraplegia Foundation, Inc., a not-for-profit organization dedicated to finding the cures for Hereditary Spastic Paraparesis and Primary Lateral Sclerosis. Additional information is available at http://www.sp-foundation.org. You can also contact SPF by mail at P.O. Box 1208, Fortson, GA 31808 or by phone at 978-256-2673.

Charcot-Disease, Spastic Spinal Paralysis, Diplegia Spinalis Progressiva, French Settlement Disease, Troyer syndrome (a variant), and Silver syndrome (a variant).

What Are the Symptoms?

The classic symptom of HSP is progressive difficulty in walking. Generally, individuals walk slowly (due to weakened muscles) and the leg muscles are taunt (spastic). It is difficult to lift the legs. Walking becomes more difficult as the disorder progresses. Additional symptoms may include balance difficulty, hyper reflexes, urinary urgency and frequency, diminished vibration sense in the feet, muscle spasms, and pes cavus (high arched foot).

Initial symptoms are usually difficulty with balance, stubbing the toe or stumbling easily. Often, these changes begin so gradually that it is other people who initially notice the change in someone's walking. Many individuals have high arched feet and hyper reflexes from birth, although these symptoms cannot diagnose HSP in the absence of other symptoms, as they can occur in the normal population. Bladder difficulties are occasionally the first symptom.

The majority of people with HSP have uncomplicated HSP, as described. There are also rare, complicated forms, which occur in about 10% of the cases. These can involve other neurological symptoms such as peripheral neuropathy, epilepsy, ataxia, optic neuropathy, retinopathy, dementia, mental retardation, deafness, or problems with speech, swallowing or breathing. It is important to realize that some of other these symptoms may be due to a separate disorder. For example a person with uncomplicated HSP may have peripheral neuropathy caused by diabetes; or could have epilepsy for unrelated reasons.

Is HSP an Ataxia?

No. The group of disorders known as ataxias (such as Friedreich's Ataxia) are spino-cerebellar disorders in which there is a disturbance either in the part of the brain known as the cerebellum or in the connections to it. HSP does not involve the cerebellum. Ataxias can be hereditary or non-hereditary (sporadic).

However, the term ataxia also means incoordination, and can also refer to a symptom in which there is a lack of muscle control resulting in a jerky or unsteady movement. People with HSP may have incoordination as a symptom. This does not mean they have one of the neurological disorders known as ataxia.

416

Why Are My Symptoms Different from Others with HSP?

Although people with HSP share the primary symptom of difficulty walking, there is enormous variability in age of onset, progression rate, and severity of symptoms as well as accompanying symptoms. One reason is that HSP is not a single disorder, but a group of genetically different disorders. Some differences may be due to having HSP caused by different genetic mutations.

However, symptoms can also differ widely among family members with the same gene mutation. It is possible for a child to show symptoms before a parent, and it's possible for some people in the family to have very mild symptoms while others have more severe symptoms.

In some families, symptoms tend to start at younger ages with each new generation. Although it is rare, HSP sometimes shows incomplete penetrance. This means that occasionally (rarely), an individual may have the gene mutation, but for some unknown reasons never develop symptoms of HSP. Such individuals can still pass HSP down to children.

Severity of symptoms can also be affected by one's individual circumstance—environment, nutrition, general health, other genes, and additional factors not yet understood.

How Severe Will My Symptoms Become?

There is no way to predict one's rate of progression, severity of symptoms, or associated symptoms. Once symptoms begin, progression generally continues slowly throughout life. In some cases, it is quite slow and people may never require the use of a cane. At the other extreme, individuals may need a wheelchair at an early age. For some childhood onset forms, symptoms may become apparent, gradually worsen, and eventually stabilize after adolescence. HSP rarely results in complete loss of lower limb mobility, although canes, walkers, or wheelchairs may become necessary.

Are Foot Problems Common?

Yes, foot problems are commonly associated with HSP. However, none should be used to determine whether a person has HSP if there are no other symptoms.

- *High arched feet (pes cavus).* High arches occur because there is more weakness in the foot extensor muscles (the muscles that extend the foot backward and flatten the arch) than in the muscles that flex the foot downward. Orthotics may help provide comfort.

417

- *Shortened Achilles tendons.* Achilles tendons are often short, and generally shorten further as HSP progresses. Physical therapy can help maintain some flexibility and comfort, but cannot stop the progression. Orthotics to keep the foot from dropping are often helpful. It is possible to have the tendons surgically lengthened, but this does not provide a long-term solution and many people report no benefit.

- *Jumping feet (clonus).* Clonus is an uncontrollable, repetitive jerking of muscles that makes the foot jump rapidly up and down. It occurs when the foot is in a particular position that causes a disruption of the signals from the brain, leading to an automatic stretch reflex. Clonus also happens in normal people, but happens much more easily and is more pronounced in people with HSP.

- *Hammer toes or bunions.* These may occur due to imbalances in the strength and tone of muscles that maintain proper alignment of joints in the feet.

- *Cold feet and/or foot swelling.* This is most likely caused by poor circulation. Normally, muscle contractions in the legs help pump blood from the legs back to the heart. If the muscles are weakened, or if the person is relatively inactive, the blood flow from the legs may be decreased, and fluids may accumulate. This can cause swelling, or a sensation of cold feet. For people who must sit for extended periods, it may be beneficial to exercise the calf muscles, and periodically elevate the legs.

Can HSP Affect the Arms?

It is unusual for people with HSP to experience problems with their arms (other than brisk reflexes, which are not uncommon). The nerves that supply the arms can be affected by HSP; however, the degeneration is very mild compared to that which occurs in the much longer nerves that supply the legs. If a person has significant symptoms in their hands or arms, but otherwise appears to have HSP, it would generally be a good idea to test for other disorders.

Is Depression Normal?

Depression and denial are not unusual for anyone with a chronic and disabling illness. Denial may help people cope and set worries aside. It is important to not let one's denial (emotional difficulty coming to terms with an illness) prevent one from receiving proper diagnosis and treatment. Some people with HSP face denial by others in their family who refuse to admit that there is a problem, which can be frustrating and stressful.

Periods of feeling down about having HSP are normal and expected. However, if the feelings linger or become overwhelming, it may help to seek out supportive services. Anti-depressant medication may help.

Why Are My Muscles Tighter When I am Stressed or Angry?

Some people find the tightness in their muscles worsens when they are angry, stressed, or upset. Even among people without HSP, stress can have this effect on the body. That phenomenon can be magnified for those with HSP. It is unknown exactly how emotions affect muscle tone, but it may involve adrenalin levels.

Can HSP Affect Sexual Function?

The short answer appears to be yes, although it is important to remember that sexual desire and/or function can be affected by many factors such as older age, stress, depression, fatigue, medical disorders or medications, which may or may not be related to HSP.

Some people report that stiffness, spasms, and cramps that are part of HSP may either inhibit (or intensify) orgasm, or that orgasm may bring on leg stiffness, spasms, or clonus. Stiffness of the legs may cause difficulty using certain positions for intercourse, so it may be helpful to try different positions.

If you have concern about a change in your sexual function or desire, it is a good idea to discuss the situation with your doctor, in order to rule out any medical causes that may be treatable.

What Is the Life Expectancy?

Life expectancy is normal for people with HSP.

What Is the Treatment/Cure?

There is currently no treatment to prevent, stop, or reverse HSP. Treatment is focused on symptom relief, such as medication to reduce spasticity; physical therapy to help maintain flexibility, strength, and range of motion; assistive devices; and supportive therapy. Individuals benefit from working closely with their neurologist and physical therapist to establish the best treatment program.

419

How Is HSP Diagnosed?

Diagnosis of HSP is a process of examining family history and exclusion of other disorders that cause spasticity and weakness in the legs. Genetic testing is available for the most common type of HSP as well as a rare form. As more genes are discovered, more testing should become available.

It is important to recognize that HSP is frequently misdiagnosed. This is because neurologists unfamiliar with HSP commonly dismiss it as a potential diagnosis when there is no evident family history. However, investigators estimate that 20% or more of individuals with HSP do not show family history. HSP is frequently misdiagnosed as cerebral palsy, multiple sclerosis, ataxia or primary lateral sclerosis, even though some tests may rule these disorders out.

Other disorders that should be ruled out are ALS, tropical spastic paraparesis (TSP), vitamin deficiencies (B_{12} or E), thoracic spine herniated disks, and spinal cord tumors. There are tests available (including magnetic resonance imaging [MRI], computer tomography [CT], spinal taps, electromyography (EMG), nerve conduction tests, electroencephalography (EEG), blood tests, and vitamin deficiency tests), that help rule these out. Evaluation for HSP and exclusion of other possible disorders should be performed by a neurologist.

What Genetic Testing Is Available and What about Prenatal Testing?

Commercial testing is available for spastin, the most common form of dominantly inherited HSP. Spastin is thought to be responsible for 40% of dominant HSP cases. It is available through Athena Diagnostics (http://www.athenadiagnostics.com). Testing is also available for a gene that causes a very rare, X-linked complicated form of HSP, the Proteolipid protein (PLP) gene. Information on that test can be found at http://www.geneclinics.org. Testing is expected to become available soon for the atlastin gene, which causes approximately 25% of dominant, childhood onset forms.

These gene tests can also be used for prenatal testing. Testing may also be possible if the family is definitely linked to a particular gene location. However, this kind of testing is only performed in research settings and is not widely available.

As more genes are discovered, it is hopeful that such information will lead to greater availability of testing.

What Is the Risk of Passing HSP to Children?

HSP has three different modes of inheritance: autosomal dominant, autosomal recessive, and X-linked. Each mode has a different risk factor for passing the disorder down to children.

Most types of HSP are autosomal dominant. That means that a person only needs to have one abnormal gene from one affected parent in order to have the disorder. The corresponding healthy gene from the other parent does not compensate for the HSP gene. The risk of a child inheriting HSP when one parent has an autosomal dominant form of HSP is 50%. This risk is the same for each pregnancy. Prenatal testing may be an option in some cases (for example, if the disorder has been shown to be due to a spastin gene mutation, discussed earlier).

Autosomal recessive HSP means a person must receive an abnormal gene from each parent in order to have the disorder. However, neither of his parents has HSP. Rather, each parent is a carrier—each one has one abnormal gene and one normal gene. When two carriers of autosomal recessive types of HSP (who do not have HSP symptoms) have a child, there is a 25% risk of the child receiving the affected gene from each parent and therefore having HSP, a 50% risk of the child being a carrier (like the parents), and a 25% chance that the child is neither a carrier nor has HSP.

It is very unlikely for individuals with autosomal recessive HSP to have children with HSP unless their spouse is also a carrier. The chance that the spouse will be a carrier is increased if both parents are related (marriages between cousins, for example).

X-linked HSP means the abnormal gene is carried on the X-chromosome. The risk of passing HSP to a child depends upon whether it is the mother or the father who has HSP, and whether the child is a boy or a girl. X-linked disorders affect males much more often and much more severely than females. Most women with X-linked gene mutations do not have significant symptoms. When a woman has an X-linked HSP gene mutation, there is a 50% chance each son will have HSP and a 50% chance that each daughter will be a carrier (unlikely to have symptoms). This risk is the same for each pregnancy. Men with X-linked HSP cannot pass HSP to their sons, and all their daughters will be carriers (but unlikely to have the disorder themselves).

What Is Happening in My Body?

HSP is caused by degeneration at the ends of the upper motor neurons. These neurons begin in the brain and their axons extend to the brainstem and down the spinal cord. They are responsible for voluntary muscle movement. They carry messages to lower motor neurons which start in the brainstem and spinal cord and extend out to the corresponding muscles.

When upper motor neurons degenerate, the impulses cannot adequately reach the lower motor neurons. Therefore, the lower motor neurons cannot transmit the correct messages to the corresponding muscles. The result is increased muscle tone (spasticity) and muscle weakness. As the degeneration occurs, spasticity and weakness increases. The legs are affected because degeneration occurs primarily at the ends of the longest axons in the spinal cord, the ones that control the legs.

Axons are surrounded by a coating known as the myelin sheath, an insulator that helps the nerves conduct impulses faster. Some disorders with similar symptoms, such as multiple sclerosis, involve demyelination of the nerves. In most cases of HSP, the primary problem is not abnormal myelin, although a rare type of X-linked HSP has been linked to a myelin protein gene mutation.

Can I Donate Blood If I Have HSP?

HSP cannot be passed to others through donation of blood. There is no medical reason why a person with HSP cannot donate blood. However, if the person is taking medications as treatment for HSP, he or she may not be able to donate for that reason, not the disorder itself. Some hospitals or organizations (such as the Red Cross) may request a letter from your doctor indicating that it is okay for you to donate.

When Was HSP Identified?

In the late 1800s, A. Strümpell, a neurologist in Heidelberg Germany, described this disorder. He observed two brothers and their father, who had gait disorders and spasticity in their legs. After the death of the brothers, Strümpell was able to show through autopsy the degeneration of the nerve fibers leading through the spinal cord. The disorder was originally named after Strümpell, and after two Frenchmen who later provided more information about the disorder, Lorrain and Charcot.

Is HSP More Prevalent in Certain Ethnic Groups?

There is no evidence that HSP is more prevalent in one ethnic group than another.

General Information about Primary Lateral Sclerosis (PLS)?

Primary lateral sclerosis (PLS) is a slowly progressive, neurological disorder. It causes increasing spasticity (stiffness) and weakness in the legs, arms, and hands. It can also cause speech and swallowing problems. Canes, forearm crutches, or walkers often become needed, and sometimes wheelchairs. In some cases, communication aids may become necessary.

There are an estimated 300–500 individuals in the United States with PLS. Age of onset is typically between 35 to 66 years of age.

What Are the Symptoms?

The classic symptoms of PLS are progressive difficulty walking and talking (slurred speech). Onset of the disorder is gradual. Generally, individuals walk slowly (due to weakening leg muscles) and leg muscles that are taunt (spastic). Problems in the legs can begin as unexplained tripping and difficulty walking. Walking becomes more difficult as the disorder progresses.

PLS usually starts in the legs and gradually spreads to involve the arms. It may also affect speech and swallowing. In some people difficulty with speaking and swallowing begin before weakness is noted in the legs.

Speech problems can begin with hoarseness, reduced rate of speaking, excessive clearing of the throat, or slurring of words when tired. As these symptoms progress, words become progressively more slurred. In some cases, an individual's speech becomes so slurred that others cannot understand it. But in other cases, speech disturbance is only mild and remains understandable.

Additional symptoms include hyperactive reflexes, a tendency for the feet to drop when walking, and muscle spasms. Individuals with PLS also experience balance problems, and have a tendency to fall.

How Severe Will My Symptoms Become?

There is no way to predict the rate at which symptoms will progress, whether additional symptoms will appear, or how severe symptoms will become.

Some individuals with PLS have reported that the progression of their symptoms seems to stop worsening and to reach a plateau for a period of time. Whether symptoms will stop worsening, and if so, for how long, cannot be predicted.

Table 38.1. A Look at Primary Upper Motor Neuron Diseases: Hereditary Spastic Paraparesis and Primary Lateral Sclerosis

	Hereditary Spastic Paraplegia	Primary Lateral Sclerosis
What is it?	A group of hereditary, degenerative, neurological disorders chiefly affecting upper motor neurons and principally causing progressive spastic weakness of the legs. Also known as familial spastic paraplegia or paraparesis (FSP) and Strümpell-Lorrain syndrome.	A group of degenerative, neurological disorders chiefly affecting upper motor neurons and principally causing progressive spastic weakness of the legs as well as the arms and bulbar muscles.
Incidence rate	Estimated at 10,000–20,000 individuals in the U.S. It may be higher. Without documented family history, it can be initially diagnosed as primary lateral sclerosis, cerebral palsy, multiple sclerosis, or ataxia. It can remain undiagnosed in mild cases.	Estimated at 300–500 individuals in the U.S. It may be lower or higher, as it can take several years for expression, making it often an uncertain initial diagnosis.
Predominant features	Insidious, progressive spasticity and weakness of the legs that often gets severe, requiring assistive devices. There is also difficulty with balance, clumsiness, and often muscle spasms.	Insidious, progressive spasticity and weakness of the legs that often gets severe, requiring assistive devices. There is also difficulty with balance, clumsiness, and often muscle spasms. In time, weakness and spasticity in the arms and hands also occurs, as well as slurred speech, drooling, and difficulty swallowing. Sometimes, symptoms begin in the upper body first.
Secondary features	Urinary urgency and frequency is common and high arched feet are often present. Very rare types can present speech problems, ataxia, mental retardation, dementia, visual or hearing dysfunctions, extrapyramidal dysfunctions, adrenal insufficiency, or ichthyosis.	

	HSP	PLS
What causes it?	HSP is hereditary, with some 30 genes thought to cause different types of HSP. Most forms are autosomal dominant, others are X-linked or autosomal recessive.	PLS is thought to be spontaneous. There is a rare, autosomal-recessive, childhood-onset form.
What is going wrong?	The upper motor neurons in the brain and spinal cord degenerate. Upper motor neurons control voluntary movement. They deliver signals to lower motor neurons, which carry messages to the muscles. Because upper motor neurons degenerate, nerve impulses cannot adequately reach the lower motor neuron, and the lower motor neuron cannot relay the correct message out to the muscles. This causes spasticity (increased muscle tone/stiffness) and weakness, which increase as the degeneration progresses	The upper motor neurons in the brain and spinal cord degenerate. Upper motor neurons control voluntary movement. They deliver signals to lower motor neurons, which carry messages to the muscles. Because upper motor neurons degenerate, nerve impulses cannot adequately reach the lower motor neuron, and the lower motor neuron cannot relay the correct message out to the muscles. This causes spasticity (increased muscle tone/stiffness) and weakness, which increase as the degeneration progresses
How is it diagnosed?	HSP is a clinical diagnosis made through exclusion of other possibilities and examining family history. Absence of documented family history cannot rule out HSP. It is estimated some 30% of individuals with HSP do not have documented family history. Gene testing can confirm dominantly inherited HSP in 45% of patients. Early stages of HSP can mimic PLS or ALS. In the absence of family history, neurologists watch for upper body symptom development to indicate PLS or lower motor neuron involvement to indicate ALS	PLS is a clinical diagnosis made through exclusion of other possibilities and examining family history. Absence of documented family history cannot rule out HSP. Early stages of PLS can mimic HSP or ALS. Neurologists watch for upper body symptoms to confirm PLS or lower motor neuron involvement to indicate ALS. EMG, nerve conduction tests and symptoms of lower motor neuron involvement distinguish mild forms of ALS from PLS.

Table 38.1. (Continued on next page)

425

Table 38.1. A Look at Primary Upper Motor Neuron Diseases: Hereditary Spastic Paraparesis and Primary Lateral Sclerosis *(continued from previous page)*

	Hereditary Spastic Paraplegia	Primary Lateral Sclerosis
Age of onset	Symptoms can begin at any age from childhood through late adulthood. Most patients experience onset of symptoms in the second through fourth decades of life.	The reported age of onset ranges from 35-66 years with a median of 50.5 years. A rare, child-onset form has been reported.
What is the prognosis?	It affects the quality of life. Difficulty walking usually gets slowly worse, often requiring canes, walkers, or wheelchairs. However, some individuals with childhood-onset of symptoms experience very little worsening. There is currently no cure.	It affects the quality of life. Difficulty walking usually gets slowly worse, often requiring canes, walkers, or wheelchairs. Speech and swallowing difficulty may become severe, as well as weakness of the arms. There is currently no cure.
What is the treatment?	There is no treatment to prevent, retard, or reverse the degenerative process. Treatment is focused on symptom relief (medications for spasticity), physical therapy and exercise, assistive devices, and supportive therapy.	There is no treatment to prevent, retard, or reverse the degenerative process. Treatment is focused on symptom relief (medications for spasticity), physical therapy and exercise, assistive devices, speech therapy, and supportive therapy.
What research is being done?	There have been few researchers working on HSP. Fortunately, there are more today and research is accelerating. At publication date, six HSP genes have been discovered and the search continues. Scientists are working to understand the genes and how mutations lead to upper motor nerve degeneration. Animal models are underway. It is hopeful that treatments or cures will be applicable to related neurological conditions such as PLS, ALS, spinal cord injury, etc. Likewise, advances made in related neurological conditions may hopefully be applicable to HSP.	There have been few researchers working on PLS. Fortunately, there are more today and research is accelerating. PLS research is currently done in conjunction with research on HSP or ALS. A gene for a rare, familial childhood form of PLS has been identified. Scientists are working to understand this gene and how mutations lead to nerve degeneration. It is hopeful that advances made in related neurological conditions (HSP, ALS, spinal cord injury, etc.) may be applicable to PLS.

Do Symptoms Become Worse with Anger, Excitement, or Emotional Stress?

Individuals with PLS have reported that their symptoms temporarily worsen when they become upset, angry, or emotionally stressed. Becoming tired can also have this effect, especially on speech.

Can PLS Be Treated/Cured?

There no treatment that can stop, reverse, or prevent PLS. Treatment is focused on symptom relief. Medication can reduce spasticity. Physical therapy helps to maintain flexibility, range of motion, and strength. Canes, forearm crutches, walkers, and wheelchairs assist in getting about, and help to prevent falls. Leg braces such as ankle-foot-orthotics provide some stability, prevent toe drop, and prevent hyperflexion injuries to the knees. Palatal lifts and injections into the area of the vocal chords sometimes improve speech. Communication aids such as computerized keyboards can speak for those with serious speech problems. Supportive therapy may be useful to deal with the psychological stresses of a progressive, disabling disorder.

Some individuals who have spasticity that is not adequately controlled by oral medication may benefit by having a pump implanted in their abdomen. The pump delivers minute quantities of Baclofen directly into fluid surrounding the spinal cord.

Individuals with PLS greatly benefit by working closely with their neurologist and physical therapist to develop the treatment program best for them.

How Does PLS Affect Lifestyle?

The combination of spasticity and weakness in the legs plus foot drop often leads to increased falling. Falls are a common hazard for individuals with PLS. Many have broken bones due to falling.

Many individuals with PLS are reluctant to begin the use of assistive devices such as canes. Many who use canes are equally reluctant to switch to forearm crutches, walkers, or wheelchairs as their symptoms progress. Those that have broken bones invariably were either not using an assistive device, or were using one inadequate for their condition.

PLS can also affect a person's ability to drive safely. Hand controls may be necessary. These can be installed in a vehicle. They allow those with leg problems the ability to continue to drive. Hand controls are designed so that able bodied drivers can drive the same vehicle without moving anything.

427

PLS may affect speech. Speech therapy is often useful. If one's speech cannot be understood, alternate ways of communicating need to be used. There are numerous communication aids available. They include electronic keyboards that "speak" the words entered into them.

Do Individuals with PLS Become Depressed?

Depression, anger, and denial are quite common in people with a chronic, disabling disorder. These feelings are normal and are to be expected, especially during the period while seeking a diagnosis, and for some time after the initial diagnosis.

Eventually, these feelings become replaced with acceptance, although this may take several years. If these negative feelings linger or become overwhelming, it may help to seek supportive services. Antidepressant medications may also help.

How Is PLS Diagnosed?

The diagnosis of PLS is a diagnosis of exclusion. This means that all other causes of the symptoms presenting in an individual must be ruled out before a PLS diagnosis can be made. Individuals showing symptoms common to PLS undergo a battery of tests to rule out these other causes. These tests include a complete neurological examination, blood tests, MRI of the brain and spine, motor and sensory nerve conduction studies, EMG, and often cerebrospinal fluid analysis.

There is usually no family history of PLS. Rarely, however, familial occurrence of PLS has been observed.

It is important to recognize that initially, it may be difficult to diagnose PLS. The symptoms of PLS that are usually present at first (difficulty walking and mild stumbling due to leg weakness and stiffness) are not specific and can also be signs of other conditions. Symptoms could develop after several years that are not consistent with PLS. It is only after a period of observation (often for a couple of years) and careful exclusion of other diagnostic possibilities that a neurologist can be certain in a PLS diagnosis.

How Does PLS Cause My Symptoms?

Motor neuron cells carry the impulses that cause muscles to move. They are responsible for all voluntary movement.

PLS is caused by degeneration of the upper motor neurons. These are cells that reside in the brain, in the motor cortex. This area of the brain is located near the top of the head—in the middle.

Upper motor neurons have long hair-like processes (axons) that leave the motor cortex. Some go to the brainstem near the top of the neck. Others travel down into the spinal cord. At the end of these axons the upper motor neurons connect to lower motor neurons.

Lower motor neurons also have axons. These axons extend from the brainstem (or spinal cord) and connect to muscle fibers.

When upper motor neurons degenerate, impulses cannot adequately reach the lower motor neurons. This interferes with the proper transmission of the impulses through the lower motor neurons to the corresponding muscles. The result is muscle weakness and increased spasticity. As the degeneration progresses, the symptoms increase.

If the axons of the upper motor neurons that degenerate extend most of the way down the spinal cord (where they connect to the lower motor neurons that connect to the muscles of the legs) then the legs

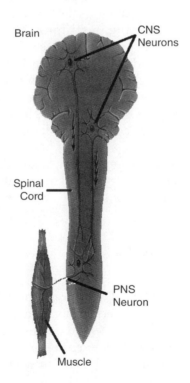

Figure 38.1. *CNS Neurons in Brain*

show symptoms. If the axons of the affected upper motor neurons extend only a short way down the spinal cord (where they connect to the lower motor neurons that connect to the muscles of the arms or hands) then the arms or hands become affected. If they extend only to the brainstem, then the muscles that control speech and swallowing become affected.

What Is Happening in HSP and PLS?

HSP and PLS are caused by degeneration of the upper motor neurons. Upper motor neurons are the nerve cells that control voluntary movement. They carry messages from the brain to the brain stem and spinal cord, where they connect to (synapse with) other nerves called lower motor neurons. The lower motor neurons carry the messages out to the muscles to tell them to move.

When there is degeneration in the upper motor neurons, messages (impulses) cannot adequately reach the lower motor neurons. This causes decreased ability to move the corresponding muscles. This nerve degeneration causes the muscles to be weak and causes muscle tone to be increased, resulting in stiffness or spasticity.

Where the degeneration occurs determines which muscles are affected. In both HSP and PLS, degeneration causes weakness and spasticity primarily in the legs. Increased muscle tone also causes hyperactive reflexes and involuntary jumping (clonus) of a joint (especially ankles and knees). For many people with HSP, there is also increased muscle tone (or conversely, decreased muscle relaxation) affecting the bladder, causing urinary urgency, and the need for frequent urination. In PLS, degeneration also occurs at higher regions in the spinal cord and brainstem, causing weakness and spasticity in the arms, slurred speech and difficulty swallowing, in addition to lower extremity symptoms.

Additional Information

The Spastic Paraplegia Foundation (SPF) is dedicated to finding the cures for Hereditary Spastic Paraparesis and Primary Lateral Sclerosis. The SPF also provides educational materials about the disorders and creates opportunities for patient support. The SPF medical advisor is John K. Fink, MD, Department of Neurology, University of Michigan. You can reach the SPF at its web site at http://www.spfoundation.org, by mail at P.O. Box 1208, Fortson, Georgia, 31808, or by phone: 978-256-2673.

Chapter 39

Spinal Cord Disease and Injury

Any damage to the spinal cord is a very complex injury. People who are injured are often confused when trying to understand what it means to be a person with a spinal cord injury (SCI). Will I be able to move my hands? Will I walk again? What can I do? Each injury is different and can affect the body in many different ways.

This is a brief summary of the changes that take place after a spinal cord injury. It tells how the spinal cord works and what some of the realistic expectations are for what a person should eventually be able to do following a spinal cord injury. Included is a chart of functional goals for specific levels of injury as well as additional information resources.

The Normal Spinal Cord

The spinal cord is a part of your nervous system. It is the largest nerve in the body. Nerves are cord-like structures made up of many

Lindsey, L; Kleibine, P; and Wells, M.J., (2000). *Understanding SCI & Functional Goals,* (SCI InfoSheet #4). Birmingham, AL: UAB Rehabilitation Research and Training Center on Secondary Conditions of Spinal Cord Injury. Available from Spinal Cord Injury Information Network website at http:// www.spinalcord.uab.edu/show.asp?durki=32060. © 2000 University of Alabama; reprinted with permission. Also included is "SCI Rehabilitation 1: Facility Section." This fact sheet is reprinted with permission from the National Spinal Cord Injury Association (NSCIA), 6701 Democracy Boulevard, Suite 300-9, Bethesda, MD 20817, 301-588-6959. For more information, visit the NSCIA website at www.spinalcord.org. © 1996.

nerve fibers. The spinal cord has many spinal nerve fibers that carry messages between the brain and different parts of the body. The messages may tell a body part to move. Other nerve fibers send and receive messages of feeling or sensation back to the brain from the body, such as heat, cold, or pain. The body also has an autonomic nervous system. It controls the involuntary activities of the body; such as blood pressure, body temperature, and sweating.

The nerve fibers that make up the communication systems of the body can be compared to a telephone system. The telephone cable (spinal cord) sends messages between the main office (the brain) and individual offices (parts of the body) over the telephone lines (nerve fibers). The spinal cord is the pathway that messages use to travel between the brain and the other parts of the body.

Because the spinal cord is such an important part of our nervous system, it is surrounded and protected by bones called vertebrae. The vertebrae, or backbones, are stacked on top of each other. This is called the vertebral column or the spinal column. The vertebral column is

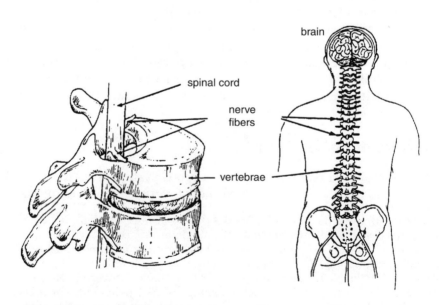

Figure 39.1. *The spinal cord goes through the center of the stacked vertebrae. These bones protect the spinal cord. The nerve fibers branch out from the spinal cord to other parts of the body.*

432

the number one support for the body. The spinal cord runs through the middle of the vertebrae [See Figure 39.1].

The spinal cord is about 18 inches long. The cord extends from the base of the brain, down the middle of the back, to about the waist. The bundles of nerve fibers that make up the spinal cord itself are Upper Motor Neurons (UMNs). Spinal nerves that branch off the spinal cord up and down the neck and back are lower motor neurons (LMNs). These nerves exit between each vertebrae and go out to all parts of the body. At the end of the spinal cord, the lower spinal nerve fibers continue down through the spinal canal to the sacrum, or tailbone. [See Figure 39.2]

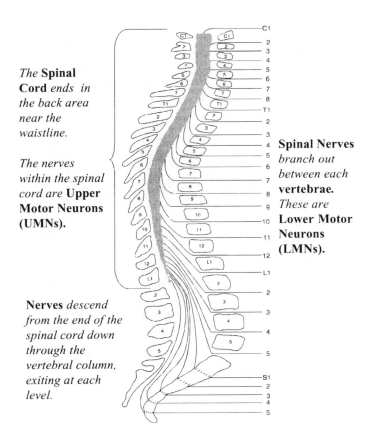

The **Spinal Cord** *ends in the back area near the waistline.*

The nerves within the spinal cord are **Upper Motor Neurons (UMNs).**

Spinal Nerves *branch out between each* **vertebrae.** *These are* **Lower Motor Neurons (LMNs).**

Nerves *descend from the end of the spinal cord down through the vertebral column, exiting at each level.*

Figure 39.2. *Spinal Nerves*

The spinal column is divided into four sections. The top portion is the cervical area. It has eight cervical nerves and seven cervical vertebrae. Moving down the back, the next section is the thoracic area. It includes the chest area and has twelve thoracic vertebrae. The lower back section is the lumbar area and has five lumbar vertebrae. The bottom section has five sacral vertebrae and is the sacral area. The bones in the sacral section are actually fused together into one bone. [See Figure 39.3]

The Spinal Cord after an Injury

Damage to the spinal cord can occur from either a traumatic injury or from a disease to the vertebral column. In most spinal cord injuries, the backbone pinches the spinal cord, causing it to become bruised

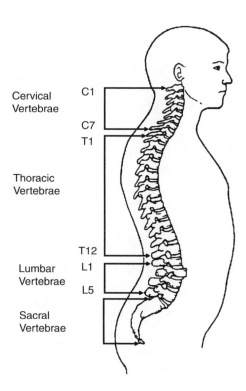

Figure 39.3. Vertebrae

or swollen. Sometimes the injury may tear the spinal cord and/or its nerve fibers. An infection or a disease can result in similar damage.

After a spinal cord injury, all the nerves above the level of injury keep working like they always have. From the point of injury and below, the spinal cord nerves cannot send messages between the brain and parts of the body like they did before the injury.

The doctor examines the individual to understand what damage has been done to the spinal cord. An x-ray shows where the damage occurred to the vertebrae. The doctor does a pin prick test to see what feeling the person has all over his body (sensory level). The doctor also asks, "what parts of the body can you move?" and tests the strength of key muscle groups (motor level). These exams are important because they tell what nerves and muscles are working.

Each spinal cord injury is different. A person's injury is described by its level and type.

Level of Injury

The level of injury for a person with SCI is the lowest point on the spinal cord below which there is a decrease or absence of feeling (the sensory level) and/or movement (the motor level).

Tetraplegia [formerly called quadriplegia] generally describes the condition of a person with a spinal cord injury that is at a level from C1 to T1. This individual can experience a loss of feeling and/or movement in their head, neck, shoulder, arms and/or upper chest.

Paraplegia is the general term describing the condition of a person who has lost feeling and/or is not able to move the lower parts of his/her body. The body parts that may be affected are the chest, stomach, hips, legs, and feet. An individual with a level from T2 to S5 has paraplegia.

The higher the spinal cord injury is on the vertebral column, or the closer it is to the brain, the more effect it has on how the body moves and what one can feel. More movement, feeling, and voluntary control of the body's systems are present with a lower level of injury. For example, a person with a C-5 level of injury has a decrease or loss of feeling and movement below the 5th cervical spinal cord segment. An injury at the T-8 level means the individual has a decrease or loss of feeling and movement below the eighth thoracic spinal cord segment. Someone with a T-8 level of injury would have more feeling and movement than someone with a C-5 level of injury.

435

Complete or Incomplete Injury

The amount of feeling and movement that an individual has also depends on whether the injury is complete or incomplete. A complete injury means there is no motor or sensory function in the S4 or S5 area, or anal area. If there is evidence of any motor or sensory function in this area, one of three incomplete injury classifications is given.

Some people with an incomplete injury may have feeling, but little or no movement. Others may have movement and little or no feeling. Incomplete spinal injuries differ from one person to another because the amount of damage to each person's nerve fibers is different. This fact makes it impossible to accurately predict how much of an individual's sensory and motor function will return. There is a greater chance of return of some or all of a person's motor and sensory function if an individual is incomplete at the time of injury.

Changes after the Initial Injury

Sometimes the spinal cord is only bruised or swollen after the initial injury. As the swelling goes down, the nerves may begin to work again. There are no tests at this time to tell how many nerves, if any, will begin to work again or when this will occur. This makes it impossible for medical staff to guarantee how much or when function may return.

Some individuals have involuntary movements, such as twitching or shaking. These movements are called spasms. Spasms are not a sign of recovery. A spasm occurs when a wrong message from the nerve causes the muscle to move. The individual often cannot control this movement.

In addition to movement and feeling, a spinal cord injury affects how other systems of the body work. An individual with SCI learns new ways to manage his/her bladder and bowel. His/her skin and lungs often need special care and attention to stay healthy. There may also be changes in sexual function.

Functional Goals

Functional goals are a realistic expectation of activities that a person with spinal cord injury eventually should be able to do with a particular level of injury. These goals are set during rehabilitation with the medical team. They help the individual with SCI learn new ways to manage his/her daily activities and stay healthy.

Achievement of functional goals can also be affected by other factors, such as an individual's body type and health-related issues. By striving to reach these functional goals, the hope is to give individuals with SCI the opportunity to achieve maximum independence.

The chart (Table 39.1), "Functional Goals for Specific Levels of Complete Injury," shows the expected functional goals for a person with a complete injury at a particular level. Motor and sensory functions improve with lower levels of injury.

Resources

Consortium for Spinal Cord Medicine. *Outcomes following traumatic spinal cord injury: Clinical practice guidelines for health care professionals.* 1999.

Corbet B, Dobbs J, and Bonin B. Spinal Network: *The Total Wheelchair Book,* 3rd Ed. 1998. [Available from: Spinal Network, P.O. Box 8987, Malibu, CA 90265-8987. 800-543-4116].

Hammond M, Umlauf R, Matteson B, and Perduta-Fulginiti S. *Yes, You Can! A Guide to Self-Care for Persons with Spinal Cord Injury.* 2nd Ed. Washington, DC: Paralyzed Veterans of America, 1993. [Cost: $12 Order from PVA].

International Standards for Neurological and Functional Classification of SCI, Rev. 1996. [Available from: American Spinal Injury Association. Online: http://www.asia-spinalinjury.org/publications/index. html].

An Introduction to Spinal Cord Injury: Understanding the Changes, 1998 Ed. [Available from: Paralyzed Veterans of America. Cost: First copy free, additional are $1.50.]

Kirshblum SC and O'Connor KC. Levels of spinal cord injury and predictors of neurologic recovery. In: Kraft GH and Hammond MC, eds. *Physical Medicine and Rehabilitation Clinics of North America, Topics in Spinal Cord Injury Medicine.* Philadelphia: W.B. Saunders Co., 2000; 11(1):1-28.

Learning about Spinal Cord Injury. 1991. Booklet. Available from Medical RRTC on Secondary Conditions of SCI. [Cost: $3 +s/h].

Locating Information About SCI, Spinal Cord Injury InfoSheet #1. Level–Consumer. [Available from RRTC on Secondary Conditions of SCI. Online: http://main.uab.edu/show.asp?durki=21478 or via FAX: 205-975-8376 / #101].

Table 39.1. Spinal Cord Injury—Functional Goals for Specific Levels of Complete Injury

Level	Abilities	Functional Goals
C1-C3	C3-limited movement of head and neck	**Breathing**: Depends on a ventilator for breathing. **Communication**: Talking is sometimes difficult, very limited or impossible. If ability to talk is limited, communication can be accomplished independently with a mouth stick and assistive technologies like a computer for speech or typing. Effective verbal communication allows the individual with SCI to direct caregivers in the person's daily activities, like bathing, dressing, personal hygiene, transferring, as well as bladder and bowel management. **Daily tasks**: Assistive technology allows for independence in tasks such as turning pages, using a telephone, and operating lights and appliances. **Mobility**: Can operate an electric wheelchair by using a head control, mouth stick, or chin control. A power tilt wheelchair also for independent pressure relief.
C3-C4	Usually has head and neck control. Individuals at C4 level may shrug their shoulders.	**Breathing**: May initially require a ventilator for breathing, usually adjust to breathing full-time without ventilatory assistance. **Communication**: Normal. **Daily tasks**: With specialized equipment, some may have limited independence in feeding and independently operate an adjustable bed with an adapted controller.
C5	Typically has head and neck control, can shrug shoulder and has shoulder control. Can bend his/her elbows and turn palms face up.	**Daily tasks**: Independence with eating, drinking, face washing, brushing of teeth, face shaving, and hair care after assistance in setting up specialized equipment. **Health care**: Can manage their own health care by doing self-assist coughs and pressure reliefs by leaning forward or side-to-side. **Mobility**: May have strength to push a manual wheelchair for short distances over smooth surfaces. A power wheelchair with hand controls is typically used for daily activities. Driving may be possible after being evaluated by a qualified professional to determine special equipment needs.

438

C6	Has movement in head, neck, shoulders, arms, and wrists. Can shrug shoulders, bend elbows, turn palms up and down, and extend wrists.	**Daily tasks:** With help of some specialized equipment, can perform with greater ease and independence, daily tasks of feeding, bathing, grooming, personal hygiene, and dressing. May independently perform light housekeeping duties. **Health care:** Can independently do pressure reliefs, skin checks, and turn in bed. **Mobility:** Some individuals can independently do transfers but often require a sliding board. Can use a manual wheelchair for daily activities but may use power wheelchair for greater ease of independence.
C7	Has similar movement as an individual with C6, with added ability to straighten his/her elbows.	**Daily tasks:** Able to perform household duties. Need fewer adaptive aids in independent living. **Health care:** Able to do wheelchair pushups for pressure reliefs. **Mobility:** Daily use of manual wheelchair. Can transfer with greater ease.
C8-T1	Has added strength and precision of fingers that result in limited or natural hand function.	**Daily tasks:** Can live independently without assistive devices in feeding, bathing, grooming, oral and facial hygiene, dressing, bladder management, and bowel management. **Mobility:** Uses manual wheelchair. Can transfer independently.
T2-T6	Has normal motor function in head, neck, shoulders, arms, hands, and fingers. Has increased use of rib and chest muscles, or trunk control.	**Daily tasks:** Should be totally independent with all activities. **Mobility:** A few individuals are capable of limited walking with extensive bracing. This requires extremely high energy and puts stress on the upper body, offering no functional advantage. Can lead to damage of upper joints.
T7-T12	Has added motor function from increased abdominal control.	**Daily tasks:** Able to perform unsupported seated activities. **Mobility:** Same as above. Health care: Has improved cough effectiveness.

Table 39.1. (continued on next page)

Table 39.1. Spinal Cord Injury—Functional Goals for Specific Levels of Complete Injury (*continued from previous page*)

Level	Abilities	Functional Goals
L1-L5	Has additional return of motor movement in the hips and knees.	**Mobility:** Walking can be a viable function, with the help of specialized leg and ankle braces. Lower levels walk with greater ease with the help of assistive devices.
S1-S5	Depending on level of injury, there are various degrees of return of voluntary bladder, bowel and sexual functions.	**Mobility:** Increased ability to walk with fewer or no supportive devices.

Spinal Cord Injury: Facts and Figures at a Glance. January 2000. National Spinal Cord Injury Statistical Center. Birmingham, AL. [Available at www.spinalcord.uab.edu/show.asp?durki=21446].

Spinal Cord Injury Patient Education Manual. 1998. [Available from Penn State Geisinger Rehabilitation Center, 500 University Dr., Hershey, PA. 17033, 717-531-8521.]

Take Control: Multimedia Guide to Spinal Cord Injury-Vol.1. 1996. [CD-Rom programs Available from Arkansas Spinal Cord Commission, 1501 N University Ste. 400, Little Rock, AR 72202, 501-296-1788, Email: arkscc@aol.com].

Spinal Cord Injury Rehabilitation Facility Selection

It is very important to be confident about the quality of care you or a loved one will receive when entering a rehabilitation program. Very few people have prior experience with rehabilitation or the effects of a spinal cord injury (SCI), thus assessing the quality of a rehabilitation program is difficult.

Although the final decision will ultimately depend upon individual circumstances such as insurance and location, all rehabilitation programs have features which can be evaluated, regardless of your prior knowledge of rehabilitation or SCI.

It is vital to select a high quality rehabilitation program with skilled professionals to help a newly injured person develop the skills needed to maintain physical and emotional health throughout his/her lifetime.

A Quick Word about Rehabilitation Programs

In order to develop and maintain quality services for individuals with spinal cord injuries, rehabilitation staff and programs *must* specialize in treating SCI. This expertise is best acquired and maintained when staff members treat people with SCI on a regular basis. High quality rehabilitation programs are often located in facilities devoted exclusively to providing rehabilitation services, or in hospitals with designated SCI units.

In-patient SCI rehabilitation programs have features which distinguish them from the hospital programs where most people receive initial treatment. Rehabilitation programs are designed to serve people with a wide variety of skills and must address complex social and community issues. A rehabilitation team comprised of specialized medical personnel is used to accomplish these goals.

Teams should include social workers, occupational and physical therapists, recreational therapists, rehabilitation nurses, rehabilitation psychologists, vocational counselors, nutritionists, and other specialists. The team is usually directed by a physiatrist, a physician specializing in physical medicine and rehabilitation. Team members are jointly responsible for working with individuals and their families to develop effective rehabilitation and discharge plans.

The team should assign a program manager who will function as a contact with the rest of the team. This contact should meet with the person undergoing rehabilitation on a regular basis to discuss the rehabilitation plan and to address personal or family concerns.

Rehabilitation programs and acute care units may also differ in their emphasis on family and patient participation. Although many factors can contribute to someone's successful return to the community following a spinal cord injury, the education and active involvement of the newly injured person and the family is crucial. Rehabilitation programs should focus on maximizing a person's ability to be independent and should assist in making decisions about treatment and goals.

The following questions were developed to assist you in your decision making process. They can be used as a checklist to obtain the information required to make an informed decision when choosing a rehabilitation program.

SCI Program Checklist

General Considerations

Peer support and contact with others who have a SCI can be extremely important in helping a person adjust to the injury. Peer support is generally most helpful and accepted when people share similar problems and issues. This is an especially important consideration when choosing programs for women. It is often difficult for women to find peer support because the incidence of SCI among women is much lower than it is for men.

1. Are the beds for people with SCI in the same area of the facility?

2. Are there people in the SCI program of the same age and sex as the person considering admission?

3. Do the people in the SCI program have similar levels and kinds of spinal cord injury e.g., quadriplegia, paraplegia, incomplete, and complete?

4. What is the average number of people admitted annually to the SCI program? (program staff should treat people with SCI on a regular basis to acquire and maintain expertise.)

5. Is the SCI program accredited by the Commission on the Accreditation of Rehabilitation Facilities (CARF) or the Joint Commission on Accreditation of Healthcare Organizations (JCAHO)? Has it been designated as a Model Spinal Cord Injury Center by the National Institute of Disability Research and Rehabilitation (NIDRR)? Is the SCI program part of a SCI rehabilitation system operated by the state?

6. Are there treatment specialists in the SCI program who speak the primary language of the individual seeking treatment?

7. Will the treatment team develop a rehabilitation plan with both short and long-term goals?

8. Will an experienced case manager be assigned to help family members obtain medical payments and other benefits from public and private insurance?

9. Will a team member be assigned to coordinate treatment and act as a contact for staff and family members?

Staffing/Rehabilitation Program Elements

1. Is the physician in charge a physiatrist? If not, what credentials does he/she have? How long has the physician in charge been directing programs specializing in SCI?

2. Is there physician coverage seven days a week? Twenty-four hours a day?

3. Do the regular nursing staff and other specialists responsible for providing treatment in the SCI program have specific training in treating SCI? Is the nursing staff employed by the hospital or employed through an outside agency?

4. Does the program ensure the availability of rehabilitation nursing and respiratory care on a twenty-four hour basis?

5. Are there consultants available at the facility or nearby medical centers? These should include neurosurgery, neurology, urology, orthopedics, plastic surgery, neuropsychology, internal

medicine, gynecology, speech pathology, pulmonary medicine, general surgery, and psychiatry.

6. How often and for how long each day will participants get treatment by specialists such as occupational and physical therapists? Treatment should be no less then three hours per day.

7. Are other specialties such as driver education, rehabilitation engineering, chaplaincy, and therapeutic recreation available if needed?

8. Are activities planned for SCI program participants on weekends and evenings?

9. How much time is spent teaching SCI program participants and their families about sexuality, bowel and bladder care, skin care, and other essential self-care activities?

10. Does the SCI program offer training in the management and hiring of personal care assistants? If so, how much time is spent by staff on this topic?

Special Programs

Pediatric Programs

Because incidence rates of SCI among children are relatively low, rehabilitation hospitals and programs usually do not maintain a separate program or unit exclusively for children with SCI. As an alternative, caregivers may consider facilities/programs which place children with SCI in rehabilitation units with other children with chronic disabilities. Hopefully, this will provide families and children with opportunities to share common experiences and information with each other, and may lead to the development of support networks in the community.

It is possible that children may be placed in units with other children who are too ill for rehabilitation. Children generally derive greater benefit if they undergo rehabilitation with other children who are actively involved in the rehabilitation process.

1. Are the beds for children with spinal cord injuries in one area or in the same location as children with similar disabilities?

2. Are children of the same sex and similar age currently in the program/facility?

3. Is the physician in charge an individual with experience in rehabilitation? Does this physician have experience with children? If not, what are his/her qualifications? Do the other staff members specialize in pediatrics?

4. How many children with SCI does the program/facility admit on an annual basis?

5. Does the program/facility offer educational programs for children and young adults undergoing treatment? If not, does the facility coordinate tutoring programs with local schools? If so, who is responsible for payment?

6. Are there child life or therapeutic recreation specialists on staff? (Child life specialists develop programs for children and families which strive to maintain normal living patterns and minimize the clinical environment. Therapeutic recreation specialists focus on teaching persons with disabilities new leisure and sports skills to maximize their independence).

7. Are young siblings and friends allowed to visit the unit?

8. Does the program/facility offer adaptive technology to help children communicate and learn?

9. Is counseling available for siblings and families members?

10. Is the equipment used by therapists, i.e. physical therapists and occupational therapists, appropriate for children?

11. Does the facility/program provide patient education materials for children and family members?

Ventilator Programs

1. Is the physician who directs the program a board certified pulmonologist or a physiatrist? Does he/she have experience with SCI?

2. Are ventilator users treated on the same unit?

3. How long has the facility been providing treatment for ventilator users?

4. If the treatment team determines that an individual cannot breathe independently, what kind of services are offered to assist them in living as independently as possible?

5. Are people in the unit similar in age to the person considering admission?

6. Will they have the opportunity to meet ventilator users who have returned to the community and maximized their independence?

Special Considerations

Psychosocial/Counseling Services

1. What types and how many hours of psychosocial services are available? These should include peer support, individual and group psychotherapy, couples, vocational and substance abuse counseling.

2. Does the facility offer sexuality and fertility counseling?

Facility Policies/Family Members

1. Do facility policies encourage family members including siblings regardless of age, to participate in rehabilitation programs?

2. Are there living arrangements for family members participating in training? What other services, parking, meals, etc. are provided?

3. Are counseling and other social services available to family members?

Discharge Planning

1. Are SCI program participants given educational self-care manuals when they are discharged?

2. Will staff members develop a formal discharge plan with program participants and their families?

3. Does the facility and discharge planner work with local Independent Living Centers? Do they incorporate referrals to these centers into their discharge planning?

4. Is there an independent living unit available for program participants and families to practice self-care skills? Can family members stay there also?

5. If the facility does not have an independent living unit do they encourage overnight therapeutic leave prior to discharge?

6. Will someone be assigned as a liaison to provide follow-up services?

7. Will a staff member visit or make arrangements for someone locally to evaluate the home for modifications?

8. Will the follow-up plan include:

   - Referral to an appropriate physician and other medical specialists in the community?
   - Regular follow-up visits with this physician or a spinal cord injury unit physician?
   - Regular urological evaluations?
   - Scheduled equipment evaluations?
   - If appropriate, a thorough vocational evaluation and referrals to a vocational rehabilitation program?
   - Referrals to other services and resources in the community, e.g. elder services?

Before Making the Final Decision

1. Were staff members helpful and friendly when information was requested?

2. Were you offered an opportunity to tour the facility? If you were able to make a tour, what were your impressions of the overall atmosphere?

3. Did you have an opportunity to speak with people currently participating in the program? If so, were they satisfied with their rehabilitation programs?

Additional Information

National Spinal Cord Injury Association
6701 Democracy Boulevard, Suite 300-9
Bethesda, MD 20817
Toll-Free: 800-962-9629
Tel: 301-588-6959

National Spinal Cord Injury Association (continued)
Fax: 301-588-9414
Website: www.spinalcord.org

American Spinal Injury Association
2020 Peachtree Road, N.W.
Atlanta, GA 30309-1402
Tel: 404-355-9772
Fax: 404-355-1826
Website: www.asia-spinalinjury.org

Paralyzed Veterans of America
801 18th St., N.W.
Washington, DC 20006
Toll-Free: 800-424-8200
E-mail: info@pva.org
Website: www.pva.org

RRTC on Aging with Spinal Cord Injury
Rancho Los Amigos Medical Center
7601 E. Imperial Hwy.
800 West Annex
Downey, CA 90242-3456
Tel: 562-401-7402
Fax: 562-401-7011
Website: www.agingwithsci.org
E-mail: rrtcsci@aol.com

Medical RRTC on Secondary Conditions of SCI
UAB Spain Rehabilitation Center
1717 6th Avenue South
Birmingham, AL 35233-3334
Tel: 205-934-3334
TTD: 205-934-4642
Fax: 205-934-4642
Website: http://main.uab.edu/show.asp?durki=8153#Contact
E-mail: rtc@sun.rehabm.uab.edu

Chapter 40

Stiff-Person Syndrome

What Is Stiff-Person Syndrome?

Stiff-person syndrome is a rare progressive neurological disorder characterized by constant painful contractions and spasms of voluntary muscles, particularly the muscles of the back and upper legs. Symptoms may occur gradually, spreading from the back and legs to involve the arms and neck. Symptoms may worsen when the affected individual is anxious or exposed to sudden motion or noise. Affected muscles may become twisted and contracted, resulting in bone fractures in the most severe cases. Individuals with stiff-person syndrome may have difficulty making sudden movements and may have a stiff-legged, unsteady gait. Sleep usually suppresses frequency of contractions. Stiffness may increase and patients may develop a hunched posture (kyphosis) or a swayback (lordosis). Researchers theorize that stiff-person syndrome may be an autoimmune disorder. Other autoimmune disorders such as diabetes, pernicious anemia (a chronic, progressive blood disorder), and thyroiditis (inflammation of the thyroid gland) may occur more frequently in patients with stiff-person syndrome.

"NINDS Stiff-Person Syndrome Information Page," National Institute of Neurological Disorders and Stroke (NINDS), reviewed 7/01/2001; and "Immunotherapy Treatment Shows Dramatic Results for Rare Neurological Disorder," NINDS news release: Wednesday, December 26, 2001.

Is There Any Treatment?

The drug diazepam, which relaxes the muscles, provides improvement in most cases. Baclofen, phenytoin, clonidine, or tizanidine may provide additional benefit. Physical and rehabilitation therapy may also be needed.

What Is the Prognosis?

There is no cure for stiff-person syndrome. The long-term prognosis for individuals with stiff-person syndrome is uncertain. Management of the disorder with drug therapy may provide significant improvements and relief of symptoms.

What Research Is Being Done?

Research on stiff-person syndrome is aimed at enhancing scientific understanding of the disorder and evaluating new therapeutic interventions.

Selected References

Barker, R, and Marsden C. Successful Treatment of Stiff Man Syndrome with Intravenous Immunoglobulin. *Journal of Neurology, Neurosurgery, and Neuropsychiatry*, 62; 426 (1997).

Bradley, W, et al (eds). *Neurology in Clinical Practice: Principles of Diagnosis and Management*, vol. II. Butterworth-Heinemann, Boston, p. 367 (1991).

Levy, L., Floeter, MK, and Dalakas, M. Stiff-person syndrome—an autoimmune disorder affecting gamma-aminobutyric acid (GABA) neurotransmission. *Annals of Internal Medicine* 131; 522-530 (1999).

McEvoy, K. Stiff-man Syndrome. *Mayo Clinic Proceedings*, 66; 300-304 (1991).

McEvoy, K. Stiff-man Syndrome. *Seminars in Neurology*, 11:3; 197-204 (September 1991).

Spada, P, and Spada, J. Stiff-man Syndrome: A Rare Disorder of the Central Nervous System. *Journal of Neuroscience Nursing*, 26:6; 364-366 (December 1994).

Thoene, J (ed). *Physicians' Guide to Rare Diseases*. Dowden Publishing Company, Inc., Montvale, NJ, p. 441 (1992).

Wyngaarden, J, et al (eds). *Cecil Textbook of Medicine*, 19th edition. W.B. Saunders Co., Philadelphia, p. 2264 (1992).

Immunotherapy Treatment Shows Dramatic Results for Rare Neurological Disorder

An immunologic therapy, intravenous immunoglobulin (IVIg), administered to patients suffering from stiff person syndrome (SPS), provides dramatic relief from disabling symptoms, according to a study appearing in the December 27, 2001, issue of *The New England Journal of Medicine*.* The study's principal author, Marinos C. Dalakas, M.D., chief of the Neuromuscular Diseases Section of the National Institute of Neurological Disorders and Stroke, says that the success of the treatment supports the theory that SPS is the result of an autoimmune response gone awry in the brain and spinal cord.

SPS is characterized by fluctuating muscle rigidity in the trunk and limbs and a heightened sensitivity to stimuli such as noise, touch, and emotional distress that can set off muscular spasms. People with SPS are often too disabled to walk or move, or are afraid to leave the house because of stimuli-triggered spasms and frequent falls. The incidence of SPS has been estimated at one in every one million persons, but according to Dr. Dalakas, "the disorder is so often misdiagnosed—as Parkinson's disease, multiple sclerosis, fibromyalgia, psychosomatic illness, or anxiety and phobia—that its actual incidence is probably much higher."

Researchers have known since the 1980s that people with SPS have elevated circulating antibodies against a particular enzyme, glutamic acid decarboxylase (GAD_{65}), involved in the synthesis of y-aminobutyric acid (GABA), an inhibitory neurotransmitter that controls muscle movement. Since GABA modulates the action of the excitatory muscular neurotransmitters, lower levels of circulating GABA allow the excitatory neurotransmitters to hijack communications between the brain and the motor system, overstimulating the muscles into stiffness and spasm.

This link between the neurological symptoms of SPS and a potential immunological culprit led to several preliminary but successful attempts to treat the symptoms of the disorder with immuno-modulating therapies, including IVIg. Dr. Dalakas and his colleagues put this anecdotal evidence to the test by designing a double-blind, cross-over study that would measure the effect of immunoglobulin therapy versus placebo in a group of patients with SPS.

The research team selected 16 patients who tested positive for GAD_{65} antibodies to receive either IVIg or placebo for 3 months. After a 1-month washout period, the patients crossed to the alternative therapy. Results were based on a stiffness scale and a heightened sense scale devised by Dr. Dalakas and his colleagues to detect changes in the severity of spasms.

Patients treated with IVIg showed a statistically significant decrease in symptoms of stiffness and spasm. The scores of the IVIg-randomized patients dropped significantly from the first month to the fourth, but rebounded when they crossed to placebo. In the placebo group, scores remained constant for the first 4 months, and then dropped after crossing to IVIg. Eleven of the 14 patients who finished the study became less stiff and more mobile, and were able to either walk unassisted, resume work activities, or remain upright without fear of falling. The current treatment standard for SPS is diazepam, but according to Dr. Dalakas, "most patients require such high dosages that they become overly sedated." IVIg treats symptoms more successfully and comes with no disabling side effects.

The mechanism of action of IVIg is not completely understood. Dalakas proposes that IVIg either blocks production of GAD65 or somehow neutralizes the circulating antibodies. What causes SPS is also uncertain. "We don't know why the body begins to produce these antibodies or how they reach the neuronal cell," says Dalakas. "It could be a virus, or something else that breaks tolerance and induces the autoimmune process. What we do know is that we have a strong indication that SPS is an autoimmune disease. As a result, we may be able to propose and test additional autoimmune modulators." The Bayer Corporation and Crescent Health donated part of the IVIg used in the study.

The NINDS, part of the National Institutes of Health in Bethesda, Maryland, is the nation's leading supporter of biomedical research on the brain and nervous system.

*Dalakas, M; Fujii, M; Li, M; Lutfi, B; Kyhos, J; McElroy, B. "A Randomized Controlled Trial of High-Dose Intravenous Immunoglobulin in the Treatment of Patients with Stiff Person Syndrome." *The New England Journal of Medicine*, December 27, 2001, Vol. 345, pp. 1870-1876.

Additional Information

National Rehabilitation Information Center (NARIC)
4200 Forbes Boulevard, Suite 202
Lanham, MD 20706
Toll-Free: 800-346-2742

Tel: 301-459-5900
Fax: 301-562-2401
Website: www.naric.com
E-mail: naricinfo@heitechservices.com

National Organization for Rare Disorders (NORD)
P.O. Box 1968
Danbury, CT 06813-1968
Toll-Free: 800-999-NORD (6673)
Tel: 203-746-6518
Fax: 203-746-6481
Website: www.rarediseases.org
E-mail: orphan@rarediseases.org

National Institute of Arthritis and Musculoskeletal and Skin Diseases (NIAMS)
National Institutes of Health
1 AMS Circle
Bethesda, MD 20892-2350
Toll-Free: 877-22-NIAMS (226-4267)
Tel: 301-496-8188
Fax: 301-718-6366
Website: www.nih.gov/niams
E-mail: NIAMSInfo@mail.nih.gov

Chapter 41

Wilson's Disease

Wilson's disease is a genetic disorder that is fatal unless detected and treated before serious illness from copper poisoning develops. Wilson's disease affects approximately one in 30,000 people worldwide. The genetic defect causes excessive copper accumulation in the liver or brain.

Small amounts of copper are as essential as vitamins. Copper is present in most foods, and most people have much more copper than they need. Healthy people excrete copper they don't need but Wilson's disease patients cannot.

Copper begins to accumulate immediately after birth. Excess copper attacks the liver or brain, resulting in hepatitis, psychiatric, or neurologic symptoms. The symptoms usually appear in late adolescence. Patients may have jaundice, abdominal swelling, vomiting of blood, and abdominal pain. They may have tremors and difficulty walking, talking, and swallowing. They may develop all degrees of mental illness including homicidal or suicidal behavior, depression, and aggression. Women may have menstrual irregularities, absent periods, infertility, or multiple miscarriages. No matter how the disease begins, it is always fatal if it is not diagnosed and treated.

The first part of the body that copper affects is the liver. In about half of Wilson's disease patients the liver is the only affected organ.

Reprinted with permission from "About Wilson's Disease," by H. Ascher Sellner, MD, President. Wilson's Disease Association International © 1997. Contact the Wilson's Disease Association at 4 Navaho Drive, Brookfield, CT 06804, 800-399-0266 or visit their website at www.wilsonsdisease.org.

The physical changes in the liver are only visible under the microscope. When hepatitis develops, patients are often thought to have infectious hepatitis or infectious mononucleosis when they actually have Wilson's disease hepatitis. Testing for Wilson's disease should be performed in individuals with unexplained, abnormal liver tests.

How Is Wilson's Disease Diagnosed?

The diagnosis of Wilson's disease is made by relatively simple tests. The tests can diagnose the disease in both symptomatic patients and people who show no signs of the disease. These tests can include:

- Ophthalmologic slit lamp examination for Kayser-Fleischer rings
- Serum ceruloplasmin test
- 24-hour urine copper test
- Liver biopsy for histology and histochemistry and copper quantification
- Genetic testing, including haplotype analysis for siblings.

It is important to diagnose Wilson's disease as early as possible, since severe liver damage can occur before there are any signs of the disease. Individuals with Wilson's disease may falsely appear to be in excellent health.

Is Wilson's Disease an Inherited Disorder?

Wilson's disease is transmitted as an autosomal recessive disease, which means it is not sex-linked (it occurs equally in men and women). At least one in 30,000 people of all races and nationalities has the disease. In order to inherit it, both parents must carry a gene that each passes to the affected child. Two abnormal genes are required to have the disease.

The responsible gene is located at a precisely known site on chromosome 13. The gene is called ATP7B. Some cases of Wilson's disease occur due to spontaneous mutations in the gene. Most are transmitted from generation to generation.

Most patients have no family history of Wilson's disease. People with only one abnormal gene are called carriers. Carriers (heterozygotes) may have mild, but medically insignificant, abnormalities of copper metabolism. Carriers do not become ill and should not be treated.

More than 300 different mutations have been identified thus far. Therefore, it has been difficult to devise a simple genetic screening test for the disease. However, in a particular family, if the precise mutation is identified, a genetic diagnosis is possible by haplotype analysis. This requires a blood sample from both the patient and a relative. The samples are compared to each other. Haplotype testing helps to find symptom-free siblings who have the disease so that they may be treated before they become ill or handicapped.

Some day a genetic test may help in prenatal diagnosis. However, at this time, there is no available test for widespread genetic screening or prenatal diagnosis.

The Likelihood of Inheriting Wilson's Disease

• One in 100 individuals in the general population carry the Wilson's disease gene. Carriers have one normal and one abnormal gene.

• 100% of a patient's children receive a Wilson's disease gene.

• 50% of a carrier's children receive the Wilson's disease gene since the carrier has one normal and one abnormal gene.

• Siblings of Wilson's disease patients have a 25% chance of having the disease. Since both of a siblings' parents are carriers, 1/4 of the siblings' children have the disease, 1/2 (2/4) are carriers, and 1/4 are disease free with no Wilson's disease gene.

• Children of patients have 1/200 chance of having the disease. From the patient, their children have a 100% chance of getting the abnormal gene. The patient's spouse, a normal person, has 1/100 chances of carrying the gene and 1/2 the time he/she will pass it on.

• Grandchildren of patients have a 1/400 chance of having the disease. From the patient's child, grandchildren have a 50% chance of getting a gene (1/2) since all patient's children are carriers. From the other parent, they have a 1/200 chance of getting the gene: 1/2 times (1/2 times 1/100) from the normal spouse = 1/400.

• Nieces and nephews of parents of siblings who do not have Wilson's disease have a 1/600 chance of having the disease. Two-thirds of unaffected siblings carry the gene. The risk of the couple both being carriers is 2/3 times 1/100 = 1/150 and the risk of each of their children having the disease is 1/4 times 1/150 = 1/600.

- Cousins have a 1/800 chance of having the disease.

*Fifty percent of aunts and uncles are carriers. Therefore, 1/2 times 1/100 = 1/200 are couples with each being a carrier and 1/4 children will be affected = 1/800.

All siblings, aunts, uncles, children, nieces, nephews, and cousins of Wilson's disease patients should be tested for Wilson's disease. People with Wilson's disease may not have any signs, symptoms, or evidence of illness. However, all of them with mild or non-apparent Wilson's disease will always become seriously ill and eventually die if they are not treated. Testing is simple and safe. There are excellent treatments available. Failure to treat Wilson's disease causes severe disability and eventually death.

How Is Wilson's Disease Being Treated?

Wilson's disease is a very treatable condition. With proper therapy, disease progress can be halted and oftentimes symptoms can be improved. Treatment is aimed at removing excess accumulated copper and preventing its reaccumulation. Therapy must be life-long. Patients may become progressively more sick from day to day, so immediate treatment can be critical. Treatment delays may cause irreversible damage.

The newest FDA-approved drug is zinc acetate (Galzin™). Zinc acts by blocking the absorption of copper in the intestinal tract. This action both depletes accumulated copper and prevents its reaccumulation. Zinc's effectiveness has been shown by more than 30 years of considerable experience overseas. A major advantage of zinc therapy is its lack of side effects.

Other drugs approved for use in Wilson's disease include penicillamine (Cuprimine, Depen) and trientine (Syprine). Both of these drugs act by chelation or binding of copper, causing its increased urinary excretion. Tetrathiomolybdate is under investigation for initial treatment of Wilson's disease and, thus far, it has not caused neurological worsening that often occurs with penicillamine and even with trientine. Zinc has far fewer side effects and the side effects are much less severe.

Patients with severe hepatitis may require liver transplant. Patients being investigated or treated for Wilson's disease should be cared for by specialists in Wilson's disease or by specialists in consultation with their primary physicians.

Stopping treatment completely will result in death, sometimes as quickly as within three months. Decreasing dosage of medications also can result in unnecessary disease progression.

Additional Information

Wilson's Disease Association, International
4 Navaho Drive
Brookfield, CT 06804
Toll-Free: 800-399-0266
Tel: 203-775-9666
Fax: 203-775-9666
Website: www.wilsonsdisease.org
E-mail: haseliner@worldnet.att.net

Wilson's Disease Association Centers of Excellence

The WDA Centers of Excellence provide physicians who are well trained in the diagnosis and treatment of Wilson's Disease, physician training, and research regarding Wilson's Disease, broad services needed by Wilson's Disease patients and their families, and technical support required by patients (including laboratory metal analysis).

University of Michigan Hospital
Department of Human Genetics
4708 Medical Science II
P.O. Box 0618
Ann Arbor, MI 48109-0618
Tel: 734-764-5499
Fax: 734-763-3784
E-mail: brewergj@umich.edu

Mount Sinai Hospital
Division of Liver Disease
P.O. Box 1633
One Gustave Levy Place
New York, NY 10029-6574
Tel: 212-241-0034
Fax: 212-996-5149
Website: www.mssm.edu/medicine/liver/web_resources.shtml
E-mail: michael.schilsky@mssm.edu

Stanford University Medical Center
Adult Hepatology
300 Pasteur Drive
Palo Alto, CA 94304
Tel: 650-498-7878
Fax: 650-498-7888
Website: www.med.Stanford.edu/shs/txp/livertxp

Stanford University Medical Center
Lucile Packard Children's Hospital Liver Clinic
Pediatric Hepatology
725 Welch Road
Palo Alto, CA 94304
Tel: 650-723-5070 (for appointments)
Fax: 650-498-5608
Website: www.lpch.org

Stanford University Medical Center
Adult and Pediatric Neurology
300 Pasteur Drive
H3160
Stanford, CA 94305
Tel: 650-723-6469
Fax: 650-725-7459
Website: www.Stanford.edu/group/neurology

University of Minnesota
Division of Pediatric Gastroenterology
13-130 Phillips-Wangensteen Building
516 Delaware Street
Minneapolis, MN 55455
Tel: 612-624-2422
Fax: 612-626-0639

Part Six

Treatments for Movement Disorders

Chapter 42

Tremor Control Therapy

More than a million Americans suffer from Essential Tremor and 500,000 have Parkinson's disease. The first new treatment approach in 30 years for disabling tremor due to Essential Tremor and tremor associated with Parkinson's disease is now available. Approved by the U.S. Food and Drug Administration (FDA), the Tremor Control Therapy uses an implanted pacemaker-like device to deliver mild, electrical stimulation to block the brain signals that cause tremor.

Tremor—the disabling, involuntary rhythmic shaking of the limbs or other parts of the body, is the only symptom of Essential Tremor and one of four major symptoms of Parkinson's disease.

"NYU Medical Center is pleased to be able to offer the benefits of Tremor Control Therapy to patients," said Dr. Patrick Kelly, Professor and Chairman, Department of Neurosurgery. "Tremor is a condition that severely impacts a patient's quality of life as well as their ability to function in life. Mistakenly, many sufferers continue to live with tremor because they assume that it is part of the normal aging process or that nothing can be done."

Essential Tremor is the most common neurological movement disorder in this country. The condition afflicts at least a million Americans, usually age 45 or older. Parkinson's disease is a progressive and degenerative neurological disease that affects approximately 500,000 people in the United States. Tremor worsens from mild to disabling

"NYU Medical Center Offers the First Completely New Approach for Treating Tremor in 30 Years," © 1999 New York University School of Medicine, Department of Neurosurgery, reprinted with permission.

at a variable rate, depending on the individual. Currently, thousands of people throughout Europe, Canada, and Australia have the system implanted to control their tremor.

The Tremor Control System includes an insulated wire lead that is surgically implanted deep within the brain's communication center, the thalamus. The lead is connected by an extension wire passed under the skin to an implanted pulse generator, similar to an advanced cardiac pacemaker, which is implanted near the collarbone. Patients control the stimulation by passing a hand-held magnet over the implanted pulse generator to turn it on or off, or to increase or decrease stimulation depending on their tremor suppression needs. To achieve maximum tremor suppression, a neurophysiologist programs the generator to deliver the precise stimulation needed for each patient.

Tremor Control Therapy: Questions and Answers

What Is Tremor Control Therapy?

Tremor Control Therapy is the first completely new approach to controlling tremor in 30 years. It is delivered by an implanted device, similar to an advanced cardiac pacemaker, that uses mild electrical stimulation to block the brain signals that cause tremor. The Tremor Control System stimulates targeted cells in the brain's thalamus via electrodes that are surgically implanted in the brain and connected to a pulse generator implanted near the collarbone. The electrical stimulation can be non-invasively adjusted to meet each patient's needs.

How Effective Is Tremor Control Therapy?

In clinical studies, more than 80 percent of Essential Tremor and Parkinsonian tremor patients had total or significant suppression of their disabling tremor and significant reduction in disability. (Medtronic Global Clinical Study Series 1992-1997)

Who Is a Candidate for This Therapy?

Tremor Control Therapy is indicated for people whose drugs are ineffective in controlling their disabling tremor due to Essential Tremor or Parkinson's disease.

What Components Make Up a Tremor Control System?

The system consists of three implantable components:

1. **DBS lead**. A thin, insulated wire lead with four electrodes at the distal tip. Using standard clinical imaging techniques and stereotactic equipment, the electrode is positioned in the brain's thalamus, and the lead is anchored to the skull.

2. **Itrel II implantable pulse generator (IPG)**. This device, which contains a battery and microelectronic circuitry, is surgically implanted under the skin near the collarbone. The pulse generator is 2 1/4 inches by 2 1/4inches by 3/8 inches and weighs 1.72 oz.

3. **Extension**. An insulated wire that is surgically passed under the skin of the head, neck, and shoulder to connect the lead to the implanted pulse generator. External components of the therapy include a console programmer and the patient's hand-held magnet.

The Itrel II device generates mild electrical pulses that are delivered by the extension and lead to the targeted cells of the thalamus. These pulses can be non-invasively adjusted by a neurologist, from a console programmer and transmitted painlessly via radio telemetry to the implanted Itrel II device.

Patients use the magnet to switch the stimulator between high, low, and off settings. For example, they can turn their stimulation level to high when their tremor increases due to stress, or they can turn the pulse generator off when they go to sleep (tremor ceases with sleep).

Physician researchers have found that the electrical pulses block faulty brain signals that cause tremor. Certain nerve cells become overactive to the point of causing uncontrollable muscle excitation in tremor patients and electrical stimulation interferes with this abnormal activity. This has been characterized as a jamming of the neural network to interrupt the tremor.

How Is the Tremor Control System Implanted?

A stereotactic headframe and imaging techniques are used to map the brain and localize the target. Imaging techniques include:

*   magnetic resonance imaging (MRI),

*   computed tomography (CT) scan

*   ventriculogram (contrast media—radio-opaque dye—is injected into the lateral ventricle in order to localize various thalamic nuclei, via their relative locations to the ventricle system)

The lead is inserted through a small opening in the bone and implanted in the thalamus, deep within the brain. Before the lead implant procedure, the patient's scalp is anesthetized, but the patient remains awake and alert, so that the doctors can test the stimulation to maximize tremor suppression and minimize side effects. To ensure proper placement of the lead, the patient must be alert during this part of the procedure for the following reasons:

- the patient must demonstrate how well tremor is suppressed, for example, by drawing a circle or by holding a cup,
- the patient needs to report any side effects, and
- anesthesia may temporarily suppress tremor independently of the Tremor Control System's mechanism of action.

If the patient's tremor is suppressed during this test stimulation, the Tremor Control System is implanted. The patient is given a general anesthetic before the pulse generator and extension wire are implanted. A small incision is made near the collarbone and the pulse generator is implanted under the skin. The extension is passed under the skin of the scalp, neck, and shoulder to connect the lead to the implanted pulse generator.

What Is the Typical Length of Hospitalization for Pre-Operative Tests and Recovery?

Pre-operative tests take approximately two days. The patient is hospitalized for approximately three days.

What Can the Patients Expect after the Implant Procedure?

Immediately following surgery, the patient may experience a thalamotomy effect, which is a reduction in tremor. When swelling subsides the tremor returns. One week after surgery, the patient returns for suture removal. Three weeks following the surgery, the patient returns for programming the stimulation parameters to tremor control and to minimize any side effects. Follow up appointments will be scheduled and the patient's medication regime will be monitored by his/her neurologist.

How Do Patients Benefit from Tremor Control Therapy?

In clinical research, tremor was usually suppressed entirely or significantly reduced as soon as the pulse generator is turned on in the operating room. Patients in clinical studies have resumed daily life activities that were previously difficult or impossible, such as writing, pouring liquids, and dressing themselves. Tremor medications have often been markedly reduced or discontinued in these patients, especially for Essential Tremor patients, although patients with Parkinsonian tremor may still need medications for other Parkinson's disease symptoms. Because brain tissue is not destroyed after the lead is implanted, patients have preserved their future options as new therapies develop. (Benabid AL, Pollak P, Gao D, et. al. Chronic electrical stimulation of the ventralis intermedius nucleus of the thalamus as a treatment of movement disorders. *Journal of Neurosurgery* 1996; (84):203-214.)

What Are the Potential Side Effects of This Therapy?

Clinical research suggests that the potential side effects of stimulation are generally mild, reversible, and well tolerated by patients. (Benabid AL, Pollak P, Gao D, et. al. Chronic electrical stimulation of the ventralis intermedius nucleus of the thalamus as a treatment of movement disorders. *Journal of Neurosurgery* 1996; (84):203-214.) The most common potential side effects include temporary tingling in the limbs (paresthesia), slight paralysis (paresis), slurred speech (dysarthria), and loss of balance (disequilibrium). These sides effects are reduced or disappear when stimulation is decreased or stopped. Risk typically associated with the surgery includes loss of effect and intracranial hemorrhage.

Does Tremor Control Therapy Cure the Cause of Tremor?

There is no cure for Essential Tremor or Parkinson's disease at this time. Tremor Control Therapy treats tremor, but does not cure the underlying condition that causes the tremor. If the therapy is discontinued, the patient's tremor will return.

How Many People Are Currently Using Tremor Control Therapy?

Thousands of people worldwide are benefiting from this therapy. It has been available in Europe, Canada, and Australia since 1995.

How Long Does the Pulse Generator Battery Last?

Battery longevity varies, depending upon the parameter settings and number of hours the pulse generator is turned on each day. Estimated longevity is about five years at typical settings, 16 hours of use per day. When the pulse generator battery needs to be replaced, the old pulse generator is replaced by an entirely new pulse generator; the extension and lead are not replaced. The replacement procedure can by done under local anesthesia.

Is Tremor Control Therapy New? What Is Its History?

This therapy is an entirely new treatment for suppression of tremor. However, electrical stimulation has been used by neurologists and neurosurgeons for more than 35 years as a way to locate and distinguish specific sites in the brain. In doing this, they discovered that by stimulating a portion of the thalamus, severe tremor could be rapidly and dramatically suppressed. The system is based upon advanced cardiac pacemaker technology adapted to neurostimulation of the brain for the suppression of tremor.

Additional Information

NYU Center for the Study & Treatment of Movement Disorders
530 First Avenue
New York, NY 10016
Tel: 212-263-1483
Fax: 212-263-8031
E-mail: anne@mcns10.med.nyu.edu

Center for Functional and Restorative Neurosurgery
Hospital for Joint Diseases
Tel: 212-598-6424
Fax: 212-598-6425
E-mail: resnick@mcns10.med.nyu.edu

Chapter 43

Managing Spasticity

Treatments

The goal of spasticity treatment is to improve some aspect of a person's life. This will differ from one person to another and over time.

The healthcare team (physicians, physiotherapists, nurses, etc.) work with the patient and caregiver to define goals for the spasticity treatment. The decision to treat spasticity should include full consideration of all aspects of the underlying condition. This can best be done through careful evaluation by the clinical team in consultation with the individual and their caregivers.

When spasticity does require treatment, a range of effective therapies that can be used alone or in combination are available.

Self Help

Dealing with Spasms

Spasms can sometimes be relieved by pushing your weight through the affected limb. For example, if it occurs in the leg, pressing your

---

The information in this chapter is reprinted with permission from Moving Forward UK, an organization committed to improving the treatment and management of spasticity. © 2002. Contact Moving Forward UK at Third Floor, 94 New Bond Street, London W1S 1SJ, United Kingdom, via email at info@movingforward.org.uk or visit their website at www.moving forward.org.uk.

hand down on your knee or standing up can break the cycle of spasm. Otherwise it is best not to fight a spasm as you will probably cause yourself further pain.

Preventing Spasms

Spasticity can be brought on by rapid movement, or by sensory stimulation. An important aspect of spasticity treatment is minimizing the types of stimuli that can trigger it: pain, pressure sores, urinary tract infection, ingrown toenails, restrictive clothing, and constipation, for example. Spasms that occur at night could be the result of poor sleeping positions—seeking advice from your physiotherapist on correctly positioning yourself in bed. Appropriate positioning in wheelchairs will also help avoid pressure areas developing.

Medicines

Oral medications are often used to treat spasticity. Side effects can occur and should be monitored, reducing the dose or changing medication may help with these. There are four major oral medicines used to reduce spasticity:

- Benzodiazepines: Diazepam (Valium®) and Clonazepam (Rivotril®)
- Baclofen: (Lioresal®)
- Dantrolene Sodium: (Dantrium®)
- Tizanidine: (Zanaflex®)

Benzodiazepines

Benzodiazepines reduce spasticity through their action on the central nervous system.

Benefits

- Improved range of movement
- Less muscle overactivity
- Fewer painful spasms
- General feeling of relaxation

Side Effects

- Drowsiness

- Unsteadiness and loss of strength
- Low blood pressure
- Stomach upsets
- Memory impairment and confusion
- Behavioral problems

Benzodiazepines can be addictive and cause withdrawal symptoms if stopped suddenly. Alcohol needs to be avoided as well as other central nervous system depressants.

Baclofen

Baclofen also works through the central nervous system to reduce spasticity.

Benefits

- Improved muscle stretching
- Improvement in passive movement
- Reduced muscle spasms, pain, and tightness

Side Effects

- Drowsiness
- Weakness
- Too much decrease in muscle tone causing limbs to become floppy
- Confusion and dizziness

Suddenly stopping baclofen may cause seizures, hallucinations, and rebound spasticity. Baclofen should not be taken with alcohol or other central nervous system depressants.

Dantrolene Sodium

Dantrolene sodium acts directly on the muscle interfering with the way the muscle contracts.

Benefits

- Improvement in range of movement
- Decreased muscle tone

471

- Reduced muscle spasms, pain, and stiffness

Side Effects

- May cause weakness in other muscles including respiratory muscles.
- Drowsiness
- Dizziness
- Diarrhea
- Increased sensitivity to sunlight

In addition, there is a potential for liver poisoning. Prior to starting treatment with Dantrolene, a liver function test is performed and compared. Dantrolene and Tizanidine are usually not prescribed together because of the increased risk to the liver.

Tizanidine

Tizanidine acts on the function of the central nervous system.

Benefits

- Less likely to cause a reduction in muscle strength than other oral anti-spasmodic drugs

Side Effects

- Drowsiness
- Low blood pressure
- Dry mouth
- Dizziness and hallucinations

It also requires regular monitoring of liver function, since a small proportion of patients experience some liver damage as a result of treatment with Tizanidine.

Physiotherapy

Physiotherapy is the treatment of disorders of movement and function caused by problems in the muscles, bones, or nervous system. Physiotherapists (physical therapists) assess and treat these disorders by natural methods such as exercise, manipulation, heat, or use of electrical and ultrasonic devices. They also advise caregivers on how to lift properly, carry out exercises at home, and how to position the person they care for. Treatment is designed to:

- Reduce excessive muscle tone
- Maintain or improve range of movement and mobility
- Increase strength and coordination
- Improve comfort

Treatment is individualized to meet the needs of the person with spasticity. Treatments may include:

Stretching

Stretching helps to maintain the full range of motion of a joint, keeping it mobile. This helps prevent contractures. To be effective, the prescribed stretching routine must be done on a regular basis, usually once or twice a day.

Strengthening

Spasticity often leads to loss of strength in both the spastic muscles and surrounding ones. Strengthening exercises are aimed at restoring strength to affected muscles, so that when tone is reduced through other treatments, maximum use of the limb is achieved.

Occupational Therapy

An occupational therapist assesses and treats people with physical disabilities to enable them to function as effectively as possible in daily life. An occupational therapist may work within the community or at the hospital. They will identify factors leading to the loss of a skill and help with acquisition of new skills or in re-establishing skills that have been lost due to illness or trauma.

Orthoses and Casts

Orthoses, or braces, allow a spastic limb to be held in a more normal position. A cast is a temporary brace. Through using a series of casts a contractured limb can be gradually stretched and returned to a more normal position.

Lycra Dynamic Splinting

Lycra dynamic splints are made-to-measure and consist of sections of Lycra stitched together using certain tensions to provide support for limbs sometimes boning is included to assist construction. The splint gives support to the wearer while allowing flexibility. It is not a rigid splint, it moves with the wearer.

Other Interventions

Intrathecal Baclofen

Intrathecal baclofen (ITB) delivers baclofen directly to the fluid surrounding the spinal cord from an implanted pump. Because the drug is administered right to its site of action, much less baclofen is needed than if it were taken by mouth. This reduces the side effects that baclofen can cause such as drowsiness and fatigue. At the same time, more of the drug actually reaches the nerve cells where it is needed most.

ITB is used to treat spasticity resistant to other treatments and is most effective against spasticity of the lower limbs. To determine whether ITB is likely to produce a beneficial response, a test dose of baclofen can be injected into the spinal fluid. This will give some indication of whether an implantation is likely to be successful. But functional gains are only likely to be seen once the continuous dose of ITB through implantation takes place, since those benefits develop over weeks or months of treatment.

The battery-powered pump used for ITB is about the size of a hockey puck, and is surgically implanted in the abdomen. The baclofen is contained within a store inside the pump. A small tube then carries the baclofen to the spine. The operation to implant the pump is performed under general anesthesia, and takes about one hour. There is likely to be some tenderness or soreness for several days after the operation, which can usually be controlled with over-the-counter painkillers.

After implantation, the pump can be reprogrammed to adjust the dose, using external controls. The pump also contains an alarm that beeps softly when the baclofen is running low or the batteries need replacing. The baclofen is refilled by injection when needed, usually every 1-3 months. When the batteries run low, the pump is removed and replaced, this usually occurs every 4-5 years.

Improvement in spasticity is usually seen within several days of the operation, but significant improvements in function require longer to occur, and will be increased with physical therapy and other forms of rehabilitation.

If infection occurs, the pump may need to be removed temporarily. Other complications include pump failure or breakage. Side effects are usually less than those receiving oral doses of baclofen and these can be managed by adjusting the dose.

Botulinum Toxin Type A (BTX-A)

Botulinum Toxin Type A (BTX-A) comes from a bacteria and is injected directly into muscles in small quantities. It is a highly effective treatment for spasticity and other conditions where there is increased muscle activity. Clinical trials have demonstrated that BTX-A is a safe and effective treatment for spasticity in properly selected patients with cerebral palsy, multiple sclerosis, stroke, spinal cord injury, or traumatic brain injury. BTX-A is produced and distributed under two different names and formulations: BOTOX® and Dysport®. As the drug does not travel more than a few centimeters from the injection site, it does not affect distant muscles and can be used to provide selective reduction in muscle overactivity.

A solution of BTX-A is injected into several areas of the spastic muscle near the nerve terminals. BTX-A works inside the nerve terminals to block release of the chemical that stimulates muscle contraction. Some nerve terminals remain unaffected by BTX-A, so that the injected muscle can still contract, but does so with less force. The target muscle is found simply by feel in larger, more accessible muscles, or by electromyography (EMG) to locate the right area in small or deep muscle groups. Small muscles may be injected in only 1-2 areas, while larger muscles may require injection in 3-4 areas. For those that are uncomfortable with needles a local anesthetic cream or general anesthetic can be used.

One important benefit of BTX-A is that the dose can be adjusted to provide the precise degree of weakness needed to overcome spasticity, while retaining some strength for normal function. Benefits depend on the patient, the location, and degree of their spasticity. Many patients also report a reduction in pain following treatment.

BTX-A is not used to treat widespread, severe spasticity, since the amount of drug required would exceed safe doses and may eventually lead to antibody formation, resistance to the drug, and eventual loss of response. The effects of BTX-A fade after 3-6 months. Re-injection is possible if it is agreed that continuing treatment is likely to be beneficial.

Phenol and Alcohol

Phenol and alcohol are used to interrupt the functioning of nerves that supply spastic muscles. In this way, the signals to those muscles are reduced allowing the muscle to relax.

Unlike BTX-A, phenol and alcohol do not provoke a reaction by the immune system. Since the level and frequency of dosing is not limited by this concern, larger muscles may be treated more effectively. This is often the treatment of choice for severe spasticity in the largest muscles, such as those of the thigh but there are a number of disadvantages in using phenol and alcohol.

The purpose of these agents is to damage the nerve or muscle near the injection site. Damage to nearby sensory nerves may cause temporary or permanent pain, requiring additional medication to control it and damage to other structures may cause tissue breakdown. In addition, the patient may need to have surgery to identify the target nerve and the subsequent injection may be painful.

Surgery

Surgical Treatments

Surgery can play an important role in the treatment of chronic long-term spasticity. It is not suitable for patients with recently acquired spasticity as changes in their muscle tone will fluctuate during this time of recovery.

For those with chronic spasticity a number of surgical options may be considered. The benefits and side effects of each procedure need to be assessed along with the likely post-operative functional gains for each individual patient. Surgery is permanent and is only likely to be considered once other methods of treating spasticity have proven ineffective in managing the condition.

Neurosurgery and/or orthopaedic surgery may be used to treat spasticity.

- Neurosurgery aims to reduce spasticity by destroying nerve cells in the spinal cord that contribute to overactivity.

- Orthopedic surgery aims to correct the effects of spasticity through procedures performed on either muscles, tendons, or bones to compensate for the effects of the spasticity.

Neurosurgery

The main neurosurgical procedure for spasticity is done on the spinal cord. This procedure is called selective dorsal rhizotomy (SDR) or selective posterior rhizotomy. Rhizotomy means cutting the sensory nerve roots that transmit nerve impulses to and from the spinal cord. Selective indicates that only selected nerve roots are cut.

Sensory nerves are targeted because of the role they play in generating spasticity. When brain or spinal cord damage occurs the sensory signals to contract/flex and stretch/extend the muscle become unbalanced. Excess sensory signaling of the sensory nerves to contract can lead to spasticity. SDR attempts to counteract this imbalance by cutting back these extra sensory signals.

SDR is used to treat severe spasticity of the lower limbs that causes problems with mobility or positioning. SDR is used when less invasive treatments are unable to control spasticity adequately.

SDR is performed under general anesthesia, the procedure lasting about 4 hours. The base of the spinal cord is exposed and nerve roots are stimulated electrically. Those that create abnormal responses are cut. Around 25-50% of all tested roots are cut away.

A week's recovery in the hospital is usually required beginning with strict bed rest, a catheter, and intravenous drip for fluid and pain medication. Gentle physical therapy should be begun after 1-2 days leading up to more vigorous activity. A 3-4 week recovery at home will normally be required before returning to normal activities.

In the weeks following surgery pain, fatigue, and changes in sleep and bladder or bowel function may occur. Long-term complications can include low back pain, spine curvature, and hip displacement. Although these may be reduced by appropriate physical therapy.

The extent of functional improvement after SDR varies from patient to patient. Factors include the pre-operative function, underlying strength and balance, undertaking regular physical therapy, and the patient's motivation during the rehabilitation process.

Orthopedic Surgery

Orthopedic surgery targets the muscle, tendon, or bone in a spastic limb. The goals of surgery may include reducing spasticity, increasing range of movement, improving access for hygiene, or reducing pain.

Contractured Release. In this procedure, the tendon of a contractured muscle is cut either partially or completely. The joint is then positioned at a more normal angle, and a cast is applied. Regrowth of the tendon in this new position occurs over several weeks. A series of casts may be used to gradually extend the joint as it mends. Following cast removal, physical therapy is used to strengthen the muscles and improve range of movement.

Tendon Transfer. A tendon transfer moves the attachment point of a spastic muscle. When the tendon is transferred to a different place,

477

the muscle can no longer pull the joint into an abnormal position. In some situations, the transfer allows improved function. In others, the joint retains passive but not active function. Ankle balancing procedures are among the most effective uses of this type of surgery.

Osteotomy. Involves a small portion of the bone being cut away. The bone is then repositioned in a way that allows a more natural position to be adopted as the bone heals. It is most likely to be used where the spasticity is unlikely to respond to less invasive treatments.

Arthrodesis. Arthrodesis is a fusing together of bones that normally move separately. This fusion limits the ability of a spastic muscle to pull the joint into an abnormal position. Arthrodesis is used most often to correct spasticity in the bones in the ankle and foot.

What Is the Right Treatment for Me?

Always follow the guidance of the medical team you are under. Ask about any aspects of your treatment you are unclear about and seek advice immediately if symptoms change or worsen. You may wish to discuss the treatment options listed here with your physician.

Chapter 44

Surgery

Chapter Contents

Section 44.1

Gamma Knife Surgery

Gamma Knife surgery is recognized worldwide as the preferred treatment for metastatic brain tumors and has successfully treated primary brain tumors and arteriovenous malformations. The Gamma Knife offers a non-invasive alternative for many patients for whom traditional brain surgery is not an option and removes the physical trauma and the majority of risks associated with conventional surgery. This effective treatment only requires an overnight hospital stay with periodic follow-up. It is proven safe over the long-term and is recognized and covered by most insurance plans.

The Gamma Knife allows noninvasive cerebral surgery to be performed with extreme precision, sparing tissues adjacent to the target. Based on preoperative radiological examinations, such as CT-scans, MR-scans, or angiography, the unit provides for highly accurate irradiation of deep-seated targets, using a multitude of collimated beams of ionizing radiation.

Gamma Knife surgery represents a major advance in brain surgery, changing the landscape within the field of neurosurgery. Its development has enhanced neurosurgical treatments offered to patients with brain tumors and vascular malformations by providing a safe, accurate, and reliable treatment option. Gamma Knife enables patients to undergo a non-invasive form of brain surgery without surgical risks or a long hospital stay.

Gamma Knife surgery is unique in that no surgical incision is made to expose the inside of the brain, thereby reducing the risk of surgical complications and eliminating the side effects and dangers of general anesthesia. The blades of the Gamma Knife are the beams of gamma radiation programmed to target the lesion at the point where they intersect. In a single treatment session, 201 beams of gamma radiation focus precisely on the lesion. Over time, most lesions slowly decrease in size and dissolve. The exposure is brief and only the tissue being treated receives a significant radiation dose, while the surrounding tissue remains unharmed.

There are numerous brain lesions for which treatment, either surgical or with radiation, is associated with considerable mortality or morbidity due to factors such as depth and inaccessibility of the lesion, its proximity to arteries, nerves and other vital structures, and the radiosensitivity of adjacent normal tissues. Even if access is possible, surgery still involves risks of hemorrhage, infection, and other post-operative complications. In addition, a lengthy hospital stay is usually required.

With the Gamma Knife, a surgical incision is not required; the attendant risks of open neurosurgical procedures (hemorrhage, infection, CSF leakage, etc.) are therefore avoided.

Published reports indicate that the Gamma Knife may be used as an alternative to standard neurosurgical operations or as an adjunctive therapy in the treatment of residual or recurrent lesions left unresected by conventional surgery. Radiosurgery can be especially useful for those patients who are not suitable for standard surgical techniques due to illness or advanced age. In many neurosurgical cases, the Gamma Knife is the only feasible treatment.

Conditions for which application of the Gamma Knife is considered most effective are:

1. Intracranial tumors such as acoustic neuromas, pituitary adenomas, pinealomas, craniopharyngiomas, meningiomas, chordomas, chondrosarcomas, metastases, and glial tumors.

2. Vascular malformations including arteriovenous malformations.

In addition to the above mentioned indications, clinical experiences exists in the treatment of functional disorders such as trigeminal neuralgia, intractable pain, Parkinson's disease, and epilepsy.

Advantages of Gamma Knife

-   Gamma Knife is a neuro-surgical tool designed exclusively for the treatment of brain disorders.

-   The lesion being treated receives a high dose of radiation with minimum risk to nearby tissue and structures.

-   The cost of Gamma Knife procedure is often 25 to 30 percent less than traditional neurosurgery.

- Patients experience little discomfort.

- The absence of an incision eliminates the risk of hemorrhage and infection.

- Hospitalization is short, typically an overnight stay. Patients can immediately resume their previous activities.

- Gamma Knife technology allows treatment of inoperable lesions. The procedure offers hope to patients who were formerly considered untreatable or at very high-risk for open-skull surgery.

Additional Information

International Radiosurgery Support Association
P.O. Box 60950
Harrisburg, PA, 17106
Tel: 717-671-1701
Fax: 717-671-1703
Website: www.irsa.org
E-mail: getinfo@irsa.org

Section 44.2

Pallidotomy for Parkinson's Disease

This section includes "Pallidotomy for Parkinson's Disease," © 1999 New York University School of Medicine, Department of Neurosurgery, reprinted with permission; and an excerpt from "Parkinson's Disease: A Research Planning Workshop," National Institute of Neurological Disorders and Stroke (NINDS), reviewed July 1, 2001.

Parkinson's disease (PD) is a neurologic disorder in which the nerve cells of the substantia nigra degenerate. These neurons are special for two reasons:

1. they are part of a brain system, the basal ganglia, which modulates movement and

2. they use the chemical dopamine to communicate with other neurons.

The death of these dopaminergic neurons leads to an imbalance in the finely tuned basal ganglia system, resulting in a number of motor disturbances. Initially, this may be manifest as a mild tremor at rest, or stiffness in one extremity. With further degeneration, symptoms worsen and become debilitating. Stiffness, slowness of movement (bradykinesia), painful muscle cramps, and freezing (akinesia) may all result, making it difficult for the patient to perform such simple tasks as eating, walking, turning over in bed, or getting dressed. People's lives are destroyed. Family members watch helplessly as their loved one, once independent and vital, becomes increasingly dependent on others.

Early on, PD responds well to medications. L-DOPA is the precursor molecule from which dopamine is formed. L-DOPA preparations such as Sinemet supplement the dopamine loss, ameliorating many Parkinsonian symptoms for many years. Pergolide and bromocriptine mimic dopamine's effects by stimulating the receptors in the brain to which dopamine normally binds. Eldepryl is believed to slow the process which leads to the death of the dopaminergic cells. These and other medications may be used alone, or in combination, depending on the patient's response, the preference of the treating physician, or other circumstances. L-DOPA therapy, however, is the mainstay of medical therapy for PD. In fact, a poor initial response to L-DOPA raises the possibility that the diagnosis of PD is incorrect.

With time, the response to L-DOPA wanes. Patients respond to the medication less consistently and for shorter periods of time. They begin to suffer from medication side effects, the so-called DOPA-induced dyskinesias (DID), and experience worsening *on-off* fluctuations. In the *off* state, these patients are rigid and immobile. They stare at the world with an expressionless mask-like face; many cannot stand without assistance from a walker or cane. In the *on* state they are freer and have less tremor, but severe dyskinesias neutralize the medication's positive effects. For many, the dyskinesias are worse than the PD, causing patients to limit the amount of medicine they take or to discontinue their medication entirely.

In the latter stages of the disease, patients may have terrible gait imbalance and recurrent falls. They respond poorly to medication and are wheelchair bound. Dopaminergic neurons in the frontal lobes of the brain may also begin to degenerate causing a decline in cognitive abilities.

What Is Pallidotomy?

Pallidotomy is a neuroablative procedure in which a small part of the globus pallidus, another part of the basal ganglia system, is destroyed. Animal models of PD have demonstrated that the loss of dopaminergic neurons causes the internal segment of globus pallidus (GPi) to become too active. This hyperactivity is believed to be responsible, in large part, for the stiffness and slowness experienced by Parkinson's patients, and may also contribute to tremor. By destroying part of GPi, the basal ganglia system is rebalanced alleviating many parkinsonian symptoms. An unexplained benefit of pallidotomy is that DID is also relieved.

Pallidotomy is not a new procedure. Neurosurgical pioneers including Irving Cooper at NYU, developed the operation in the 1950s and 60s. While their results were encouraging, the complication rates were quite high, and the procedure was abandoned in the late 1960s with the introduction of L-DOPA therapy. Over the past years technological advances such as magnetic resonance imaging (MRI), microelectrode recording (MER), advanced stereotactic frames, and, of course, the computer revolution, have made it possible for neurosurgeons to refine the pallidotomy technique, yielding excellent therapeutic results and low complication rates. These advances, combined with the understanding that L-DOPA will not work forever, have led to renewed interest in pallidotomy.

Indications for Pallidotomy

Pallidotomy is not for everyone. The primary goal of the work at the Center for Movement Disorders at New York University School of Medicine has been to refine the indications for the procedure, thereby reducing complications and avoiding surgery for those who will not improve.

Good candidates typically have had PD for 5-10 years during which time they have been responsive to L-DOPA. Their PD is asymmetric (i.e. one side of their body is affected more than the other). They have a predominance of stiffness, slowness, and muscle cramping; tremor is not their primary problem. In the *on* state they suffer from DID. Younger patients tend to respond better than older patients; however, no one is eliminated from consideration based solely on their age.

Midline symptoms do not usually respond well to pallidotomy. These include low voice volume, swallowing difficulty, unsteadiness, falls, and freezing. Resting tremor improves in some patients, but this is not the best indication for the operation.

Keep in mind that the above descriptions of good and poor indications are presented for the sake of comparison. Most individuals suffer from a combination of symptoms some of which will improve with pallidotomy. A detailed discussion between the patient and surgeon is critical so that the surgeon understands which symptoms are most bothersome to the patient and the patient understands just what the operation will and will not do. Only then can an informed decision be made. This decision, of course, is made in light of our clinical evaluation, the neuropsychological testing, and positron emission tomographic (PET) results.

The Preoperative Work-Up for NYU

Patients who are interested in undergoing pallidotomy at NYU must be evaluated by our Parkinson's neurologists, and by our neurosurgeons. A recent MRI of the head must be available to rule out significant brain atrophy or other brain lesions. Such findings may eliminate a patient from consideration. If the team agrees that the patient is potentially a good candidate for pallidotomy, arrangements are made for preoperative neuropsychological testing and a PET scan.

485

Neuropsychological testing is performed at the Hospital for Joint Diseases. The tests typically take 2-3 hours to complete. These are performed in order to rule out subtle memory loss, an early sign of the dementia which may accompany PD. We have found that individuals with even subtle cognitive deficits are at increased risk for having more severe cognitive difficulties following pallidotomy. If these early changes are discovered, we will not proceed with surgery.

The final hurdle is the PET scan. NYU is the only center in the world that employs PET scan results in its clinical decision making. In true PD, PET scanning reveals the hyperactivity in GPi. We have demonstrated that patients without this hyperactivity will not respond to pallidotomy and should not have this surgery. Most important, if the PET scan reveals too little activity in the region of GPi, the patient may have one of the so-called Parkinson's Plus syndromes, rarer disorders which resemble PD but involve more than the dopaminergic system. NYU experience has shown that Parkinson's Plus syndromes do not improve with pallidotomy.

Once a patient is deemed a good candidate for the surgery, they are sent for medical clearance and presurgical testing. Assuming the patient has no medical problems which make surgery unsafe, we proceed with the pallidotomy.

The Surgery

Pallidotomy patients are admitted 2 days prior to surgery for a complete preoperative motor evaluation. On the day prior to surgery, a full evaluation is performed with the patient off and on medications. This evaluation includes the performance of timed motor tasks and stabilometry, a machine which assesses the patients stability and motor responsiveness.

The pallidotomy must be performed with the patient off medications for at least 12 hours so that on the evening prior to surgery, Parkinson's medications are again stopped. The operation is usually performed in the morning so that the time off medications is minimized. All told, the operation takes 4-5 hours to perform, but there are only 2-3 hours of actual operating time.

The first step is to apply the stereotactic frame, a simple procedure which takes 5 minutes to perform. This frame is rigidly fixed to the skull at 4 points. Each site is anesthetized. The frame is necessary to achieve the millimeter accuracy required to perform pallidotomy safely.

An MRI is then obtained with the frame and the images are transferred to the computer planning system. The operation is planned on the computer and the initial coordinates for the target are selected. The scalp is then shaved where the operation is to be performed, and the operation is begun. Accuracy is everything; therefore the patient's head is fixed in position for the operation. Every effort is made to make the patient as comfortable as possible. This includes placement of an air pillow behind the neck, pillows below the knees, and a nurse who will massage any cramps the patient experiences. For those who urinate frequently, a catheter is placed in the bladder to drain urine during the operation. It is promptly removed after surgery.

The operation is performed through a 1/4 inch incision and a tiny hole that is drilled through the skull. The microelectrode is then inserted into the brain. Each recording session takes 20-30 minutes to complete. Typically only one or two trajectories are required, but sometimes 3 or 4 passes are needed in order to assure proper placement of the lesion. During microelectrode recording, the patient must remain perfectly still and quiet. This tends to be the most difficult part of the operation for most patients and every effort is made to keep them comfortable during this time.

When recording has revealed the desired trajectory and target point, the microelectrode is replaced by the lesioning electrode and test stimulation is performed. The brain is stimulated with very low voltages to determine the proximity to critical structures which we want to preserve. These structures are the internal capsule and the optic tract. Damage to the former can cause paralysis while injury to the latter can cause partial blindness. The patient's cooperation during this phase of the operation is critical to the safety of the procedure. The final safety check is to make a test lesion. This is performed by warming the electrode so that the surrounding tissue is stunned but not destroyed. The patient is then examined, looking for any new signs of weakness.

Once all of the safety checks are complete, the lesions are made. Typically, 4-5 lesions are made at 2 mm intervals along the lesioning trajectory. Each lesion takes 1 minute to perform. After lesioning, the electrode is removed and the incision closed with a single suture. The stereotactic frame is removed and a head wrap applied. The patient is then taken to CT scan to rule out a hemorrhage. Assuming no hemorrhage occurred, the patient is taken to ICU where he or she will spend the night. In most cases, the patient is in ICU by lunch time. They may eat immediately and their Parkinson's medications are resumed.

Post-Operative Care

Patients are observed in the ICU overnight for the sake of precaution. In most instances, the patient can be discharged home the next day or the day after.

Patients return to NYU one week post-op for suture removal and a post-operative MRI which demonstrates the exact location of the lesion.

What Can You Expect?

The response to pallidotomy is dependent on the patient's symptoms. A relief from stiffness is often noted on the operating table while the lesions are being made. Dyskinesias secondary to the medication are almost universally eliminated, something which the patient notices after taking 1 or 2 doses in the ICU. Family members may note enhanced facial expression.

There is often an emotional let down in the first week after surgery. In the hospital, patient's often feel euphoric due to their new found freedoms and their delight at having survived awake brain surgery. Once the newness of it all has worn off, there can be a slight let down which is often mistaken for a return of symptoms. It is important to keep in mind that there are dramatic physiologic changes occurring in the patient's brain which take 3-4 months to complete. During this time, as is always the case with PD, some days will be better than others. Try to keep a long-range perspective and not get discouraged by 1 or 2 bad days. It is our experience that the full effects of the pallidotomy cannot be assessed until 6 months post-operatively.

Concluding Remarks

Thanks to many technological advances, modern pallidotomy is much safer and accurate than the procedure which was performed 35 years ago. Pallidotomy's continuing success has provided an invaluable therapeutic option for many PD patients whose response to medications is waning. The keys to a successful pallidotomy are careful patient selection and attention to details while performing the surgery.

NINDS Note on Pallidotomy

Preliminary studies of microelectrode-guided pallidotomy show that all signs and symptoms of Parkinson's disease respond to pallidotomy to some extent. The wide variety of symptoms relieved by pallidotomy is difficult to reconcile with current models of basal ganglia function and suggests more complex functions within this brain region than described by theoretical models. Many patients who receive pallidotomy show bilateral improvement in symptoms even if only one side of the brain is lesioned. Patients receiving pallidotomy so far have shown no permanent dyskinesia or other motor impairments. A related procedure called thalamotomy (destruction of a part of the thalamus that participates in motor control) may be more effective in treating tremor, but pallidotomy is generally safer than thalamotomy, especially in older patients. Patients' age and location of the lesion affect the outcome of pallidotomy, and effects on motor symptoms are much more dramatic than effects on cognitive and psychological symptoms. Some patients do continue to deteriorate after the procedure, especially in the unlesioned side of the brain.

While apparently successful in the short-term, pallidotomy has several drawbacks, including partial loss of vision in about 11 percent of initial patients, potentially impaired cognition, and increased risk of hemorrhage and stroke. Careful monitoring and surgical expertise are necessary to reduce these risks. Pallidotomy also fails to stop the underlying disease progression, and patients usually need medication long-term.

Experiments with pallidotomy show that effective therapies for Parkinson's do not necessarily need to target the dopamine neurotransmitter system directly and suggest that current models of basal ganglia function are inadequate. A better understanding of the normal motor control pathways is badly needed. The findings also suggest that hypokinetic (slowed movement) and hyperkinetic (excessive movement) disorders result from opposite changes in activity of the basal ganglia and thalamocortical regions. These findings suggest many areas for future research. Scientists must now evaluate the long-term effectiveness of pallidotomy in treating symptoms and define how the effects of unilateral and bilateral lesions differ. A related surgical procedure called ansotomy, which consists of interrupting axon connections to the globus pallidus, also has been shown effective in animals and may soon be ready for testing in human trials.

Section 44.3

Stereotactic Thalamotomy

Definition

Precision placement of a destructive lesion in the thalamus for the treatment of movement disorders such as Parkinsonian resting tremor, intention tremor, or dystonia.

Indications

- Resting tremor of Parkinson's disease
- Intention tremor
  - Multiple Sclerosis
  - Post-traumatic
  - Familial (Essential)
  - Post Cerebrovascular Accident (Stroke)
- Dystonia of arm or leg
- Dystonia Musculorum Deformans
- Post-traumatic

Contraindications (Exclusion Criteria)

- Dementia: memory or thought disturbance
- Poorly controlled high blood pressure
- Gait disturbance
- Significant speech problems

Surgical Procedure

- Data Base acquisition
  - Head Frame Placement

- Stereotactic CT Scan
- Stereotactic MRI
- Stereotactic Ventriculogram
- Microelectrode Recording
- Speech Monitoring
- Radiofrequency Lesioning

The National Institute of Neurological Disorders and Stroke notes that Thalamotomy (destruction of a part of the thalamus that participates in motor control) may be more effective in treating tremor, but pallidotomy is generally safer than thalamotomy, especially in older patients.

Section 44.4

Following Surgery

"Following Surgery," © 1999 New York University School of Medicine, Department of Neurosurgery, reprinted with permission.

Intensive Care Unit Observation

Since all of the surgical procedures done for movement disorders are performed under local anesthesia (with some sedation in some cases), there is no need for post-anesthesia recovery room as is customary following most other surgical procedures which are performed under general anesthesia. Patients are taken directly from the operating room to the Intensive Care Unit where they are observed for 24 hours following surgery. The purpose of this period of observation is to carefully monitor neurological function and vital signs. In particular, blood pressure will be recorded frequently and controlled by medication if elevated.

What about Families?

There usually is a comfortable waiting area on the neurosurgical floor in which families and friends can relax while the patient is undergoing his/her procedure. Following surgery, the surgeon will speak to relatives either by telephone from the operating room or in person to let them know how things went and how the patient is doing. Families are free to visit the patient in the Intensive Care Unit at visiting hours which have been set by the nursing staff.

After the ICU?

If all is stable on the morning following surgery the patient will be moved to a private or semiprivate room for one to two days additional hospitalization. This will allow for final adjustment of medications and for the patient to get comfortable with the activities of daily living before discharge.

How Will You Feel?

This will depend on the type of surgery performed but you should note an improvement in your symptoms almost immediately after the surgery.

Following a successful thalamotomy, which is almost always done for the treatment of tremor, the results are dramatic even before the patient gets off the operating table. The tremor is gone! There is occasionally a mild headache or mild discomfort at the sites of stereotactic frame attachment. Medication can be given for this if necessary. On the next day or two there may be a very slight clumsiness of the treated limb due to swelling around the lesion. This resolves.

The immediate postoperative effects following Pallidotomy are more subtle to appreciate. Many patients report an immediate improvement in rigidity and leg cramps on the side opposite the side of surgery and later notice a reduction in drug induced dyskinesia after they receive their first dose of Sinemet following surgery. Of course, they won't appreciate an improvement in gait until they actually start walking a day or so postoperatively. There is occasionally a mild headache or mild discomfort at the sites of stereotactic frame attachment. Medication can be given for this if necessary. In rare cases, patients may notice some mild weakness of the arm the night of or day following surgery due to swelling around the lesion site. This resolves within a few days.

In most cases, the postoperative medications and dosages will be unchanged from preop and will remain at these schedules for several weeks. Some drugs may be discontinued or their doses reduced at the discretion of the neurologist when the patients are examined postoperatively.

After Discharge from the Hospital

Following discharge from the hospital patients are told to refrain from strenuous physical activity or heavy lifting for a total of three weeks. Sutures are typically removed from 7 to 10 days following surgery. In some cases patients may return to sedentary work 1-2 weeks following surgery. Patients who do heavy physical activity in the course of their employment are considered totally disabled for disability insurance purposes for up to three months postoperatively.

Chapter 45

Dystonia Treatments

Chapter Contents

Section 45.1

Medications

Treatment Options

Treatment for dystonia is designed to help lessen the symptoms of spasms, pain, and disturbed postures and functions. Most therapies are symptomatic, attempting to cover up or release the dystonic spasms. No single strategy will be appropriate for every case.

The goal of any treatment is to achieve the greatest benefits while incurring the fewest risks. It is to allow you to lead a fuller, more productive life by reducing the effects of dystonia. Establishing a satisfactory regimen requires patience on the part of both the affected individual and the physician.

The approach for treatment of dystonia is usually three-tiered: oral medications, botulinum toxin injections, and surgery. These therapies may be used in alone or in combination.

Complementary care, such as physical therapy and speech therapy, may also have a role in the treatment management depending on the form of dystonia. For many people, supportive therapy provides an important adjunct to medical treatments.

Although there is currently no known cure for dystonia, we are gaining a better understanding of dystonia through research and are developing new approaches to treatments.

Oral Medications

Medication treatments may lessen the symptoms of pain, spasm, and abnormal posturing and function. These treatments have different mechanisms of action, so benefits and side effects may be difficult to predict. One drug may work for one patient and not for another. Sometimes the benefit is only short-lived. The treatment of dystonia must be tailored to the individual patient. There are several possible categories of medications used in the treatment of dystonia:

Anticholinergics

Anticholinergics include such drugs as Artane (trihexyphenidyl), Cogentin (benztropine), or Parsitan (ethopropazine) which block the acetylcholine. In most people the dosage is limited by central side effects such as confusion, drowsiness, hallucination, personality change, and memory difficulties, and peripheral side effects such as dry mouth, blurred vision, urinary retention, and constipation.

Benzodiazepines

Benzodiazepines, such as Valium (diazepam), Klonopin (clonazepam), and Ativan (lorazepam) block the Gaba-A receptor in the central nervous system. The primary side effect is sedation, but others include depression, personality change, and drug addiction. Rapid discontinuation can result in a withdrawal syndrome. Some dystonia patients may tolerate very high doses without apparent adverse effects.

Baclofen

Baclofen (Lioresal) stimulates the Gaba-B receptor. Intrathecal (spinal infusion) forms of Baclofen are also available.

Dopamine

Some patients with primary dystonia respond to drugs which increases dopamine such as Sinemet (levodopa) or Parlodel (bromocriptine); however, many patients respond to agents which block or deplete dopamine, such as standard anti-psychotics like Clozaril (clozapine), Nitoman (tetrabenazine), or Reserpine.

Can You Explain How You Start a Person on a New Medication?

Generally, a person starts on a medication at a low dose and slowly increases the dosage. It may take weeks to months to undergo an adequate trial of one medication. Drug trials require tremendous patience in deciding whether one medication will work or not.

It is important to stay in contact with your physician because of the risk of the side effects and to report on how the trial is going.

During a drug trial, you may have to wait at a certain dose level or slowly taper off to discontinuation depending on the severity of side

497

effects. Remember there is no magic level which you must obtain. Some people will experience benefits at a relatively low dose without side effects while others will require higher dosages. This is the reason physicians slowly increase the medicine because should you have benefits at a level that is acceptable, then that will probably be your level.

Overall, medication benefits between 40-60% of the dystonia patients, but medications have dose limitations because of side effects. Some reasons for medication failure are the lack of benefit and the occurrence of side effects. Other reasons include inadequate trials, not all possible medications tried, too many medications at one time, rapid increase in dose, or abrupt discontinuation.

What Are the Effects of These Drugs on Longevity?

The medications that are used for dystonia do not shorten life expectancy and can be used, as far as we know, indefinitely. The side effects may force us to reduce them, but the side effects are reversible.

What Can Be Done for Patients with Drug-Induced Dystonia? Can It Be Counteracted?

There are several types of dystonia that can be induced by drug. One type is called an acute dystonic reaction and manifests itself as a dystonic state resulting after a one-time exposure to a medication. The medications that are most likely to induce dystonic reactions are the so-called neuroleptic drugs which have as a common mode of action to block the effects of the neurotransmitter dopamine in the brain. These reactions are generally self-limited but can be quite frightening. Acute dystonia induced by anti-psychotic or anti-emetic agents may be relieved by intravenous Benadryl (diphenhydramine), anticholinergics, or benzodiazepines.

Another type of drug-induced dystonia is called tardive dystonia. Tardive dystonia is produced by the long-term ingestion of drugs such as neuroleptics. The more common type of tardive syndrome is tardive dyskinesia wherein the movements are generally quick movements without sustained postures. Tardive dystonia is similar where many of the movements involve sustained posturing. It is generally considered to be a severe form of tardive dyskinesia. Tardive dystonia, induced by anti-psychotics or anti-emetics may be treated by withdrawal or the offending agents or by anticholinergics, benzodiazepines, baclofen, or clozapine; however this condition may be relatively resistant to treatments.

Tardive dyskinesia and tardive dystonia are very difficult to treat. Once initiated, they can be life-long problems although it is possible that they may spontaneously remit. There are a variety of therapeutic programs that have been suggested to be useful for treatment of tardive dystonia and while some are clearly successful in some patients, there is no therapy that is so uniformly successful that it might be considered a standard of care. Patients who are affected by tardive dystonia need to work closely with their doctors to try to find a successful regimen.

What Drugs Can Cause Tardive Dystonia?

Drugs belonging to a class called dopamine receptor blocking agents, also referred to as neuroleptics, can cause dystonia. The following is a list of such drugs that can cause dystonia (trade name listed in parenthesis):

- Acetophenazine (Tindal®)
- Amoxapine (Asendin®)
- Chlorpromazine (Thorazine®)
- Fluphenazine (Permitil®, Prolixin®)
- Haloperidol (Haldol®)
- Loxapine (Loxitane®, Daxolin®)
- Mesoridazine (Serentil®)
- Metoclopramide (Reglan®)
- Molindone (Lidone®, Moban®)
- Perphenazine (Trilafon ® or Triavil®)
- Piperacetazine (Quide®)
- Prochlorperazine (Compazine®)
- Promazine (Sparine®)
- Promethazine (Phenergan®)
- Thiethylperazine (Torecan®)
- Thioridazine (Mellaril®)
- Thiothixene (Navane®)
- Trifluoperazine (Stelazine®)
- Triflupromazine (Vesprin®)
- Trimeprazine (Temaril®)

Is Thorazine (Chlorpromazine) a Cause of or Treatment for Dystonia?

Thorazine is a dopamine receptor blocker. Many forms of dystonia (especially dopa-responsive dystonia) are associated with the role of dopamine in the brain. By blocking dopamine, Thorazine is capable of causing tardive (i.e. drug-induced) dystonia. In some instances dopamine blockers may help dystonia. It is generally best for people with dystonia to avoid medications that block dopamine receptors.

Are Some Drugs Better Suited to Treat Secondary Rather Than Primary Dystonia?

Wilson's disease requires a very specific treatment; therefore in a case of secondary dystonia caused by Wilson's disease (which is a copper abnormality), the dystonia will be alleviated by treating the Wilson's disease. Tetrabenazine, a dopamine depleter, may be appropriate to treat tardive dystonia. For the most part, many of the drugs of choice for secondary dystonia also work well for primary dystonia and vice versa.

Can Artane (Trihexyphenidyl), and/or Klonopin (Clonazepam) Be Used during Pregnancy?

They are not recommended. Treatment for dystonia during pregnancy is very individual. In some cases doses can be reduced; in other cases the woman may (gradually) stop taking oral drugs completely. There is no single recommendation for all women patients.

Section 45.2

Botulism Toxin Injections

The introduction of botulinum toxin as a therapeutic tool in the late 1980s revolutionized the treatment of dystonia offering significant relief of symptoms to many people with dystonia. Botulinum toxin, a biological product, is injected into specific muscles where it acts to reduce the involuntary contractions that cause the symptoms of dystonia. The injections weaken muscle activity sufficiently to reduce a spasm but not enough to cause paralysis.

Botulinum toxin is a complex protein produced by the bacterium *Clostridium botulinum*. It is a nerve blocker that binds to nerve endings and prevents the release of acetylcholine, a neurotransmitter that activates muscle contractions. If the message is blocked, muscle spasms are significantly reduced or eliminated.

Forms

Seven serotypes or forms of botulinum toxin have been isolated, and they are A, B, C, D, E, F, and G. Each one has different properties and actions. No two are exactly alike. Of these subtypes, botulinum toxin type-A is currently the most studied and most widely used. Clinical applications of other toxins, including B and F, are also being investigated.

Botulinum toxin type-A is commercially available as BOTOX® from Allergan, Inc. and as Dysport® from Ipsen, Ltd. in England. Pending approval by the U.S. Food and Drug Administration, botulinum toxin type-B is being marketed for treatment of cervical dystonia (spasmodic torticollis) by Athena Neurosciences.

Botulinum toxin preparations are not all the same. They possess different amounts of protein per effective dose and are likely to have a different duration of action. The activities of botulinum toxin are measured in terms of a biologic unit (mouse unit). The mouse units vary among the commercially produced toxins and different types act on different proteins at the neuromuscular junction. The effectiveness and duration of weakness induced in the muscles may vary from product to product

Methods

Injections of botulinum toxin should only be performed by a physician who is trained to administer this treatment. The physician needs to know the clinical features and study the involuntary movements of the person being treated. The physician doing the treatment may palpate the muscles carefully, trying to ascertain which muscles are over-contracting and which muscles may be compensating for the over-contracting. In some instances, such as in the treatment of laryngeal dystonia, a team approach, including other specialists, may be required.

For selected areas of the body, and particularly when injecting muscles that are difficult or impossible to palpate, guidance using an electromyograph (EMG) may be necessary. For instance, when injecting the deep muscles of the jaw, neck, or vocal cords, an electromyographically guided injection may improve precision since these muscles cannot be readily palpated.

Injections into the overactive muscle are done with a small needle, with one to three injections per muscle. Discomfort at the site of injections is usually temporary, and a local anesthetic may be used to minimize any discomfort associated with the injection.

History

In the late sixties, Alan B. Scott, MD, of the Smith-Kettlewell Eye Research Foundation and Edward J. Schantz, PhD, Director of Food Microbiology and Toxicology at the University of Wisconsin were researching a substance to relax certain eye muscles causing strabismus (crossed-eyed). Botulinum toxin type-A was developed as a therapeutic agent for this disorder along with blepharospasm, hemifacial spasm, and other disorders characterized by inappropriate muscle spasms.

Botulinum Toxin Type-A

In 1989, botulinum toxin type-A was approved by the Food and Drug Administration and is commercially available under the trade name BOTOX®. It has been widely used as an effective treatment for dystonia, reducing the spasms or sustained muscle contractions in the eyelids, neck, vocal cords, hands, and limbs. The American Academy of Neurology, American Academy of Ophthalmology, and National Institutes of Health have recognized BOTOX® as a valuable treatment.

Effects of the treatment generally start to show within five to ten days with benefits lasting three to four months after which a gradual decline occurs until the injection needs to be repeated. Side effects are usually transient and mild to moderate in nature. Some people notice temporary weakness of muscles or discomfort at the injection site. Symptoms may vary throughout the course of the condition, and so the degree of relief and duration of effect varies from person to person. Changes occurring with subsequent BOTOX® injections may be less dramatic than the first injection.

Since the effects of botulinum toxin usually last only a few months, permanent impairment would be highly unlikely and no such complications have been reported. Treatment with BOTOX® can typically be repeated indefinitely. Acceptable safety in long-term treatment has been well established.

The effects of BOTOX® may be increased with the use of certain antibiotics or other drugs that interfere with neuromuscular transmission. The BOTOX® guidelines recommend the discontinuation of use during pregnancy and nursing.

A small percentage of people have become unresponsive to the treatment of BOTOX®. There are a number of possible reasons for this lack of response. First, it's possible that the pattern of muscles involved may have changed over time and that different muscles need to be injected. Second, doses may need to be altered, especially if the pattern of muscles involved has changed. Third, consistent clinical outcomes require sufficient precision in the injection technique to ensure the medication was delivered accurately to the target muscle(s). Finally, it's possible that a person may have formed antibodies to BOTOX®. Botulinum toxins contain proteins. In certain circumstances, when foreign proteins enter the body, the natural response is to form antibodies to the protein. When antibodies are formed, the effect may be that one is no longer able to respond to the therapy.

If a person develops antibodies, botulinum toxin won't exert its effects in any of the muscles in the body. This observation forms the basis of a simple clinical test that can be used to determine whether the patient has developed antibodies that prevent the toxin from working. In this test, botulinum toxin is injected into the middle of one eyebrow. If the toxin is still working, the patient will not be able to frown the eyebrow on the side that was injected because botulinum toxin will have relaxed the frown muscles. In contrast, if the person frowns equally on both sides, it suggests that antibodies may have formed to the toxin.

One important factor that can affect the development of antibodies is exposure to large amounts of toxin's complex protein. In certain circumstances, when foreign proteins such as botulinum toxin enter the body, the immune system responds by forming antibodies to the protein. Minimizing exposure to toxin's complex protein is likely to help reduce the potential for antibody formation. One way to minimize the amount of toxin's complex protein exposure is by having treatment no more frequently than about every three months. BOTOX® has approximately 5 mg of neurotoxin complex proteins per 100 unit vial, a relatively low amount of protein, which may help to further minimize the potential to form antibodies.

Allergan, the manufacturer of BOTOX®, sponsors a comprehensive reimbursement program for patients and providers called the BOTOX Advantage™ Program. The BOTOX Advantage™ Program includes a reimbursement hotline and patient assistance program to assist patients who are receiving BOTOX® injections. The BOTOX® reimbursement hotline is designed to respond to your reimbursement questions and help access BOTOX®, even when you do not have insurance coverage. For more information about this program log on to www.botox.com or call 800-530-6680.

Botulinum Toxin Type-B

Botulinum toxin type-B has been shown to be a safe and effective treatment for individuals with cervical dystonia (spasmodic torticollis) as reported in clinical trials which included double-blind studies (in patients who have responded to botulinum toxin type-A and patients who developed resistance to it). This includes patients who are resistant to botulinum toxin as well as those who continue to respond to botulinum toxin. This form of botulinum toxin is being marketed for the treatment of cervical dystonia (spasmodic torticollis) by Athena Neurosciences pending approval from the Food and Drug Administration.

Botulinum toxin type-B and botulinum toxin type-A have slightly different chemical structures as well as primary mechanisms of action. Potentially, different serotypes of botulinum toxin may be different antigenically (viewed by the body defense mechanism as different substances) from one another. In this way, people who develop antibodies to one type of botulinum toxin may respond to another type of botulinum toxin. However, there may be cross antigenicity among the different serotypes.

Further research is needed to determine whether botulinum toxin type-B will cause resistance in people who are being treated over long periods of time. In addition, there is currently no data to suggest if people receiving injections of botulinum toxin type-B will be either more or less likely to develop antibodies than botulinum toxin type-A.

Section 45.3

Surgery

Surgery may be considered when patients are no longer receptive to other treatments. It should be noted, surgery may lose its effect over the years, but it can possibly provide some relief.

Surgery is undertaken to interrupt, at various levels of the nervous system, the pathways responsible for the abnormal movements. Some operations intentionally damage small regions of the thalamus (thalamotomy), globus pallidus (pallidotomy), or other deep centers in the brain. Recently, chronic deep brain stimulation (DBS) has been tried with some success. Other surgical approaches include cutting nerves going to the nerve roots deep in the neck close to the spinal cord (anterior cervical rhizotomy) or removing the nerves at the point they enter the contracting muscles (selective peripheral denervation).

There are a number of factors that may influence the success of the operation. Each patient is unique, and the muscles involved vary from one patient to another. It is for this reason that pre-operative evaluation by a movement disorders expert is essential.

Are Pallidotomy and Thalamotomy Appropriate for Dystonia?

With the considerable success from pallidotomy for the treatment of Parkinson's disease it was only a matter of time before this procedure was tried for dystonia. As was true for Parkinson's, pallidotomy was actually first performed in the 1950s for dystonia. Pallidotomy was rapidly replaced by another surgery, thalamotomy, which continues to be performed even today for severe, poorly responsive forms of dystonia.

Although there are only a small number of reported cases from several centers in the U.S. and abroad, pallidotomy is again being tried in severe cases. The results are encouraging, even in several cases where bilateral surgery has been performed.

Pallidotomy and thalamotomy target regions of the brain that are involved in movement generation. By destroying one or the other of these small brain regions, these surgeries attempt to re-balance movement and posture control. Adverse effects can be significant and include swallowing difficulty, speech difficulty, and cerebral hemorrhage.

As for all movement disorders, surgery should be performed at established centers with a movement disorders specialist, a neurosurgeon trained in functional techniques, and supporting staff of neuropsychologists and nurses.

What Is Deep Brain Stimulation and What Role Does It Play in the Treatment of Dystonia?

Physicians are taking a second look at older forms of brain surgery for movement disorders such as Parkinson's disease and dystonia for several reasons. One is the obvious and frustrating lack of effective long-term drug treatment for many people. Another is the considerable progress in understanding the underlying causes of these disorders, proving a clearer rational for them.

For example, it is now clear that Parkinson's disease and dystonia result from abnormal and excessive or reduced neuronal activity respectively, in specific nuclei (e.g., the globus pallidus) in the basal ganglia. A final reason for the resurgence in surgical approaches are the substantial advances in neuroimaging (e.g., MRI) and physiologic mapping (e.g., microelectrode recording) that enable the surgeon to more accurately pinpoint the desired target.

Recently, the technique of deep brain stimulation (DBS) has been used in place of the conventional approach of lesioning or ablation. DBS entails placing a permanent radiofrequency stimulating electrode in the brain which is connected to a pulse generator implanted in the chest wall. Where as ablation causes permanent destruction of the targeted area, DBS acts reversibly to inactivate the area. It offers the further advantage of being adjustable in terms of frequency and amplitude of the current pulses, thus specifying the area influenced. DBS was FDA approved in 1999 for the treatment of tremor, but not for other sites or disorders.

Although the thalamus has been the most common target to ablation in dystonia, the pallidum has been targeted recently because of the successes with Parkinson's disease. The preliminary results are encouraging. Now, several centers are exploring the use of DBS in the pallidum for dystonia. A feasibility study of people with intractable dystonia is currently being performed.

What Is Selective Peripheral Denervation?

In 1976, Dr. Claude Betrand developed a new surgical technique called selective peripheral denervation (SPD) for patients with cervical dystonia (spasmodic torticollis/ST). The best type of ST for eventual surgical treatment is a pure rotatory ST, which may be combined with a mild lateral inclination and/or extension. The worst type of ST is a retrocollis, in which the head is bent backward. It is essential to identify the muscles involved by inspection, palpation, video, and most importantly, electromyographic (EMG) study.

In SPD surgery, the aim is to abolish the abnormal movement in all the muscles involved in producing the movement, while preserving the innervation of normal muscles. That is what the word selective refers to. The word peripheral refers to something that is outside of the brain and spinal canal. Denervation means cutting the impulse to certain muscles.

Physiotherapy, starting very soon after surgery, is essential in order to recover a full range of motion. The brain must relearn a new position.

Are Ramisectomy and Rhizotomy Surgeries Still Performed for Cervical Dystonia?

Ramisectomy and rhizotomy involve cutting the nerve or nerves supplying overactive muscles. These surgeries are also rarely performed today. Nonetheless, they may be effective in properly chosen patients. They are most commonly performed for cervical dystonia patients who have developed resistance to botulinum toxin injections. Possible adverse effects include permanent weakness and difficulty swallowing.

507

What Is the Difference between Rhizotomy and Selective Peripheral Denervation?

The rhizotomy procedure, in contrast to SPD, is inside the spine. That means the destruction of muscle is more generalized. There is also a greater degree of weakness. With selective peripheral denervation, patients don't have permanent weakness. Morbidity and complications are also greater with rhizotomy.

Please Explain the Various Myectomy Operations?

Limited Myectomy

Limited myectomy operations were performed by removing the excess skin and underlying orbicularis muscle in the upper eyelids. While healing was predictable with this operation and nearly all patients were improved short term, with time, virtually all patients had symptoms recur. Botulinum treatment was not available at this time and either myectomy or neurectomy surgery were the best treatments.

Full Myectomy

To combat this reoccurrence of symptoms, the full myectomy was developed, where nearly all of the squeezing muscles of the upper eyelids were removed. These muscles were removed through a brow incision and an eyelid crease incision.

Following the routine use of botulinum toxin as the first-line treatment for blepharospasm, the patients presenting for myectomy became a more difficult group of patients, as they were failures of botulinum toxin.

The failures of botulinum toxin must be differentiated into three groups. First, it must be determined whether botulinum A toxin actually is failing to cause weakness in the eyelids or if other problems are preventing the patient from obtaining an adequate result. Many patients who feel they are failures of botulinum toxin actually have weakness in the squeezing muscles of the eyelids, but droopiness of the eyelids, inability to open the eyelids, or excess baggage in the eyelids prevents the patient from obtaining a good result.

Easiest Patients to Treat

The first and easiest group of patients to treat with myectomy surgery are those in whom botulinum A toxin weakens the squeezing muscles, but have developed excess baggage in the eyelids, stretching of the tendon that raises the upper eyelids (ptosis), droopy brows, and, on some occasions, malpositions or in-turning or out-turning of the eyelids and the lashes.

In the first group of patients, these functional and cosmetic deformities are corrected and a limited myectomy is performed by removing the orbicularis muscle in the upper eyelids and in the lateral raphe and temporal regions.

This operation is performed through an upper eyelid crease incision, which is the same incision used for cosmetic surgeries of the upper eyelids. This group of patients predictably achieves good results and is the most satisfied group of patients, as they achieve the benefit of both botulinum A toxin and surgery, which improves their function and cosmesis. The post-operative use of botulinum toxin is needed in virtually all cases as an adjunct to this treatment.

Apraxia of Lid Opening

In the second group of patients, botulinum A toxin also is working at weakening the squeezing muscles, and they may have the associated cosmetic and functional deformities of the first group. However, in addition, these patients are unable to adequately open the eyelids, even when the eyelids are not in spasm or squeezing.

This group is treated with a limited myectomy similar to that described in group 1, but more tightening and advancement of the levator aponeurosis or tendon of the elevating muscle is required.

True Failures of Botulinum A Toxin

The third group of patients are the true failures of botulinum A toxin, for the drug fails to weaken the squeezing muscle of the eyelids. There is a small percentage of patients in which Botox® (botulinum toxin type A, Allergan) has virtually no effect initially, and in other cases it may lose its effect with time.

Postoperative Botulinum A Toxin

Patients in all three groups require botulinum A toxin less frequently with fewer units and fewer injection sites after the limited myectomy.

Best Functional Surgical Improvement

The myectomy can provide functional surgical improvement for patients suffering from blepharospasm. Eliminating most of the negative side effects makes this surgery a much more desirable option to consider when botulinum A toxin is not providing adequate relief of blepharospasm, or if functional or cosmetic deformities of the eyelids are present that prevent the patient from achieving an optimal result.

Chapter 46

Cerebral Palsy and Spasticity Treatment Questions

Botox

What Are the Risks?

There are minimal risks to using Botox when administered by competent professional staff. There is some chance of being allergic, but there have been no reported allergies to Botox in over 30 years of usage. There is always the chance of a small blood clot and/or infection occurring from the needle stick, which in our experience has never occurred (1,000s of injections). Although Botox (Botulinum toxin) is the most deadly substance known to man, when used in small dosages in the right muscles, it has essentially no threat to the body in general. The reason people have been injured or died from Botulinum toxin in the past (botulism) is that they consumed excessive amounts of the substance from spoiled food unknowingly, causing a life-threatening overdose and poisoning. We tell our patients that there is some comparison to simple aspirin. If one takes just two aspirin for their headache, then there is no problem. If one takes a whole bottle of aspirin, then it becomes a poison and causes a life-threatening situation. In simple words, Botox taken in small dosages (not more than 10 to 12 mouse units per kilogram body weight) is very safe.

The information in this chapter is reprinted with permission from "Cerebral Palsy & Spasticity—Frequently Asked Questions," © 2001 Miller-Dwan Medical Center. For additional information, contact Miller-Dwan Medical Center at 502 East Second Street, Duluth, MN, 55805, 218-727-8762. Information is also available at www.miller-dwan.com.

What Are the Benefits?

Botox injections can be completed within about five minutes in the cooperative patient. Injections are generally placed into no more than two or three different muscle groups at a time, creating a significant local effect. This causes spasticity reduction in the muscles injected for approximately three months, allowing improvements in range of motion and function. If significant stretching occurs during this three-month period, then tissue lengthening can occur and there can be a permanent improvement in range of motion function even after the Botox wears off. Children and adults can go to therapy, play in sporting activities, or participate in other extracurricular activities the same day of their injections. Botox is also FDA approved and quite helpful for individuals with spastic torticollis and some other less controllable movement disorders.

Why Choose Botox over Intrathecal Baclofen (the Baclofen Pump-ITB) or Selective Posterior Rhizotomy (SPR)?

Botox is only chosen for two or three select muscle groups at a time. Commonly, Botox is injected into the hamstring groups and/or the calf muscles on both sides to improve walking and/or sitting and self-care skills. The Baclofen pump and selective posterior rhizotomies are for treating more diffuse muscle spasms and essentially all the muscles of the trunk and lower extremities at the same time in a more wide-spread manner. One cannot inject this many muscles at a single time with Botox without causing undue harm to the individual. Thus, Botox is for just two or three select muscles at a time, whereby the other treatments discussed (ITB and SPR) are more for diffuse spasticity and muscle involvement.

How Much Does It Cost?

Botox is quite expensive. When we purchase the substance from Allergan Pharmaceuticals, the cost is at least $365 per milliliter. It is not uncommon that 3 or 4 milliliters are used at any one time in an individual.

What about Outpatient Therapy after Botox?

There is often physical therapy and/or occupational therapy two to three times per week after local Botox muscle injections. This is basically for intensive stretching to increase tissue lengthening and improve function during the time the Botox is active (the first three months). Often outpatient therapy can include serial casting of the feet or hands into a maximum stretched position. This includes changing the cast every week with increased stretch through the soft tissues in an effort to increase the length of the muscle gradually over time. It is not uncommon to prescribe new foot orthotics and/or modification in addition to hand splints to the extremity, post Botox injections, to improve function. This would be a decision between your physician, family, and therapy staff.

Baclofen Pump (Intrathecal Baclofen–ITB)

What Are the Risks?

If administered by competent professional staff, the risks associated with intrathecal Baclofen (ITB) are minimal. In our opinion, there is less than one percent chance of serious lifelong harm if all team members perform their duties correctly. Specifically, there is a less than one percent chance of delivering excessive intrathecal Baclofen (overdose) causing over sedation, depressed breathing, and sometimes requiring an Intensive Care Unit stay on a ventilator until the medication clears the body (about 24 hours). There is a less than one percent chance of having an infection to the spine and/or brain causing meningitis or encephalitis and further physical and mental limitations. There is a less than one percent chance of a serious seizure compromising the airway and/or breathing mechanisms, creating further impairments. There is about a five percent chance of having an infection of the pump that requires immediate removal without spread to the brain and spine and without further injury. In this case, a new Baclofen pump is often replaced in about three months after there are no clear signs of recurrent infection. There is about a ten percent chance of having the catheter kink as it enters the spine, creating a lack of flow of Baclofen into the spinal fluid. This can cause increased spasticity again and a loss of function temporarily until the catheter has been repaired. In our experience, this has not been a major problem but certainly an inconvenience. There is some chance of having a Baclofen withdrawal reaction and a seizure (less than one percent in our experience) when the catheter kinks.

What Are the Benefits of the Baclofen Pump (ITB)?

The Baclofen pump only takes about 50 minutes for the experienced surgeon to implant with no major incisions into the spine and/or body

513

cavities. In comparison, the operative time for selective posterior rhizotomy (SPR) can be four to six hours, depending upon the number of nerve rootlets severed. The children and adults generally recover more quickly from the more minor surgery, allowing for more aggressive early therapy and home dismissals. The Baclofen pump is completely reversible, and thus even if it does not work to one's best perceptions, it can always be removed. One can gradually increase the pump dosage over time, taking away as much tone or spasticity as is best for the patient's function. This allows the patient to gradually strengthen as appropriate over time, not creating excessive weakness or low tone post surgery. If the child eventually goes through a growth spurt a year or two later, then one can simply increase the dosage of the pump to help the tissues stretch out and keep up with the more accelerated bone growth. The dosage within the pump can also be adjusted for night spasms and/or other episodes of increased tone on a 24-hour clock. Many people have an increased intrathecal Baclofen dosage during the sleepful hours when spasms become more prominent and less of a dose during the more wakeful hours when they need more spasticity in the legs to walk or transfer. For this reason, the Baclofen pump is felt to be much more flexible and compatible with multiple lifestyles. It is surprisingly durable within common-sense environments.

Why Choose the Baclofen Pump (Intrathecal Baclofen–ITB) over Selective Posterior Rhizotomy (SPR)?

Most people feel that because the Baclofen pump requires less surgery and is entirely reversible with a less than one percent chance of a serious lifelong problem, it is the reasonable first choice. It is most important the child and/or adult receiving the Baclofen pump is able to frequently attend the rehabilitation center for follow-up visits post surgery. If the social and family situation is difficult with minimum follow-up and poor compliance on record for office visits and therapy sessions, then the Baclofen pump should not be implanted. The Baclofen pump is the only choice for adults with spasticity having no serious contractures and failing other more conservative treatment options.

How Much Time Do You Spend in the Hospital?

Generally, people having the Baclofen pump implanted are home and receiving outpatient therapy within the first seven to ten days after surgery. The week immediately following surgery is often involved with intensive rehabilitation and nursing interventions. Frequently, overall hospital therapy and costs can exceed $20,000 within the first year. The Baclofen pump is FDA approved and, thus, most third-party payors have authorized payments.

What about Outpatient Therapy after Leaving the Hospital?

Generally, there is intensive physical and occupational therapy for the first three to six months after surgery. This can involve physical therapy three to five times per week and occupational therapy two to three times per week. In addition, there can be improvements noted with swallowing and communication functions requiring the services of a speech therapist up to two to three times per week. Generally, the outpatient therapy program tapers more toward a baseline of two to three times per week interventions for physical therapy and one to two times per week for occupational and speech therapy between six months to a year after surgery. The therapy services, although intensive and requiring pediatric specialists, are somewhat less in our opinion than those required for individuals having selective posterior rhizotomy (SPR).

Selective Posterior Rhizotomy (SPR)

What Are the Risks?

The main risks with SPR include cutting excessive nerve rootlets entering the spine, creating undue weakness to the trunk and lower extremities, and a greater loss of feeling to the legs. If well-experienced professionals do the surgery, this risk is less but still present. People have also reported bladder problems after SPR, including wetness and inability to void. There is also a slight risk of scoliosis associated with a laminectomy (bony uncovering of the spine) with future growth. One still can develop spasticity and tightness in the legs over time with future growth spurts that can be amenable to stretching, bracing, and even Botox injections.

What Are the Benefits?

SPR can be a single intervention in the lifetime of a young person with cerebral palsy, facilitating more functional ambulatory skills and self-care if done correctly. There is no implantation of artificial devices and no problems with maintenance of these devices over time such as with the Baclofen pump. Cosmetically, one does not have to have an implantable device in the lower abdominal region in addition to a catheter that tracts around the abdomen and into the back. People enjoy having just one major intervention and not having to return to the hospital every two to three months for refill of their Baclofen pump and subsequent dose adjustments of intrathecal Baclofen.

Why Choose SPR over Intrathecal Baclofen (the Baclofen Pump)?

In addition to benefits previously mentioned, for those families who live a long distance from medical centers and whereby follow-up can be difficult, SPR appears to be a better choice. Candidates for SPR tend to be more strong and selective in their lower extremities and trunk, all ambulatory and wishing to improve their walking skills over time. Both intrathecal Baclofen (the Baclofen pump) and SPR are costly, and comparable over the first year in expenses when taking into account all hospital, surgical, and therapy services (over $20,000 easily in the first year).

How Much Time Do You Spend in the Hospital?

Often children with SPR have longer acute hospital stays (immediately after surgery) than those receiving ITB (the Baclofen pump). The hospital stay can be up to four to six weeks depending upon whether inpatient rehabilitation services are provided in the same center or elsewhere. The children can be quite weak immediately after SPR, requiring intensive re-education, strengthening, and therapy services in general to help relearn basic motor and functional skills.

What about Therapy after the Hospital Stay?

Children receiving SPR frequently have at least a year of intensive physical therapy after their operation. This includes physical therapy at least three to five times per week, in conjunction with occupational therapy two to three times per week, depending upon functional gains and goals. Often the therapy is quite sophisticated, requiring trained pediatric specialists to deliver basic neurodevelopmental exercise at progressive functional levels. These therapy services can require a lot of transportation to and from the rehabilitation center and/or school.

516

Continence and Neurogenic Bladder

What Are the Most Common Causes of Bladder Incontinence?

The lack of adequate accessibility to bathrooms, toilets, and personal assistants in transfers and donning and doffing garments continues to be, in our opinion, the major source of incontinence in adults with Cerebral Palsy. Additional causes of incontinence include about a 10 percent incidence of neurogenic bladder in children and adults creating urgency and frequency of voiding with small volume bladders and high voiding pressures. This condition of neurogenic bladder appears to be more common in individuals with bilateral involvement of cerebral palsy (both sides). It can also be associated with an increased incidence of urinary tract infections as can other forms of incontinence in cerebral palsy.

What Is a Neurogenic Bladder?

A neurogenic bladder is one that is affected through the spinal nerves lacking sufficient inhibition from higher control centers in the brain and/or brainstem region. This can cause excessive spasticity flowing to the bladder creating small volumes and higher pressures with urgent and frequent voiding and subsequent incontinence. Frequently adults and children will be voiding every one to two hours with very little time to make it to the bathroom and frequent wetness with transfers. It is a correctable situation in most instances.

What Is the Treatment?

Most of the time continence in cerebral palsy can be achieved by reasonable access to toileting environments including public bathrooms and personal care attendants providing assistance with transfers and donning and doffing of garments. It is important to have unisex bathrooms (universal) in a public setting so care attendants of the opposite sex can assist the individual.

Individuals having a spastic, low volume, neurogenic bladder can, over 90 percent of the time, become continent on anticholinergic medication such as Ditropan and/or Levsinex. Frequently these medications will relax the bladder and cause it to grow to a more normal, age-appropriate volume allowing for comfortable three-to-four hour voiding intervals or more. If the bladder cannot grow toward a more normal size and volume on medication, then surgical options may be offered. This could include taking a loop of bowel (colon) and sewing it on top of the bladder creating larger volume and lower pressures and more comfortable voiding over time. This is called a colonic patch cystoplasty or surgical augmentation of the bladder, which is performed by a trained specialist in the field (pediatric or adult urologist).

What Are the Risks of Having a Neurogenic Bladder?

A neurogenic bladder with high pressures and low volumes that is left neglected over time can cause future medical problems. This might include frequent urinary tract infections or reflux of urine upward into the kidneys (back-flow) causing swelling of the kidneys (hydronephrosis). If reflux and hydronephrosis should develop over time there is a potential for kidney stones, kidney infections, high blood pressure and/or developing renal failure in the worst-case scenario. Most adults in our experience, have not been bothered by upper tract and kidney problems over time unless they had inadequate drainage of urine to the outside. Sometimes individuals can be seated in a wheelchair for 10-12 hours or more with inability to discharge their urine to the outside creating harmful back pressure and swelling of the kidneys (hydronephrosis). In these individuals we see some kidney stone infections and early renal failure develop. An intermittent clean catheterization program (ICC) or an even indwelling Foley catheter or suprapubic catheter can provide adequate drainage and minimize risk over time.

What Should I Do If I Experience Frequent Voiding and/or Incontinence?

Symptoms such as these should be brought to the attention of your local physician and/or medical care specialist. A referral to a physiatrist who does bladder studies and/or a urologist (surgeon), would be reasonable. Many times the medical specialist will not know much about cerebral palsy and/or the presence of a neurologic bladder. Often urologists are trained more for surgical conditions of which the described neurogenic bladder is generally not. For this reason some frustrations may occur with contact of the medical care delivery system. If you should find extreme frustrations in this regard, please feel free to contact us and we will try to make an appropriate referral in your local area as helpful. It is important to remember that neurogenic bladder occurs across a life span (in children and adults) and across all educational and living circumstances.

Chapter 47

Plasmapheresis: Removal of Plasma from Blood Cells to Treat Autoimmune Disease

Many diseases, including myasthenia gravis, Lambert-Eaton syndrome, Guillain-Barré syndrome, and others are caused by a so-called autoimmune, or self-immune, process. In autoimmune conditions, the body's immune system mistakenly turns against itself, attacking its own tissues. Some of the specialized cells involved in this process can attack tissues directly, while others can produce substances known as antibodies that circulate in the blood and carry out the attack. Antibodies produced against the body's own tissues are known as autoantibodies.

Treatment with medications that suppress the activities of the immune system and/or reduce inflammation of tissues has been the most common approach to autoimmune disease for more than 30 years. Many new immunosuppressants have become available since the 1960s, but all the medications used to treat autoimmune disease have serious side effects when taken in high doses for months or years.

In the 1970s, with the support of the Muscular Dystrophy Association, researchers developed a new approach to the treatment of autoimmune conditions. Instead of trying to change the immune system with medication alone, they thought that it might be possible to mechanically remove autoantibodies from the bloodstream in a process similar to that used in an artificial kidney, or dialysis, treatment.

"Facts about Plasmapheresis," © 1999 Muscular Dystrophy Association. Reprinted with permission of the Muscular Dystrophy Association.

The procedure became known as plasmapheresis, meaning plasma separation. It's also known as plasma exchange.

Medications that suppress the immune system or reduce inflammation are often combined with plasmapheresis, but they can usually be given in lower doses than when used alone.

Today, plasmapheresis is widely accepted for the treatment of myasthenia gravis, Lambert-Eaton syndrome, Guillain-Barré syndrome, and chronic demyelinating polyneuropathy. Its effectiveness in other conditions, such as multiple sclerosis, polymyositis, and dermatomyositis is not as well established.

What Is Plasmapheresis?

Plasmapheresis is a process in which the fluid part of the blood, called plasma, is removed from blood cells by a device known as a cell separator. The separator works either by spinning the blood at high speed to separate the cells from the fluid or by passing the blood through a membrane with pores so small that only the fluid part of the blood can pass through. The cells are returned to the person undergoing treatment, while the plasma, which contains the antibodies, is discarded and replaced with other fluids. Medication to keep the blood from clotting (an anticoagulant) is given through a vein during the procedure.

What's Involved in a Plasmapheresis Treatment?

A plasmapheresis treatment takes several hours and can be done on an outpatient basis. It can be uncomfortable but is normally not painful. The number of treatments needed varies greatly depending on the particular disease and the person's general condition. An average course of plasma exchanges is six to ten treatments over two to ten weeks. In some centers, treatments are performed once a week, while in others, more than one weekly treatment is done.

Plasmapheresis removes the fluid part of the blood, the plasma, from blood cells. The cells are returned to the person undergoing treatment, while the plasma is discarded. The procedure takes several hours and can be uncomfortable, although it is normally not painful.

A person undergoing plasmapheresis can lie in bed or sit in a reclining chair. A small, thin tube (catheter) is placed in a large vein, usually the one in the crook of the arm, and another tube is placed in the opposite hand or foot (so that at least one arm can move freely during the procedure). Blood is taken to the separator from one tube, while the separated blood cells, combined with replacement fluids, are returned to the patient through the other tube. The amount of blood outside the body at any one time is much less than the amount ordinarily donated in a blood bank.

Are There Risks Associated with Plasmapheresis?

Yes, but most can be controlled. Any unusual symptoms should be immediately reported to the doctor or the person in charge of the procedure. Symptoms that may seem trivial sometimes herald the onset of a serious complication.

The most common problem is a drop in blood pressure, which can be experienced as faintness, dizziness, blurred vision, coldness, sweating, or abdominal cramps. A drop in blood pressure is remedied by lowering the patient's head, raising the legs, and giving intravenous fluid.

Bleeding can occasionally occur because of the medications used to keep the blood from clotting during the procedure. Some of these medications can cause other adverse reactions, which begin with tingling around the mouth or in the limbs, muscle cramps, or a metallic taste in the mouth. If allowed to progress, these reactions can lead to an irregular heartbeat or seizures.

An allergic reaction to the solutions used to replace the plasma or to the sterilizing agents used for the tubing can be a true emergency. This type of reaction usually begins with itching, wheezing, or a rash. The plasma exchange must be stopped and the person treated with intravenous medications.

Excessive suppression of the immune system can temporarily occur with plasmapheresis, since the procedure isn't selective about which antibodies it removes. In time, the body can replenish its supply of needed antibodies, but some physicians give these intravenously after each plasmapheresis treatment. Outpatients may have to take special precautions against infection.

Medication dosages need careful observation and adjustment in people being treated with plasmapheresis because some drugs can be removed from the blood or changed by the procedure.

How Long Does It Take to See Improvement?

Improvement can sometimes occur within days, especially in myasthenia gravis. In other conditions, especially where there is extensive tissue damage, improvement is slower but can still occur within weeks.

Does MDA Pay for Plasmapheresis?

MDA supported pioneering research to develop plasmapheresis. However, payment for this procedure is not among the many services included in MDA's program. A number of health insurance plans do cover the procedure.

Where Are Plasmapheresis Treatments Offered?

Plasmapheresis is performed at many major medical centers across the country. MDA clinic directors can offer advice about the availability of this treatment and its use for specific conditions.

Chapter 48

Hippotherapy: A Treatment Tool to Improve Neuromuscular Function

What Is Hippotherapy?

Hippotherapy is a term that refers to the use of the movement of the horse as a treatment tool by physical therapists, occupational therapists, and speech-language pathologists to address impairments, functional limitations, and disabilities in patients with neuromusculoskeletal dysfunction. Hippotherapy is used as part of an integrated treatment program to achieve functional outcomes.

In hippotherapy, the patient engages in activities on the horse that are enjoyable and challenging. In the controlled hippotherapy environment, the therapist modifies the horse's movement and carefully grades sensory input. Specific riding skills are not taught (as in therapeutic horseback riding); but rather a foundation is established to improve neurological function and sensory processing. This foundation can be generalized to a wide range of daily activities.

Terminology

The term therapeutic riding has been used for many years to encompass the variety of equine activities in which people with disabilities

This information is reprinted with permission from the American Hippotherapy Association (AHA) website at www.narah.org/sec_aha/default.asp; cited January 2002. The American Hippotherapy Association is a section of NARHA (North American Riding for the Handicapped Association), more information is available on the NARHA website at www.narha.org.

participate. Though still commonly used, this umbrella term has caused confusion among the medical community. When the therapist uses the movement of the horse as a treatment tool to improve neuromuscular function, it is important to consistently use the correct terminology and refer to it as hippotherapy.

Why the Horse?

The horse's walk provides sensory input through movement, which is variable, rhythmic, and repetitive. The resultant movement responses in the patient are similar to human movement patterns of the pelvis while walking. The variability of the horse's gait enables the therapist to grade the degree of sensory input to the patient, and then use this movement in combination with other treatment strategies to achieve desired results. Patients respond enthusiastically to this enjoyable experience in a natural setting.

General Indications for Hippotherapy

- Population—children and adults with mild to severe neuromusculoskeletal dysfunction

  Impairments that may be modified with hippotherapy are:

- Abnormal tone
- Impaired balance responses
- Impaired coordination
- Impaired communication
- Impaired sensorimotor function
- Postural asymmetry
- Poor postural control
- Decreased mobility
- Limbic system issues related to arousal, motivation, and attention

  Functional limitations relating to the following general areas may be improved with hippotherapy:

- Gross motor skills such as sitting, standing, walking
- Speech and language abilities
- Behavioral and cognitive abilities

Medical Conditions

The primary medical conditions, which may manifest some or all of the listed problems and may be indications for hippotherapy, follow. However, hippotherapy is not for every patient. Specially trained health professionals must evaluate each potential patient on an individual basis.

- Cerebral Palsy
- Cerebral Vascular Accident
- Developmental Delay
- Down Syndrome
- Functional Spinal Curvature
- Learning or language disabilities
- Multiple Sclerosis
- Sensory Integrative Dysfunction
- Traumatic Brain Injury

Part Seven

Quality of Life Assistance

Chapter 49

Be Independent: Activities of Daily Living

Activities of daily living include tasks such as bathing, grooming, dressing, preparing food, eating, and caring for the home. Walking and general mobility—getting from place to place—are also important aspects of a person's life. Individuals with declining abilities may have difficulty caring for themselves. People with Parkinson's disease often have tremors, rigidity, and slowness of movement, all of which may interfere with their ability to care for themselves.

This chapter contains suggested techniques and useful aids which can help people to remain independent and assist with activities of daily living. The adaptive devices mentioned can be purchased at a surgical supply store or through the catalogues listed in the reference section. There are many things that can be done to increase independence and safety in self-care and mobility. For further information, consult your physician, occupational therapist, or physical therapist.

The Bedroom

The bedroom should be kept free of clutter and be large enough to allow free access to the bed, bureau, closet, and hallway doors. Scatter rugs increase the risk of falling and should be avoided. If they are used, they must be taped or tacked to the floor even if they have nonskid

The information in this chapter is reprinted from *Be Independent*, a booklet published by The American Parkinson Disease Association, 1250 Hylan Boulevard, Suite 4, Staten Island, NY 10305. © 1999 American Parkinson Disease Association. Reprinted with permission.

rubber pads beneath them. Casters should be removed from furniture, since objects that roll provide unstable handholds. Shoes and other small objects should be kept off the floor, especially at night.

Special equipment and aids can be used in the bedroom to help maintain independence and safety while increasing comfort.

Bedroom Equipment

1. Bed pulls can be attached to the frame at the end of the bed. They are useful to assist in rising to a seated position or turning in bed, and can be either purchased or made at home. To make: Braid three pieces of tightly woven fabric, such as sheeting, together in a length that reaches from the base of the bed to your hand when you are lying down. Sew a large wooden curtain ring to the end to serve as a grasp. Then sew a small binder clip near the ring so that the bed pull can be clamped to the bedding and remain within your reach. Bed pulls can also be attached to the sides of the bed to assist in turning.

2. A trapeze installed over the head of the bed can help individuals to change position. It may be purchased at a surgical supply store and can be mounted to most standard beds.

3. A sturdy cardboard box can be placed under the covers at the foot of the bed. This "bed cradle" keeps feet and lower legs free of the sheets while turning.

4. A urinal may be kept within reach on a bed table, or a commode may be placed at the bedside for nighttime use. The urinal or commode helps reduce walks to the bathroom.

5. Disposable incontinence garments are designed to address the problem of accidental urination and may be especially helpful at night.

6. A chair with armrests and a firm seat should be part of the bedroom furniture. Dressing can be accomplished while sitting in the chair, thus eliminating the risk of falling. Try to avoid sitting in a low chair. A firm pillow, secured to the chair, makes it easier to rise from a low surface.

7. The bed should be no lower than knee height for ease in getting in and out. If the bed is too high, a carpenter can cut two

or three inches off the legs. If the bed is too low, use a thicker mattress or mattress padding.

8. A railing can be installed on a bedroom wall ten inches higher than the level of the bed, and the bed placed against the wall under the railing. The railing becomes an assist for rising from and turning in bed. Commercially made bed rails are available and can be mounted on most beds. Satin sheets are smooth and can also facilitate turning.

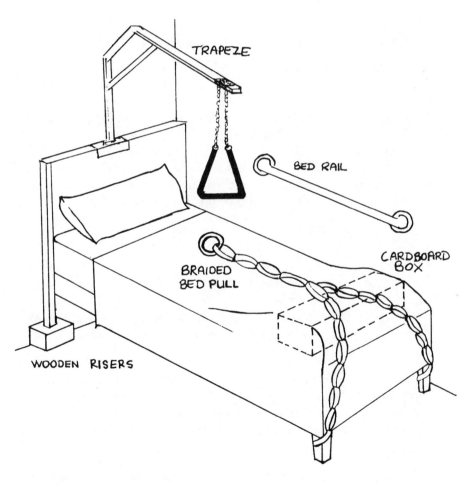

Figure 49.1. *Bedroom Ideas*

9. For difficulty in sitting up in bed, place a foam wedge cushion under the mattress at the head of the bed, or place wooden risers under the legs at the head of the bed.

10. Nightlights should be installed in a wall socket near the bedroom door, in the hallway leading to the bathroom, and in the bathroom. They are indispensable in helping you avoid accidents.

11. A communication device such as a bell or intercom system may be needed to ensure safety at night, especially if you have decreased voice volume.

The Bathroom

Safety is essential in the bathroom. It is the most dangerous room in your house. The tile floor is slippery and the surfaces of the shower or tub are extremely slick, especially when wet. The average bathroom is often small and furnished with porcelain fixtures that jut out from the walls and restrict walking space. A call for help may go unheard, especially if the water is running or the door is closed.

It is important that the bathroom be made as safe as possible. Adequate equipment and awareness of danger increases the ease and safety of bathing and grooming. Bathing is easier if you are organized and keep everything that you need arranged safely within or near the tub.

Bathroom Safety

1. Non-skid decals or strips, attached to a tub or shower floor, or the use of a rubber mat, help to eliminate falls. Small bathroom rugs are easy to trip over, and should not be used. Use a large rug that covers most of the floor, wall-to-wall carpeting, or bare flooring. Do not wax the floor.

2. Grab bars or tub rails placed in strategic locations provide balance and support for getting in and out of the tub or shower. Never use towel racks or wall soap holders as grab bars. They are not designed for this and may break away under pressure.

3. Tub seats or shower chairs make bathing easier and safer. A flexible shower hose or a hand-held shower massage allows

for safer bathing while seated. A shower nozzle with a turn-off knob is more convenient than a free-flow nozzle.

4. A raised toilet seat makes sitting on and rising from the toilet easier. Arm rails attached to the toilet, or a grab bar installed on the wall adjacent to the toilet, provide convenient hand holds.

5. If you have difficulty holding objects, do not use glass tumblers. Paper or plastic cups are safer.

6. A nightlight should always be installed in a bathroom wall socket.

7. The hot water heater in your house should be turned down to prevent accidental scalding.

Grooming

1. Soap on a rope keeps soap conveniently within reach while showering or taking a tub bath.

2. A suction nailbrush makes grooming easier and safer. It can be secured to the tub, reducing the risk of injury from falling.

3. A long-handled sponge reaches the lower legs, feet, and back. It helps eliminate bending and is necessary if you have a problem with balance. A curved bath sponge can be useful for washing your back.

4. Wash mitts are terry cloth gloves that eliminate the need for holding onto a washcloth.

5. An electric razor should be used for safety, particularly if you have hand tremor. A variety of electric razor holders, which make grasp easier, are commercially available.

6. Round-headed faucets require a twisting motion to operate. This is difficult for people with impaired strength or coordination. They can be replaced with a lever-type handle or a single arm control faucet. The round-headed faucet can be improved by adding tap-turner adaptations.

7. Adding a commercial built-up handle, a bicycle handle, or a wrist cuff makes your tooth brush, hairbrush, or comb handles

larger and easier to grip. Extension handles may be helpful if your shoulder or arm movement is limited.

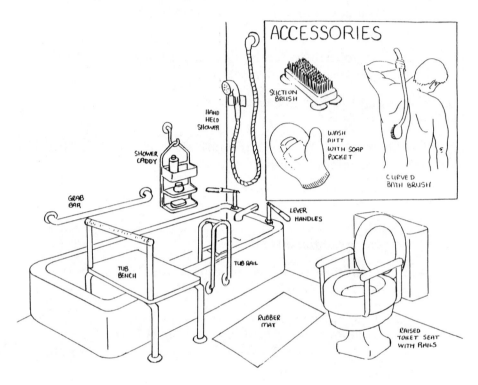

Figure 49.2. *Bathroom Ideas*

Dressing

The fine hand coordination and strength needed for dressing is sometimes impaired. Pain and stiffness in the limbs can also complicate putting on and taking off clothing, particularly underwear, socks, and slacks. There are many simple and useful aids that can help people remain independent.

Try to choose clothing that is easy to manage. Loose fitting, stretchy clothes with simple fastenings are easier to put on and take off. For some people, pullover tops may be more convenient. They eliminate

534

the need for buttoning. Front-closing garments are easier to manage than zipper and button-back garments.

Knee-length stockings can be worn instead of panty hose only if they have wide elasticized tops to prevent constriction of circulation. **Never** wear stockings rolled down and secured with a rubber band or garter. This impairs circulation.

Clothing should be placed, in order of wear, on a chair near the individual. Take time and, if possible, do not allow anyone to rush the care recipient. Try to maintain their independence.

Dressing Devices

1. Velcro closures are excellent substitutes for buttons and zippers. Sew tabs of Velcro over the buttonhole and on the underside of the button. Press the Velcro strips together to fasten your shirt.

2. A button hook or button aid slips through the buttonhole and pulls the button back through it. The handles of these tools are more easily grasped than a small button when fine hand coordination is impaired.

3. Large, easily grasped zipper pulls or rings make opening and closing trouser flys, jackets, and coats less difficult.

4. Small cuff buttons can be difficult to manipulate. Use elastic thread to sew buttons onto cuffs. Keep them buttoned all the time and slide your hand through. You can also join the cuff with a Velcro closure.

5. A dressing stick or reacher is useful for pulling pants and undergarments up over your legs. It allows you to remain seated while dressing and reduces the risk of falling. Reachers are also useful for picking up objects that have dropped to the floor.

6. Elastic shoelaces need to be tied only once, thus converting laced shoes to slip-on shoes. Standard tie shoes can be closed with Velcro strips. A shoemaker can stitch them on.

7. A front-closing bra is easier to put on and take off. You can adapt a back-closing bra by sewing up the rear closure, cutting the front open and attaching Velcro strips.

8. A long-handled shoehorn and a sock donner reduce bending and straining when putting on socks and shoes.

535

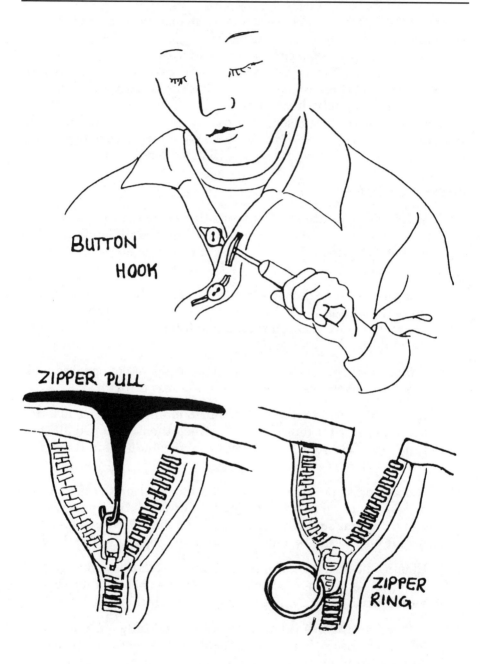

Figure 49.3a. Dressing Ideas

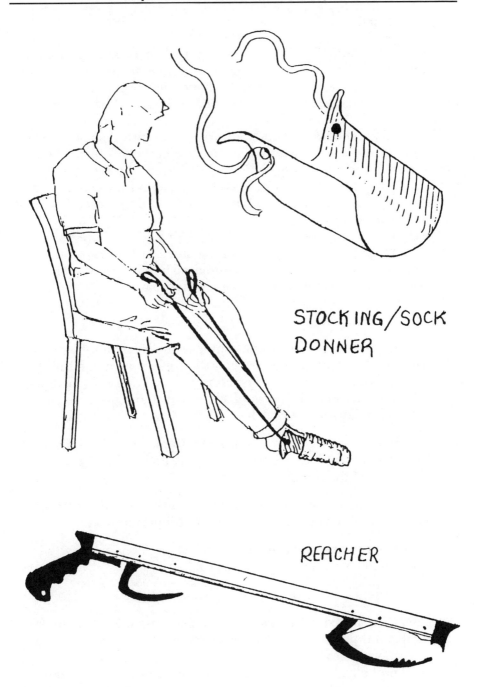

STOCKING/SOCK DONNER

REACHER

Figure 49.3b. *Dressing Ideas*

537

The Kitchen

Decreased strength, range of motion, and coordination problems can limit your ability to perform kitchen activities such as: meal preparation, food storage, eating, cleaning, and clearing up after meals. Many ingenious aids have been devised to improve safety and efficiency in the kitchen.

The kitchen should be kept well organized with dishes, utensils, and foods stored near to where they are used and within easy reach. Coffee and tea for instance, should be stored as close as possible to the tea kettle. Store utensils you rarely use behind those used everyday. If there is wall space, install a pegboard at an accessible height and hang utensils there.

Pace yourself during kitchen activities and plan before you start to avoid unnecessary energy-consuming steps. If you have impaired balance, slowness of movement, or decreased hand coordination, meal preparation is safer and easier if done while seated.

Kitchen Equipment

1. A Lazy Susan, placed in the center of the kitchen table or on a counter, holds numerous frequently used items and eliminates the need to gather each one before meals. The Lazy Susan can also be used as a shelf organizer to reduce the need to reach for objects at the back of the shelf.

2. Reachers can be used in the kitchen to pick up light objects that fall to the floor. Heavy objects should be placed in counter-height cabinets.

3. A rubber pad or wet dishcloth can be placed under bowls and pans to stabilize them while you are preparing food.

4. Electric can openers are useful and convenient, especially if fine hand coordination is impaired.

5. A jar opener eases the problem of opening jars.

6. A cutting board with a raised edge prevents diced vegetables and small pieces of meat from scattering off the board. A nail hammered into the board skewers food while dicing or cutting. The nail also helps when buttering bread or toast. Suction cups can be attached to the bottom of your cutting board to prevent it from sliding.

7. A microwave, used instead of a stove, reduces the risk of injury from burns.

8. A long-handled dustpan enables you to collect floor sweepings without bending to the floor. A sponge mop should be kept

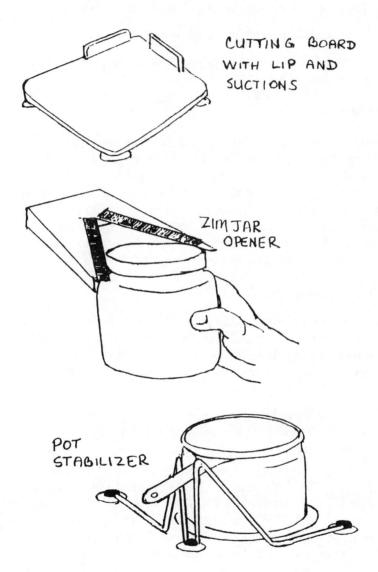

CUTTING BOARD WITH LIP AND SUCTIONS

ZIM JAR OPENER

POT STABILIZER

Figure 49.4. Kitchen Ideas

539

accessible as spills should be wiped up immediately to reduce the chance of falling.

9. Your strength and hand function should affect your choice of pots and pans. If you have limited strength, use aluminum pots and pans and lightweight dishes. Make sure that the shape and size of the handles are suited to your grasp strength. A long pot handle allows for two-handed lifting.

10. A pot stabilizer keeps the handle steady when you stir.

11. Kitchen scissors can help you to open plastic packages and boxes that are difficult to rip.

Mealtime

There are many attractive and durable commercially available mealtime aids. They have been designed to enable people to continue to eat with as much independence as possible.

If a special or adapted piece of silverware is used at home, take it along when dining in a restaurant. If a person has difficulty cutting food, ask the waiter to have the food cut in the kitchen before it is presented. This prevents someone from having to reach across the table to assist. Take time while eating and try not to rush.

Mealtime Equipment

1. Attachable plate guards provide a rim on one side of the plate. Food, especially small vegetables, can be pushed against the guard, where they fall onto the fork. Plate guards also prevent spills. Scoop dishes contoured with raised edges serve the same purpose.

2. Silverware with built up plastic handles is more easily grasped. Tubular foam padding can be attached to the utensil to widen the grip.

    Soup spoons can be used instead of forks when eating small pieces of food. Sporks are a combination spoon and fork. This one utensil can spear as well as hold food. A rocking knife may be used instead of a straight knife if you have problems with co-ordination. Weighted utensils may help to decrease hand tremors, thus allowing the utensil to reach your mouth more easily.

3. If you have a tremor, flexible plastic straws help you to drink.

4. A mug with a large handle for easy grasp should be used if your tremor is severe. An insulated mug with a lid reduces the risk of burns from spills when drinking hot liquids.

5. A rubber pad or a moist paper towel can be placed under plates, cups, and serving dishes to keep them from sliding.

Walking

The ability to get from one place to another inside or outside the home is very important. There are a number of assistive devices that can help a person with decreased balance, coordination, or mobility to walk safely.

Canes can be used to compensate for minor balance problems. They come in a variety of shapes and sizes and increase an individual's base of support.

The standard J-Handle cane offers some stability as well as a sense of security. An ortho-cane or a quad cane may also be used. Each offers an increasing degree of support and balance.

If more assistance than a cane is needed, a walker can be prescribed. A walker that folds is good if you need to store or transport it in limited space—for example, in a car. Wheels can be added if you have difficulty coordinating the advancement of the walker or are unable to lift it off the floor. A braking mechanism which locks with downward pressure can be attached to the front or back wheels. It is important to note, however, that although the rolling walker is easier to advance, it can be unsafe on rugs and other uneven surfaces.

If you are unable to walk, or can walk only short distances in your home, a wheelchair provides more functional mobility.

In order to best suit your individual needs, a physical therapist should be consulted so that the appropriate ambulatory device or wheelchair is provided.

Negotiating Stairs

Stairs often become a major barrier to a person who has limited strength, balance, and mobility. The following guidelines make stair climbing easier.

If there is a handrail available, use it as long as it is well secured. Hold onto the handrailing with one hand and an assistive device, if needed, in the other hand. Both hands can also be placed on the handrail to sidestep up and down the stairs one at a time.

541

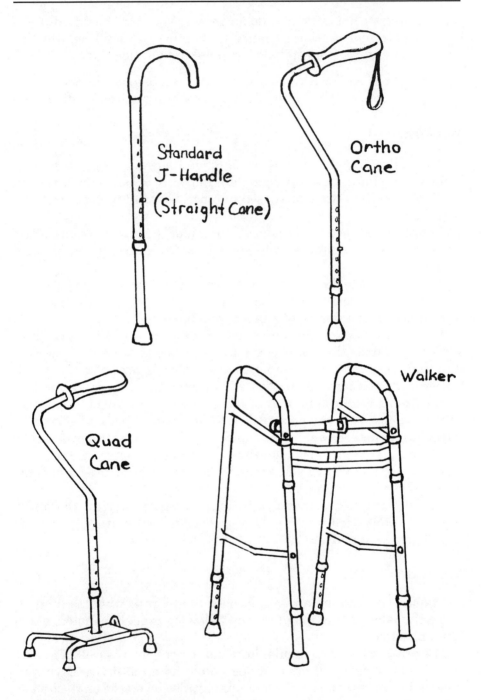

Figure 49.5. *Walking Ideas*

If you are unable to go up or down the stairs safely in a step-over-step manner, negotiate the stairs one step at a time. Place one foot on the step; place the second foot on that same step before you move on to the next.

If someone is assisting you, that person should stay by your side. The assisting person should stagger their feet so that their lead foot is one step down from yours. This maintains good balance.

If you cannot safely climb stairs, you can be carried up and down in a wheelchair. A lift may be installed, but it is expensive.

Specific instructions for walking up and down the stairs or being assisted in a wheelchair can best be given by a physical therapist.

Getting In or Out of a Car

There are ways to make getting in or out of a car easier. First, the car must be parked far enough away from the curb so that you can step onto the level ground before you go into or get out of the car. To get into a car turn so that you back in for the last steps. Your buttocks should lead. Then sit down and swing your legs in.

To exit the car, swing both legs out together and stand up. Sit in the front or back seat, whichever gives you more room. Use pillows to make it easier to get up from a low car. Specific techniques should be taught by and practiced with a physical therapist or occupational therapist.

Miscellaneous Tips

If you have a problem with shuffling, small steps, and stopping while walking, arrange the furniture so as to avoid congested areas. Keep hallways free of obstacles. Plan a route through the house so that there is always a safe handhold available in case you lose your balance.

Railings can be installed on the walls to provide support. Your family should consult with you before they rearrange the furniture so that you do not lose familiarity with your surroundings.

Avoid low couches and chairs as it is often extremely difficult to rise from them without help. A straight back chair with armrests and a firm seat is easier to get up from. A firm cushion can be used to acquire the height that is suitable for you. Pneumatic lifter seats can assist someone who has severe difficulty rising from a chair.

Handrails should be installed on all staircases, especially those outside.

Use a carpet sweeper instead of a vacuum. It is lighter and easier to manipulate.

The "Fone Holder" is a long, flexible shaft that attaches to most tables and can be positioned to hold the telephone receiver so a person can use the handset without having to move or even touch it. Another device adapts huge push buttons to the small touch-tone buttons of a standard phone to make dialing easier.

Handwriting can be a serious problem for persons with Parkinson's disease. Various pens, pencils, and writing devices are available to stabilize your grip. A weighted pen may help reduce tremors and improve writing.

A door knob turner fits over the door handle and converts the round knob into a lever. This makes it easier to open.

A Word to the Family

In order to preserve independence in activities of daily living, people should do all that they can for themselves. Because of tremor, rigidity, and slowness of movement, each activity may take more time than it used to.

It is tempting to do or to complete tasks for people. It saves time and, perhaps, frustration. However, this may lead to dependence, because it decreases people's motivation to help themselves.

The physical ability of persons with Parkinson's disease varies throughout the day in response to anti-Parkinson's medication. Tremor, rigidity, and slowness of movement may be more pronounced in the morning than in the afternoon. People's ability to dress or to eat may be impaired at one time and not another.

To decrease misunderstanding and further frustration, families should be aware that their relatives are not malingering but that it is the variability of the disease that causes fluctuation in independence. People may require help some of the time, but not all of the time.

It is vitally important for the families of people with Parkinson's disease to help them remain as independent as possible.

Resources for Independent Living

Please refer to Chapter 55 "Directory of Resources for People with Movement Disorders," for information on some companies that feature products, equipment, and clothing designed to make self-care skills easier.

Chapter 50

Mobility Aids

Whether it is to the grocery store, to work, or to the ballgame, your ability to move around is an important factor in determining your quality of life.

Using assistive technology devices to improve your personal mobility means using something to do the work typically done by another part of your body. For the most part, this means taking work away from your legs. Options include items such as canes, crutches, and walkers, which help transfer weight to the arms and upper body. If standing or using your arms is not an option, wheelchairs (manual or electric) or scooters are usually the next best choice. Power for movement is provided either manually or by some type of motor. Controlling an electric wheelchair is most commonly done with the arms and hands, but can also be done by mouth, head movement, or breath.

It may be necessary to have more than one kind of device to help with personal mobility. It can be helpful to have different devices for different places. Some disabilities can be highly variable in terms of severity—maybe a wheelchair is good one day, maybe another day you will need crutches. Chances are the devices you use most for personal

This chapter includes, "Mobility Aids," "Illustrated Tour—Technology for Mobility," "Seating Technology—Illustrated Tour," and "About Seating and Positioning." Reprinted with permission from the Washington Assistive Technology Alliance, a consumer advocacy network that includes the University of Washington Center for Technology and Disability Studies and the AT Resource Center at the Easter Seal Society in Spokane, Washington. © 1999 Washington Assistive Technology Alliance. For additional information, visit the WATA website at www.wata.org.

mobility will eventually break down—having a backup is a good way to keep up your mobility while waiting for repairs.

About Seating and Positioning

People with disabilities often spend more time sitting than other people. Devices related to the seat are often referred to as the seating system. Seating can be considered the interface between a mobility device and the user. Seating devices allow a person to operate at their highest functional level, helping in a wide range of activities including body support, reach, interaction with others, and breath support. Devices for support range from a piece of plywood under a foam cushion to a custom mold that conforms exactly to the consumer.

Often a specialized assessment by a wheelchair seating specialist is recommended so that sizing and positioning of seat, back, and footrests is appropriate. Typical areas involved in evaluating for seating device selection include physical function (strength and range of motion), muscle tone, reflexes, fatigue, and endurance. Choosing appropriate support surface materials and upholstery, as well as cushioning, are critical and many options exist to enhance sitting posture, comfort, and safety.

In terms of seating system needs, three broad kinds of systems are often considered: flat (planar), pre-fit (or contoured), and custom fit (contoured). Wheelchairs typically come with an attached seat and back that are generally flat (or planar) with little or no cushioning. Cushions may be secured to the seat and or back for comfort, and this seating system approach is often enough for those individuals who have good sitting balance and posture and who can easily move about and take pressure off of the bottom, back, and feet.

For the individual who has some challenge in posture and sitting balance, the seating system can be used to improve the ability to be comfortable while sitting. This is done by creating curves or contours in the seat that shape to the body. An additional method is to add support to the trunk, hips and thighs, legs, arms, and/or head. Special hardware is often necessary to mount contoured seats, backs, and other attachments. Pre-contoured seat and back systems can be selected when the individual has a common size and shape.

Custom contouring is often used when the individual has a deformity of the back, pelvis, or lower limbs. In this approach, either or both the seat and back are shaped to the person by way of special molding techniques. Custom contouring should always involve seating specialists in decision making and molding procedures. As you might expect, the custom contouring seating approach is the most expensive and necessitates careful follow-up and follow-along to assure good fit, use, and adjustment.

A precaution with contouring and additions of other seating components like trunk pads, hip, and thigh supports, is that freedom of movement is further restricted and great attention needs to be paid to relieving pressure on the skin. Individuals sitting in wheelchairs need to relieve pressure on skin surfaces, particularly the buttock and thighs. Lifting the bottom off the seat surface by using the arms to do a push-up, or by leaning sideways or forward are methods often taught to individuals to relieve pressure. If they are unable to perform these moves, the wheelchair might need to be reclined or leaned back to take pressure off of the bottom. Recline or tilt-back systems are another assistive technology component of wheelchairs that can be considered.

Technology for Mobility

Canes

Canes come in a variety of styles. Other than the common straight cane, there also are collapsible canes that are easier to transport. A straight up and down shaft and "L" shaped handle is pretty standard. Some canes have four legs, which means better stability and contact with the ground, with four legs, it can also stand on its own, which is helpful because you don't have to hold it all the time. The extra legs also increase the weight of the cane and the coordination necessary for moving it.

Crutches

The difference between canes and crutches is the point of weight bearing. Crutches allow some of the weight to be borne by the shoulders and the wrists. With common crutches weight can be supported by the upper body, or just below the armpits, or both. A platform crutch uses a padded support to allow your elbows and forearms to bear weight. A forearm crutch has a handle to grab for supporting weight and a cuff for increased forearm stability.

Walkers

Walkers are typically metal frames that provide more stability than canes or crutches. The standard model has rubber tips on the feet to give better traction, but it would need to be picked up to move. Small rubber grips on the handle make it easy to push, but don't give any additional support. Many walkers have wheels on the front legs, making movement of the walker easier but control more difficult. Wheels on any of the legs are a common addition for almost any walker. Another type of walker provides many other options. It has four big wheels that make it easy to move it around. There are hand brakes on the handlebars, a seat for sitting, and a basket on the front. While this walker may provide more options and flexibility, it will not provide equal support of weight and will require more consumer ability to control it.

Wheelchairs and Scooters

Manual Wheelchairs

A standard, non-lightweight chair often works well as a back-up chair or for someone who does not need a chair for a lot of activities.

A lightweight version besides actually being lighter (easier to push or lift), has a lower backrest, a footrest that does not stick out from the chair (not good if you have problems bending your knees) and the brakes are located under the seat rather than off to the side (not good if you have problems bending over).

A racing model wheelchair pays little attention to things like back and foot support. The wheels are huge and extend to the level of the backrest. The lone front wheel is also big. This chair is designed for one reason—to go fast.

Power Wheelchairs

The work of pushing a chair is not practical for many people. In these situations electric wheelchairs or scooters may be the next best option for personal mobility. Most electric wheelchairs involve some sort of machine attached to a chair that takes the place of human power. Steering is usually accomplished by a joystick placed where the person can best reach and control it. Steering can also be accomplished by using breath and head or mouth movement. Some power wheelchairs have big wheels in the front and small ones in the back. Some people find this gives better power and traction. Others have big wheels in the back and a bigger motor. The bigger motor may provide more power, but also increases the weight of the chair. The seat on other chairs can raise the user to a fully standing position. You wouldn't want to drive standing up (bad balance), but being able to change position is an effective way to stretch or alter pressure, without actually standing up on your own.

Scooters

Scooters are platforms with a seat on the back, a motor, a steering column, and three or four wheels. The strength to move the steering column (and steer the scooter) must be provided by the user, which is different from electric wheelchairs. It is much easier to store items (groceries, mail) in front of a scooter user. As with other electrical mobility products the speed and power of scooters will vary.

Scooters range from the basic scooter with a relatively small motor and minimal padding to one with a much larger motor and generous padding so that it can go faster and handle bigger hills. A deluxe model offers lots of lower back support and a headrest along with a basket on the front and rear view mirror on the left side. Four wheels offer more balance than three, but more room is required to turn around and maneuver.

Chapter 51

A Wheeler's Best Friend: Service Animals

Service dogs enhance the lives of their handlers—owners—on many levels. They can tow your chair, pick up objects, bring the phone when it rings, even help you dress and undress. They can redirect comments like, "What happened to you?" to "Wow, cool dog!" They are great conversation starters and even help with making acquaintances. Having a bad day, bad spasms, bowel or bladder problems? A dog's unconditional love puts everything into perspective: "What's the big deal?" they seem to say. "How about a hug and a walk?"

"Having Kasten has turned my disability into an asset," says Ruthie Rudek, 22, of Palo Alto, Calif., who was diagnosed with MS at 16. Kasten is the female golden retriever service dog she has had for the past two years. "The treatments for MS suck—they're painful, miserable, and it's very frustrating. Kasten has helped me more than any drug or doctor. When I ask for help, she helps, no questions asked, and she makes me happy."

Nancy Sawhney, 55, from Sacramento, Calif., has had a motor-neuron disease since age 30. Sawhney's service dog, Union, is a golden retriever/lab mix. "Union picks things up for me, anything from a can of soda to an onion to a dime, and brings me the telephone when it rings. And she pulls my wheelchair. When I'm with her I don't get any of those condescending 'God bless people like you' pats on the head, which is a great relief."

Rules of the Game

No official certification is required for a disabled handler/service dog team to enjoy public access rights. What is required is that the handler be considered disabled under ADA guidelines. Also, the dog must be trained to perform a task or tasks that help mitigate the disability and must be well-behaved and under control at all times. It's helpful if the dog wears an identifying harness or backpack.

If a service dog does any damage in a public establishment, the owner of the dog is liable. "A dog's work ethic and training have to be developed to an incredible level. It should not have to be 'managed' in public," says Shari Dehouwer, dog trainer and founder of Discovery Dogs. Dehouwer has strong feelings about authentic service dogs. "When I see how hard a person works to train a dog, and then I see somebody trying to pass their pet dog off as a service dog when the dog is yapping and barking and doesn't even know how to heel, that's just plain scary. It's worse than able people using bogus parking placards."

It isn't easy to train a service dog. Pete Rapalus, public relations coordinator for Canine Companions for Independence in Santa Rosa, Calif., says, "Our rate of success from birth to graduation with a handler is about 35 to 40 percent. Not all dogs make it for the same reason not all people make into the Olympics. It takes a very talented dog. It costs about $15,000 to $25,000 to feed and train a finished dog that graduates. So every time there's a half-trained 'service dog' out there it makes it tougher for everybody who has a well-behaved service dog."

Unfortunately, not everyone plays by the rules. There are stories of people who mysteriously develop bad backs because there's a no dog policy where they rent and they want to keep their pet dog. But the rules are clear: If you are not disabled, or if your dog hasn't been trained as a service dog and doesn't behave the way a service dog should, it isn't a service dog.

Worth the Wait

Most people receive fully trained service dogs from one of the many nonprofit organizations such as CCI. Cost to the person receiving the dog is at most a nominal application fee; quite often there is no cost at all. According to Rapalus, CCI dogs (golden and Labrador retrievers or a cross of both) are between two and two-and-a-half years old when placed and have learned a list of 40 basic commands. To get on the recipient list a person must have been disabled for at least one year and have a stabilized disability. An application form must specify what task or tasks a dog will be asked to do to improve independence.

Waiting time can be a hang-up. Rudek was on a waiting list for two years before she got Kasten from CCI. "But it was well worth it. I can ambulate but have trouble with my balance," says Rudek. "Kasten has a special harness that helps me balance. She also helps me get up if I fall, and if I can't get up she runs and barks for help, just like in the Lassie and Rin-Tin-Tin movies."

A service dog can even lessen embarrassment. "Once, in a really expensive French restaurant," says Rudek, "I fell and took a table cloth and the contents of the entire table down with me. I was mortified and everybody around me was freaked out. Kasten just looked at me as if to say, 'What are you doing on the floor? Get up, we have places to go.'"

Old Dogs, New Tricks

An alternative to being on a long waiting list is working with a program that will either train and place a dog with you for a fee or support you in training your own dog. Discovery Dogs charges a fee to cover portions of training costs. Many of their clients find creative ways to fund their training costs, including writing Social Security PASS (Plan for Achieving Self-Support) plans, getting vocational re-hab funding, and soliciting donations from local service organizations.

Some people don't want a fully-trained dog because they already have a dog they love. Paul Knott, 47, from Davis, Calif., became a C6-7 quad 16 years ago. Before his accident he owned a 18-month-old Australian shepherd named Bear. Knott had never trained dogs, but he hooked up with a trainer that specialized in search and rescue dogs. Knott worked with Bear and the trainer every day for four months, then asked CCI if they would test Bear. They skeptically agreed, and Bear passed the test on his first try.

Knott credits Bear's pulling ability for enabling him to stay in a manual chair on the University of California campus in Davis. "Plus, Bear was a great way to meet cute girls. He helped me feel more comfortable with my injury."

Although rare, run-ins with people who don't understand the rights of service dogs do happen. "We went to rent an apartment," says Knott, "and the manager looked at Bear and said, 'No pets.' I said, 'This isn't a pet, he's a service dog,' and showed her a copy of the legislation. She said, 'Well, I guess I don't have a choice, do I?' A week later I was out-side brushing Bear and some kids asked if they could play with him and I said OK. Later there was a knock at the door and it was the manager. I thought, 'Here we go again.' It turns out the kids were her grandkids and they had told her what a great time they had playing with the dog. She was bringing a bag of dog treats as a thank you."

Although difficult, it is possible to train your own service dog. Candace Cable, 47, from Truckee, Calif., is a Paralympic athlete and corporate spokesperson. When she and her boyfriend, Michael Byxbe, were put on a five-year waiting list, they decided to get a dog and train it themselves. They chose a yellow lab they named Homey, read up on how to train dogs and went to work.

"Working together as a team, being committed to the training, and being consistent is what made this work," says Cable. Homey is now 5 years old, fully trained in voice and hand signals. He can take the garbage bag out, put it in the trash can, retrieve Cable's chair if it rolls away, pick things up, pull on command, and close the door after he enters the house.

He also makes it easier for Cable to feel secure. "One day after I'd had Homey about a year," she says, "I was at an ATM and realized that for a long time I'd had this sense of vulnerability, but with him at my side I felt safe. I also noticed that when panhandlers see him, they back off."

The right to own a service dog is one of the benefits of having a disability. They can do a lot to mitigate a disability and enhance your life. The public is becoming more aware of service dogs and rights, but just like any other ADA right, owning a service dog comes with responsibility. Well-trained service dogs help their handlers, help educate the public, and advance the power of the ADA. They also make cool companions.

Additional Information

Assistance Dogs International
980 Everett St.
Lakewood, CO 80215-5458
Tel: 303-238-5711
Website: www.assistance-dogs-intl.org.
E-mail: info@adionline.org

Canine Companions for Independence
P.O. Box 446
Santa Rosa, CA 95402
Tel: 707-577-1700

TDD: 707-577-1756
Website: www.caninecompanions.org
E-mail: info@caninecompanions.org

Discovery Dogs
P.O. Box 6050
San Rafael, CA 94903-0050
Tel: 415-479-9557
Fax: 415-472-4431
Website: www.discoverydogs.org.
E-mail: DiscoveryDogs@DiscoveryDogs.org

International Association of Assistance Dog Partners
38691 Filly Drive
Sterling Heights, MI 48310
Tel: 586-826-3938
Website: www.iaadp.org.
E-mail: info@iaadp.org

U.S. Department of Justice
950 Pennsylvania Ave., N.W.
Washington, DC 20530
Toll-Free Information Line: 800-514-0301
TDD: 800-514-0383
Website: www.usdoj.gov/crt/ada/qasrvc.htm
E-mail: askdoj@usdoj.gov

Contact for answers to commonly asked questions about service dogs.

Chapter 52

Assistive Technology: What It Is and How to Find Funding

Choosing Appropriate Technology

People with disabilities can use technology to develop new skills, keep old ones, and live more independently. However, choosing the right technology is often a difficult task. This chapter offers strategies and tips to use when considering a technology solution.

Being informed about purchases is important. Funding sources want to make sure any device they purchase with dwindling resources is fully utilized. So, whether you are using your own precious resources, or third-party payer funds, consumers need to ensure that they spend money wisely.

This chapter includes, "The Right Stuff: Choosing Appropriate Technology," © Illinois Assistive Technology Project. Reprinted with permission from Illinois Assistive Technology Project, 1 W. Old State Capitol Plaza, Suite 100, Springfield, IL, www.iltech.org. Also included are "Funding Tips in General," and "Insurance, Medicare and Medicaid Funding for Assistive Technology." These are reprinted with permission from "Finding the Money," by Candace Bennett, Managing Editor, Infinitec, Inc. Infinitec, a joint project of United Cerebral Palsy Association of Greater Chicago and United Cerebral Palsy Associations, Inc., is a non-profit corporation dedicated to helping individuals with disabilities and their families access life-enhancing technologies. Reprinted with permission of the author and UCP of Greater Chicago, © 1999. For additional information, visit www.infinitec.org.

Basic Principles

These principles are universal—no matter what the technology, where it is used, or the age of the user. Applying these principles will ensure that the device helps you do the job.

A Team Approach Is Always Best

Even when you are choosing a very simple, low-tech piece of equipment, talking it over with another user, or a person who knows you well, will offer another perspective. He/she may also see some pitfalls that weren't obvious to you.

Technology assessment teams usually come from different disciplines and can vary from team to team depending on the user's abilities and needs. Traditionally, the user, a family member or significant other, medical personnel, rehabilitation specialists and occupational, physical, and/or speech therapists are members of the team. Try adding nontraditional team members if you think it will improve the group's problem solving skills. A custodian, shop teacher, local handyperson, or someone good at crafts, or even a classmate will look at the issues differently and often have valuable insights. Don't be afraid to be a courageous problem solver. It will make for a much more elegant solution.

Considerations for Choosing Technology

Personal Considerations

Does it help me do what I want/need to do? If it doesn't, don't get it! This may sound like an elementary question, but many people receive technology and from day one it does not work for them. When this happens, you can be sure the user was not an integral part of the assessment team. More than likely the team told the user what would work for him/her. As a consumer of technology and services, you should never allow that to happen. Speak up for yourself and your needs.

Are there any limitations or risks? Users often see the benefit of AT, but don't bother looking at the other side, and there is nearly always another side. While the technology may help you do what you want to do, it may also limit other aspects of your life.

For example, a user is considering purchasing a standing wheelchair to improve circulation and movement. He/she should also know that standing wheelchairs can weigh up to three times more than a lightweight manual chair. While it may improve movement and circulation, the weight could cause exhaustion. Does that mean a standing wheelchair is not a good product? Not at all, it just means that the user will need to measure the pluses and the minuses. Maybe he/she will want to keep his/her old lightweight chair and use one or the other when it's appropriate.

Is it comfortable to use? Have you ever worn a shirt a half-size too small? If you have, when it was time to wear it again, you probably thought twice about it. If there was at least one other clean shirt in your closet, the small one would just sit there. The same applies to any technology you use. If it is not comfortable, you will eventually discard it. Better to speak up during the assessment process than wait until it's over and the device is in the closet, and you are no closer to your goal than you were before the process began.

May I have a trial period to see if it works for me? Let the buyer beware. Don't get caught in the trap of thinking you have to purchase the device outright before you agree to use it. Ask for a trial period. Most reputable vendors will allow you to rent the device for a month or two and then apply the rental payments toward the purchase. Others have a 30-60 day return policy on the device if it does not work for you.

It's common for users to successfully use a device in an insulated clinical setting (when evaluating or learning about the device) and still be unable to use it in a real world setting. A child may be able to use a communication device in formal speech therapy sessions, but be unable to use it to order lunch at McDonald's. It's not until you try it in the real world that you can be sure the device will work for you!

Training Considerations

Is it ready to use? Imagine this. A user receives his/her technology at home or office. The box is placed in the center of the room and the delivery person leaves. The user did not ask about set up procedures or support. He/she can't open the box. Even if the box were open, he/she would not know how to set the device up. By asking this question ahead of time, a user can eliminate these problems once the device arrives.

What skills do I need to learn? Let's assume a user and his/her team decide a specific computer and software package is just the thing to help a child benefit from his/her educational program. However, he/she has never used a computer alone before. He/she will need many skills before the device really helps. Until that day comes, the team

559

needs to have alternate plans in place. The child needs to become proficient in using the technology. By asking this question, you ask the team to consider technology's appropriateness and any learning curve the user may need to get comfortable with a device.

How does it work? The device you are trying out may seem simple enough to use, but it may have taken the evaluator three days to program it so that you could use it. Ask about set up, what you will need to know about it, what other functions it has, and how can you access those too.

Where do I get training? Will the person who conducts the assessment also provide your training? Do you have a good rapport with him/her? Will the training come from the sales representative? Is there a 24-hour support line available should you need it? How long will that be available to you?

Is training included in the purchase price? Wow, what a shock to learn you're responsible for training, when you assumed the price included it. Unfortunately, some folks don't ask ahead of time. Also, decide who needs training. Certainly the user will need it, but what about others? Teachers, family members, roommates, spouses are just a few examples of others who may need to know the device as well, or better than the user.

Access Considerations

Where can I use the AT? Think about what uses you have for a specific device. If you will use it in multiple settings, how well will it travel? Is there room for it there? Is it noisy? Will it disturb others around you? Will it need to be reprogrammed to use it in different settings? Who will do that? Will that limit the use?

Is it bulky? A device that works well in a stationary setting, may be just fine, unless you need to lug it to the library twice a week. Imagine all the settings you will be using the device in and consider how portable it needs to be.

Can I use it indoors or out? How does moisture affect functioning? Climate changes can affect how a device works. If you will be operating the device at the bus stand and it starts to rain, or you drool, you may need to be concerned about this issue. Ask!

What is the battery life? Battery life is a huge issue when considering technology. If you don't stop to ask this question prior to the purchase, you may have a non-functioning device when you need it. If the device requires recharging after every three hours of use, and you will use it twice that amount of time, obviously you'll need extra batteries. But if you don't ask, you won't know. Batteries eventually wear out. Find out how soon you will need new ones.

If powered, can you plug it in, or is there a power source where you want to use it? You can often conserve battery life by plugging in. So, think about the places you can hook your technology to an electric outlet. For example, consider sitting next to the wall outlet when you take a laptop to class. You will have more battery life for times when no outlet is convenient.

Repair and Maintenance

Is it reliable? The best place to get this information is to ask other users. They have experience with the device, its quirkiness, features, and reliability. To find other users, contact a local independent living center, or other disability related social service agency. Ask them to help you find someone who has used the device. Remember that the vendors and manufacturers are there to sell products, not necessarily to be candid about product reliability.

What is the life expectancy? Nothing lasts forever and at some point your technology will reach the end of its natural life. Knowing the life expectancy of a device will help you decide if it's time to repair or replace the device. Funding sources should also be aware that eventually, replacing the device is far more cost effective or efficient than repairing it.

What is average use? All technology has a lifespan. Not all devices can be used constantly. Find out what the manufacturer considers an average amount of use for the device. For example, you plan to purchase a device and anticipate using it every 25 seconds. However, average use is once every 10 minutes. The device is going to wear out much quicker than usual. Again, if you don't ask, you don't know.

What does the guarantee/warranty cover? Some manufacturers provide a bumper-to-bumper warranty, others provide a sort of cash and carry/as is coverage for their device. Finding out what the guarantee/warranty covers after the purchase, is too late. Remember to ask.

What is the service record of the manufacturer/vendor? Again, to be a good self-advocate, you must check the sales/service record of the manufacturer and vendor of the device. You could find a device that works very well for you, but unfortunately, other users have had nothing but problems with the vendor's reliability with follow-up and regular maintenance. Unless you ask other people who have worked with them, you don't know.

Is repair service convenient? Find out where the device will need to go for maintenance and repair. If you need to send it to outer Mongolia, it's going to take a long time to get there and get back. Perhaps another device can do the same job and repairs will be closer. Also, find out if the vendor has loaner equipment available while your device is in the shop.

What is considered regular maintenance? You may be able to perform some of the maintenance yourself. Other maintenance may need specialized training. Find out what kind of maintenance your device needs and to prolong the life of the device, follow the directions carefully.

Financial

What is the total final cost? Some devices come all in one piece, others come with add-ons that will up the cost of the device. Be sure to get the total cost of the item with all the add-ons you need. Are there package deals? Will you need a specifically designed mounting system? Will you need two battery packs instead of one? It's frustrating to finally get the device and then find out that you need another item to make it work for you.

Are there training costs? Is training included in purchase price? If you don't ask these questions prior to purchase, you may find training costs will make the device unattainable. Purchasing it and being unable to use it because you lack training is a discouraging experience.

Who will fund maintenance and repairs? Imagine how you will feel if your device needs repair, and you find out that you are responsible for the cost of repairs and you didn't know it. Ask before the purchase!

Are rental/lease plans more cost effective? If you are going to use the device on a short-term basis, you may want to consider renting or leasing options. It's also a good idea to try out the device before you invest much money in it. Most reputable dealers have rental/lease options that either will let you apply the money toward the purchase price, or offer a 30-60 day return policy. You'll need to ask so you know the specific details of the trial period. If you are working with a vendor that does not allow that type of option, look elsewhere. They may not be there after the purchase if they are so uncompromising prior to it. Will I need to change devices or upgrade soon? If you are gaining and/or losing skills because of the type of disability you have, consider how much time you will be using the device. Measure these factors into the equation about whether the device will work, really work for you.

562

Will I get a trade-in/upgrade allowance? With the rapidly changing world of technology, things you purchase may be obsolete in a year. As long as the device still works for you, that's fine. However, you need to realize that it will have very little market value if you need another device or decide to upgrade.

Parting Words

Consumers with disabilities need to become advocates for their own needs. Relying on professionals alone to figure out what you need means you will not get the best device for you. You need to use professionals to help figure out the kinds of devices that will help you perform certain tasks; however, you alone will ultimately decide if a device works for you. If you are not comfortable with a device for any reason, speak up! It will be better in the end if you express your opinions prior to the purchase. Complaining to a funding agent that a device doesn't meet your needs months after the fact, is upsetting and disheartening for the funder and you.

Finally, it's important to realize that often the best technology solution is a simple-tech solution. Consider how environmental adaptations can meet your needs prior to purchasing any device. Environmental changes are long lasting and usually don't require ongoing repair and maintenance. However, environmental changes aren't the answer for all the barriers people with disabilities face. After deciding that an environmental change won't work, technology may be the most practical option however, always keep in mind that the technology solution should be appropriate for the task and meet your need as well as your own sense of who you are.

Finding the Money

Funding Tips in General

The number one tip is to know your rights under the law. Research, read, attend workshops, talk to knowledgeable people. Laws passed by the national and state legislatures, court decisions, and agency regulations all have an impact on assistive tech funding.

Learn about the best strategies for approaching funding sources. Recognize that you must become your own best advocate or the best advocate for your child, patient, employee, friend, etc., and that knowledge is power. The deeper your personal involvement, the better chance you have of finding funding.

Know your technology needs—specifically, exactly. You will need the help of a professional or cross-disciplinary team of professionals who can assess need, suggest an appropriate device, and clearly describe in writing how that device meets a specific need. You are looking for an occupational therapist, physical therapist, speech pathologist, or rehabilitation engineer (or all of the above) who is qualified by his or her training in and experience with assistive technology. You can find these experts by asking other people in situations similar to yours, asking at school, asking your doctor or hospital, contacting a professional society, asking at parent support groups. Local, state, and national non-profit disability organizations also may provide referrals.

During the process of assessing and prescribing, ask all the questions you can think of and offer plenty of input. A trial of a recommended device is essential. If you can, borrow the device for a real life trial at home, school, or work. (There are technology resource centers which loan equipment and some equipment suppliers or manufacturers also make *try before you buy* equipment loans.) You must become an expert on what a device does and what difference it can make in your life, or in the life of the person with a disability with whom you are involved.

If it seems one piece of equipment works better for you than another, document the superiority of the device you prefer. Take notes, take photos, make a video. You also should document functioning with and without the recommended device, to show how it makes a difference. You may need this evidence when seeking funding.

Sources of funding for assistive technology may be public or private. Public sources include all agencies which are funded and operated by national, state, or local governments. Private sources include private insurance companies and special no- or low-interest loan programs from private lenders arranged for you by a government agency or by a technology manufacturer.

In addition to the most common sources of funding for assistive technology, other options might include the U.S. Veterans Administration which serves armed forces veterans; the Social Security Administration's PASS (Plan To Achieve Self-Support) program for people receiving SSI or SSDI; your state's Workers Compensation program, if the disability was caused by a work-related injury; non-profit disability organizations; and civic or service organizations serving your community (Lions Club, VFW, Rotary Club, etc.). Some families have had success in working with local service groups, churches, labor unions, or school organizations to stage fund-raisers in their communities.

It's possible to fund the purchase of an assistive device by relying on more than one source. In fact, sometimes this is the best or only way.

The way in which you plan to use a device will dictate your funding options. If a device is necessary to a student's highest functioning in the least-restrictive school setting, then the school should write the need for the device into the student's IEP (individualized education plan) or IFSP (individualized family service plan for families with children in an early intervention program) and fund the device. If the device is necessary for work, your state's department, office, or division of vocational rehabilitation should help. If the device is medically necessary (essential to attaining or maintaining health or to replace lost or non-functioning body parts), private insurance, Medicare, or Medicaid comes into play. If a device is necessary to enable a person to live outside an institution, a different government program may be the source of funding. There are many areas of overlap between these funding sources, and arguments can be made (and often should be made) in any direction. But you'll have better luck if, for example, you ask a school, rather than your insurer, to fund an education-related device.

Each source of funding has its own definitions, requirements, and eligibility rules. Learn the rules and follow them. Funding can be denied simply because an applicant forgot to sign a form. If you find a funding source's rules confusing, seek help from an experienced advocate or insist on a fuller explanation from the source.

Supplement funding application forms with additional information, such as a brochure about the requested device, a video you've made, photos, etc. Turn in everything at the same time. It may be a good idea to turn in your application package in person, and have an agency or insurance company employee (get the person's name) check your submission to make sure you've covered everything.

Call regularly to check on the process of your application for funding. Keep a journal of all contacts with the funding agency. Write down the date, the name of the person with whom you spoke, and what was discussed. Keep copies of all correspondence. If an appeal process becomes necessary, your records will be important. Be patient, but make it clear you are very involved and serious about your application.

Be persistent. If a funding request is denied, ask the agency or insurance company for the reason for denial in writing. If the denial was based on a mistake, misunderstanding, or lack of information, clear that up and resubmit your application. If you still are denied, determine what you must do to appeal the denial, and stick with the process. If needed, work with an advocate. If you are dealing with a government agency, you may contact your legislators (state or federal) and ask them to contact the funding agency on your behalf.

Find an outside advocate, especially if you are new to the funding game. Many assistive technology manufacturers employ funding co-ordinators who can be quite helpful. Disability groups, advocacy groups, parent support groups, other people with disabilities or their family members, teachers, and therapists can help you determine your best course of action and, if necessary, help you find someone to speak on your behalf to funding sources. If you feel a funding source is not giving you a fair hearing and that your rights are being violated, obtain legal counsel.

If you cannot afford an attorney, contact your local Legal Aid Society. In the best of all possible worlds, the process of finding funding for assistive technology would not become adversarial, but in reality, sometimes it does. Do not be intimidated. Get someone on your side who knows the law relating to assistive technology funding.

Insurance, Medicare, and Medicaid Funding for Assistive Technology

The health care system is a major source of technology for people with disabilities. In the main, private insurance, Medicare, and Medicaid cover medical equipment. An often used term is durable medical equipment, meaning items that are intended for long-term use, such as a wheelchair. However, these funding sources can provide a range of devices that can be defined as assistive technology. There is a great deal of flexibility as well as confusion in this area; most insurance policies are silent about technological devices and neither the Medicare nor Medicaid rules address assistive technology. Also, the trend towards managed care and other medical cost-cutting moves can cloud the picture.

Private Insurance

Insurance companies still are largely unregulated when it comes to assistive technology. Insurance plans and policies usually don't even refer to funding assistive technology devices and services, but they fund specific equipment such as wheelchairs or scooters, other medical equipment, and even things like air conditioners, when they are medically necessary. For instance, a person with acute asthma may require an air conditioner at home. Private insurance companies require documentation and/or prescriptions so be sure to provide them.

Private insurance companies also challenge or deny claims because the equipment costs more than what is termed standard and customary. When this happens, call around to medical equipment dealers in your area that sell the same piece of equipment and get three quotes; you will most likely find that standard and customary costs considerably more than what an insurance company says it should cost, granting the policy-holder a much higher reimbursement! It could mean the difference of $600 or more reimbursement if you are persistent and do your homework! (A woman who bought a used wheelchair for $1000.00 was told by her insurance provider that used wheelchairs normally cost about $150.00 in her area. So she called around and got quotes of up to $1400.00, so she re-submitted her claim and was reimbursed $850.00. This is a very typical scenario.)

Medicare

Medicare is a federal health care funding program available to people older than age 65 and those younger than 65 who have been entitled to receive Social Security disability benefits for 24 months. The scope of Medicare's coverage for assistive technology devices is very limited.

Medicaid

Medicaid is a joint federal/state program that provides health care services to people with low incomes. To be funded by Medicaid, assistive devices must specifically address medical problems and be prescribed by a physician, so he or she is the starting point for accessing assistive technology through Medicaid.

The physician must provide a medical diagnosis, define the technology as medically necessary treatment and as the least costly of treatment alternatives. This can include prosthetics, orthotics, and certain speech-language and rehabilitation services.

Complicating Medicaid is the fact that the states differ widely in the range of Medicaid services they provide. The law requires states to cover a set of mandatory services, but also lists optional services which states may or may not provide through Medicaid. States also define services differently and put different cost or duration limits on services which sometimes seem arbitrary (with no or little relation to diagnosis). Still, many people have secured assistive technology through Medicaid, most commonly, augmentative communication devices.

567

Persistence in dealing with health care providers is important. Insurance companies, Medicare, and Medicaid all have appeals processes. Never accept an initial denial as the final word.

Additional Information

Please refer to "Assistive Technology Funding Resources," in Chapter 54 for further information.

Part Eight

Additional Help and Information

Chapter 53

Glossary of Terms Related to Movement Disorders

Akinesia. Decreased body movements.[3]

Apgar score. A numbered score doctors use to assess a baby's physical state at the time of birth.[2]

Apraxia. Impaired ability to carry out purposeful movements in an individual who does not have significant motor problems.[2]

Asphyxia. Lack of oxygen due to trouble with breathing or poor oxygen supply in the air.[2]

Autosomal dominant disorder. A non-sex-linked disorder that can be inherited even if only one parent passes on the defective gene.[3]

Basal ganglia. A region located at the base of the brain composed of four clusters of neurons, or nerve cells. This area is responsible for body movement and coordination. The neuron groups most prominently and consistently affected by HD [Hungington's Disease]—the pallidum and striatum—are located here. See neuron, pallidum, striatum.[3]

Definitions in this chapter were compiled from several sources. Terms marked "1" are from *Stedman's Medical Dictionary, 27th Edition*. Copyright © 2000 Lippincott Williams & Wilkins. All rights reserved. Reprinted with permission. Terms marked "2" are from "Cerebral Palsy: Hope Through Research," National Institute of Neurological Disorders and Stroke (NINDS), updated June 2000. Terms marked "3" are from "Huntington's Disease—Hope Through Research," National Institute of Neurological Disorders and Stroke (NINDS), reviewed July 1, 2001.

Caudate nuclei. Part of the striatum in the basal ganglia. See basal ganglia, striatum.[3]

Cerebral. Relating to the two hemispheres of the human brain.[2]

Chorea. Irregular, spasmodic, involuntary movements of the limbs or facial muscles, often accompanied by hypotonia. The location of the responsible cerebral lesion is not known.[1]

Chromosomes. The structures in cells that contain genes. They are composed of deoxyribonucleic acid (DNA) and proteins and, under a microscope, appear as rod-like structures. See deoxyribonucleic acid (DNA), gene.[3]

Computed tomography (CT). A technique used for diagnosing brain disorders. CT uses a computer to produce a high-quality image of brain structures. These images are called CT scans. [3]

Congenital. Present at birth.[2]

Contracture. A condition in which muscles become fixed in a rigid, abnormal position causing distortion or deformity.[2]

Cortex. Part of the brain responsible for thought, perception, and memory. Huntington's disease affects the basal ganglia and cortex. See basal ganglia.[3]

Creatine kinase (CK). An enzyme catalyzing the reversible transfer of phosphate from phosphocreatine to ADP, forming creatine and ATP; of importance in muscle contraction. Certain isozymes are elevated in plasma following myocardial infarctions. Syn: creatine phosphokinase.[1]

Deoxyribonucleic acid (DNA). The substance of heredity containing the genetic information necessary for cells to divide and produce proteins. DNA carries the code for every inherited characteristic of an organism. See gene.[3]

Disability. 1. According to the "International Classification of Impairments, Disabilities and Handicaps" (World Health Organization), any restriction or lack of ability to perform an activity in a manner or within the range considered normal for a human being. The term disability reflects the consequences of impairment in terms of functional performance and activity by the individual; disabilities thus represent disturbances at the level of the person. 2. An impairment or defect of one or more organs or members.[1]

Dominant. A trait that is apparent even when the gene for that disorder is inherited from only one parent. See autosomal dominant disorder, recessive, gene.[3]

Dopamine (DM). An intermediate in tyrosine metabolism and precursor of norepinephrine and epinephrine; it accounts for 90% of the catecholamines; its presence in the central nervous system and localization in the basal ganglia (caudate and lentiform nuclei) suggest that dopamine may have other functions. Depletion of dopamine produces Parkinson disease. Syn: decarboxylated dopa, 3-hydroxytyramine.[1]

Dysarthria. Problems with speaking caused by difficulty moving or coordinating the muscles needed for speech.[2]

Dystonia. A state of abnormal (either hypo- or hyper-) tonicity in any of the tissues resulting in impairment of voluntary movement.[1]

Electroencephalogram (EEG). A technique for recording the pattern of electrical currents inside the brain.[2]

Electromyography. A special recording technique that detects muscle activity.[2]

Essential tremor. An action tremor of 4-8 Hz frequency that usually begins in early adult life and is limited to the upper limbs and head; called familial when it appears in several family members.[1]

Failure to thrive. A condition characterized by lag in physical growth and development.[2]

Gait analysis. A technique that uses camera recording, force plates, electromyography, and computer analysis to objectively measure an individual's pattern of walking.[2]

Gamma knife. A minimally invasive radiosurgical system used in the treatment of benign and malignant intracranial neoplasms and arteriovenous malformations.[1]

As a preliminary to use of the gamma knife, the lesion to be ablated is precisely located by imaging techniques such as MRI, CT, PET, and angiography. Beams of gamma rays from 200 cobalt-60 sources are then directed by a computer so that they converge on the lesion. A series of exposures are made during a period of about 1 hour. Lesions larger than about 3 cm cannot be treated. The mechanism is bulky and costly, but the procedure has shown a success rate of about

85% in the treatment of arteriovenous malformations and 50-95% for neoplasms. Besides avoiding the risks and complications of open surgery, the gamma knife permits treatment of lesions whose location prohibits any attempt at surgical removal. In addition, patient discomfort is minimal and most patients remain in the hospital for only 1 night; many return home, or even to work, on the day of treatment. The gamma knife is expected to prove useful in the treatment of other disorders, such as tumors of the eye and the pituitary gland, trigeminal neuralgia, epilepsy, parkinsonism, and other movement disorders.[1]

Gastrostomy. A surgical procedure to create an artificial opening in the stomach.[2]

Gene. The basic unit of heredity, composed of a segment of DNA containing the code for a specific trait. See deoxyribonucleic acid (DNA).[3]

Hemianopia. Defective vision or blindness that impairs half of the normal field of vision.[2]

Hemiparetic tremors. Uncontrollable shaking affecting the limbs on the spastic side of the body in those who have spastic hemiplegia.[2]

Huntingtin. The protein encoded by the gene that carries the Huntington's disease defect. The repeated CAG sequence in the gene causes an abnormal form of huntingtin to be formed. The function of the normal form of huntingtin is not yet known.[3]

Hypertonia. Increased tone.[2]

Hypotonia. Decreased tone.[2]

Hypoxic-ischemic encephalopathy. Brain damage caused by poor blood flow or insufficient oxygen supply to the brain.[2]

Jaundice. A blood disorder caused by the abnormal buildup of bile pigments in the bloodstream.[2]

Kindred. A group of related persons, such as a family or clan.[3]

Lumbar puncture. A puncture into the subarachnoid space of the lumbar region to obtain spinal fluid for diagnostic or therapeutic purposes. Syn: Quincke puncture, spinal puncture, rachicentesis, rachiocentesis, spinal tap.[1]

Magnetic resonance imaging (MRI). An imaging technique that uses radiowaves, magnetic fields, and computer analysis to create a picture of body tissues and structures.[2]

Marker. A piece of DNA that lies on the chromosome so close to a gene that the two are inherited together. Like a signpost, markers are used during genetic testing and research to locate the nearby presence of a gene. See chromosome, deoxyribonucleic acid (DNA).[3]

Mitochondria. Microscopic, energy-producing bodies within cells that are the cells' power plants.[3]

Movement. The act of motion; said of the entire body or of one or more of its members or parts.[1]

Muscle. A primary tissue, consisting predominantly of highly specialized contractile cells, which may be classified as skeletal muscle, cardiac muscle, or smooth muscle; microscopically, the latter is lacking in transverse striations characteristic of the other two types; one of the contractile organs of the body by which movements of the various organs and parts are effected; typical musculus is a mass of musculus fibers (venter or belly), attached at each extremity, by means of a tendon, to a bone or other structure; the more proximal or more fixed attachment is called the origin, the more distal or more movable attachment is the insertion; the narrowing part of the belly that is attached to the tendon of origin is called the caput or head. Syn: musculus [TA].[1]

Mutation. In genetics, any defect in a gene. See gene.[3]

Myoclonus. One or a series of shock-like contractions of a group of muscles, of variable regularity, synchrony, and symmetry, generally due to a central nervous system lesion.[1]

Neonatal hemorrhage. Bleeding of brain blood vessels in the newborn.[2]

Neurologist. A specialist in the diagnosis and treatment of disorders of the neuromuscular system: the central, peripheral, and autonomic nervous systems, the neuromuscular junction, and muscle.[1]

Neuron. Greek word for a nerve cell, the basic impulse-conducting unit of the nervous system. Nerve cells communicate with other cells through an electrochemical process called neurotransmission.[3]

Neurotransmitters. Special chemicals that transmit nerve impulses from one cell to another.[3]

Occupational therapy (OT). Therapeutic use of self-care, work, and recreational activities to increase independent function, enhance development, and prevent disability; may include adaptation of tasks or environment to achieve maximum independence and optimum quality of life.[1]

Orthotic devices. Special devices, such as splints or braces, used to treat problems of the muscles, ligaments, or bones of the skeletal system.[2]

Pallidotomy. A destructive operation on the globus pallidus, done to relieve involuntary movements or muscular rigidity.[1]

Pallidum. Part of the basal ganglia of the brain. The pallidum is composed of the globus pallidus and the ventral pallidum. See basal ganglia.[3]

Palsy. Paralysis, or problems in the control of voluntary movement.[2]

Paresis or plegia. Weakness or paralysis. In cerebral palsy, these terms are typically combined with another phrase that describes the distribution of paralysis and weakness, e.g., paraparesis.[2]

Parkinsonism. 1. A neurologic syndrome usually resulting from deficiency of the neurotransmitter dopamine as the consequence of degenerative, vascular, or inflammatory changes in the basal ganglia; characterized by rhythmic muscular tremors, rigidity of movement, festination, droopy posture, and mask-like faces. Syn: Parkinson disease, shaking palsy. 2. A syndrome similar to parkinsonism appearing as a side effect of certain antipsychotic drugs.[1]

Physical therapy (PT). 1. Treatment of pain, disease, or injury by physical means; Syn: physiotherapy. 2. The profession concerned with promotion of health, with prevention of physical disabilities, with evaluation and rehabilitation of persons disabled by pain, disease, or injury, and with treatment by physical therapeutic measures as opposed to medical, surgical, or radiologic measures.[1]

Plasmapheresis. Removal of whole blood from the body, separation of its cellular elements by centrifugation, and reinfusion of them suspended in saline or some other plasma substitute, thus depleting the body's own plasma without depleting its cells.[1]

Positron emission tomography (PET). A tool used to diagnose brain functions and disorders. PET produces three-dimensional, colored images of chemicals or substances functioning within the body.

These images are called PET scans. PET shows brain function, in contrast to CT or MRI, which show brain structure.[3]

Prevalence. The number of cases of a disease that are present in a particular population at a given time.[3]

Putamen. An area of the brain that decreases in size as a result of the damage produced by HD.[3]

Receptor. Proteins that serve as recognition sites on cells and cause a response in the body when stimulated by chemicals called neurotransmitters. They act as on-and-off switches for the next nerve cell. See neuron, neurotransmitters.[3]

Recessive. A trait that is apparent only when the gene or genes for it are inherited from both parents. See dominant, gene.[3]

Reflexes. Movements that the body makes automatically in response to a specific cue.[2]

Rh incompatibility. A blood condition in which antibodies in a pregnant woman's blood can attack fetal blood cells, impairing the fetus's supply of oxygen and nutrients.[2]

Rubella. Also known as German measles, rubella is a viral infection that can damage the nervous system in the developing fetus.[2]

Selective dorsal root rhizotomy. A surgical procedure in which selected nerves are severed to reduce spasticity in the legs.[2]

Senile chorea. A relatively mild and rare disorder found in elderly adults and characterized by choreic movements. It is believed by some scientists to be caused by a different gene mutation than that causing HD.[3]

Spastic diplegia. A form of cerebral palsy in which both arms and both legs are affected, the legs being more severely affected.[2]

Spastic hemiplegia (or hemiparesis). A form of cerebral palsy in which spasticity affects the arm and leg on one side of the body.[2]

Spastic paraplegia (or paraparesis). A form of cerebral palsy in which spasticity affects both legs but the arms are relatively or completely spared.[2]

Spastic quadriplegia (or quadriparesis). A form of cerebral palsy in which all four limbs are affected equally.[2]

Spasticity. One type of increase in muscle tone at rest; characterized by increased resistance to passive stretch, velocity dependent, and asymmetric about joints (i.e., greater in the flexor muscles at the elbow and the extensor muscles at the knee). Exaggerated deep tendon reflexes and clonus are additional manifestations.[1]

Stereognosia. Difficulty perceiving and identifying objects using the sense of touch.[2]

Strabismus. Misalignment of the eyes.[2]

Striatum. Art of the basal ganglia of the brain. The striatum is composed of the caudate nucleus, putamen, and ventral striatum. See basal ganglia, caudate nuclei.[3]

Thalamotomy. Destruction of a selected portion of the thalamus by stereotaxy for the relief of pain, involuntary movements, epilepsy, and, rarely, emotional disturbances; produces few, if any, neurologic deficits or undesirable personality changes.[1]

Trait. Any genetically determined characteristic. See dominant, gene, recessive.[3]

Transgenic mice. Mice that receive injections of foreign genes during the embryonic stage of development. Their cells then follow the instructions of the foreign genes, resulting in the development of a certain trait or characteristic. Transgenic mice can serve as an animal model of a certain disease, telling researchers how genes work in specific cells.[3]

Tremor. 1. Repetitive, often regular, oscillatory movements caused by alternate, or synchronous, but irregular contraction of opposing muscle groups; usually involuntary. 2. Minute ocular movement occurring during fixation on an object.[1]

Ultrasonography. A technique that bounces sound waves off of tissues and structures and uses the pattern of echoes to form an image, called a sonogram.[2]

Ventricles. Cavities within the brain that are filled with cerebrospinal fluid. In Huntington's disease, tissue loss causes enlargement of the ventricles.[3]

Chapter 54

Directory of Movement Disorder Organizations

Government Agencies and Organizations

Brain Resources and Information Network (BRAIN)

P.O. Box 5801
Bethesda, MD 20824
Toll-Free: 800-352-9424
TTY: 301-468-5981
Website: www.ninds.nih.gov

National Heart, Lung, and Blood Institute

National Center on Sleep
Disorders Research
Two Rockledge Center
Suite 10038
6701 Rockledge Drive, MSC 7920
Bethesda, MD 20892-7920
Tel: 301-435-0199
Fax: 301-480-3451
Website: www.nhlbi.nih.gov/
about/ncsdr
E-mail: ncsdr@prospectassoc.com

This chapter includes excerpts from "Parkinson's Disease—Hope Through Research," National Institute of Neurological Disorders and Stroke (NINDS), reviewed July 1, 2002; and from ABLEDATA at www.abledata.com, sponsored by the National Institute on Disability and Rehabilitation Research (NIDRR). All contact information was verified and updated in August 2002.

National Institute of Arthritis and Musculoskeletal and Skin Diseases (NIAMS)
National Institutes of Health
1 AMS Circle
Bethesda, MD 20892-2350
Toll-Free: 877-22-NIAMS (226-4267)
Tel: 301-496-8188
Fax: 301-718-6366
Website: www.nih.gov/niams
E-mail: NIAMSInfo@mail.nih.gov

National Information Center for Children and Youth with Disabilities
P.O. Box 1492
Washington, DC 20013-1492
Toll-Free: 800-695-0285
Tel: 202-884-8200
Fax: 202-884-8441
Website: www.nichcy.org
E-mail: nichcy@aed.org

National Institute of Child Health and Human Development
Building 31, Room 2A32
Bethesda, MD 20892-2425
Toll-Free: 800-370-2943
Tel: 301-496-5133
Website: www.nichd.nih.gov
E-mail: nichdclearinghouse@mail.nih.gov

National Organization for Rare Disorders (NORD)
55 Kenosia Avenue
P.O. Box 1968
Danbury, CT 06813-1968
Tel: 203-744-0100
Voice Mail: 800-999-NORD (6673)
Fax: 203-798-2291
Website: www.rarediseases.org
E-mail: orphan@rarediseases.org

National Rehabilitation Information Center (NARIC)
4200 Forbes Boulevard
Suite 202
Lanham, MD 20706
Toll-Free: 800-346-2742
Tel: 301-459-5900
Fax: 301-562-2401
Website: www.naric.com
E-mail: naricinfo@heitech services.com

U.S. Department of Justice
950 Pennsylvania Ave., N.W.
Washington, DC 20530
Toll-Free Information Line: 800-514-0301
TDD: 800-514-0383
Website: www.usdoj.gov/crt/ada/qasrvc.htm
E-mail: askdoj@usdoj.gov

Organizations Focused on Specific Movement Disorders and Concerns

Alliance of Genetic Support Groups
4301 Connecticut Ave., N.W.
Suite 404
Washington, DC 20008-2304
Toll-Free: 800-336-GENE (4363)
Tel: 202-966-5557
Fax: 202-966-8553
Website: www.geneticalliance.org
E-mail: info@geneticalliance.org

ALS Association of America (ALSA)
27001 Agoura Road, Suite 150
Calabasas Hills, CA 91301-5104
Toll-Free: 800-782-4747
Tel: 818-880-9007
Website: www.alsa.org

American Speech Language Hearing Association (ASHA)
10801 Rockville Pike
Rockville, MD 20852-3279
Toll-Free: 800-638-8255
Tel: 301-897-5700
Fax: 301-571-0457
Website: www.asha.org
E-mail: actioncenter@asha.org

Ataxia Telangiectasia Children's Project
688 S. Military Trail
Deerfield Beach, FL 33442
Toll-Free: 800-543-5728
Website: www.atcp.org
E-mail: info@atcp.org

Center for Neurologic Study
9850 Genesee Avenue, Suite 320
LaJolla, CA 92037
Tel: 858-455-5463
Fax: 858-455-1713
Website: www.cnsonline.org
E-mail: cns@cts.com

Benign Essential Blepharospasm Research Foundation, Inc.
637 North 7th Street, Suite 102
P.O. Box 12468
Beaumont, TX 77726-2468
Tel: 409-832-0788
Fax: 409-832-0890
Website: www.blepharospasm.org
E-mail: bebrf@ih2000.net

Disabled Sports USA
451 Hungerford Drive, Suite 100
Rockville, MD 20850
Tel: 301-217-0960 or 301-217-9736
Fax: 301-217-0968
Website: www.dsusa.org
E-mail: dsusa@dsusa.org

Dystonia Medical Research Foundation
1 East Wacker Drive, Suite 2430
Chicago, IL 60601-1905
Toll-Free in Canada: 800-361-8061
Tel: 312-755-0198
Fax: 312-803-0138
Website: www.dystonia-foundation.org
E-mail: dystonia@dystonia-foundation.org

Epilepsy Foundation
4351 Garden City Drive
Suite 500
Landover, MD 20785-2267
Toll-Free: 800-EFA-1000 (332-1000)
Tel: 301-459-3700
Fax: 301-577-2684
Website:
www.epilepsyfoundation.org
E-mail: postmaster@efa.org

Facioscapulohumeral Dystrophy (FSHD) Society
3 Westwood Road
Lexington, MA 02420
Tel: 781-860-0501
Fax: 781-860-0599
Website: www.fshsociety.org
E-mail: info@fshsociety.org

Families of S.M.A. (Spinal Muscular Atrophy)
National Headquarters
P.O. Box 196
Libertyville, IL 60048-0196
Toll-Free: 800-886-1762
Tel: 847-367-7620
Fax: 847-367-7623
E-mail: info@fsma.org

Family Caregiver Alliance
690 Market Street
Suite 600
San Francisco, CA 94104
Tel: 415-434-3388
Fax: 415-434-3508
Website: www.caregiver.org
E-mail: info@caregiver.org

Forbes Norris ALS Research Center
California Pacific Medical Center
2324 Sacramento Street
San Francisco, CA 94115
Tel: 415-923-3604
Fax: 415-673-5184
Website: www.cpmc.org/services/als

Friedreich's Ataxia Research Alliance (FARA)
2001 Jefferson Davis Hwy.
Suite 209
Arlington, VA 22202
Tel: 703-413-4468
Fax: 703-413-4467
Website: www.frda.org
E-mail: fara@frda.org

Genetic Alliance
4301 Connecticut Avenue, N.W
Suite 404
Washington, DC 20008-2304
Toll-Free: 800-336-GENE (4363)
Tel: 202-966-5557
Fax: 202-966-8553
Website: www.geneticalliance.org
E-mail: info@geneticalliance.org

Hereditary Disease Foundation
11400 W. Olympic Blvd.
Suite 855
Los Angeles, CA 90064-1560
Tel: 310-575-9656
Fax: 310-575-9156
Website: www.hdfoundation.org
E-mail: cures@hdfoundation.org

Huntington's Disease Society of America (HDSA)
158 West 29th Street
7th Floor
New York, NY 10001-5300
Toll-Free: 800-345-HDSA (345-4372)
Tel: 212-242-1968
Fax: 212-239-3430
Website: www.hdsa.org
E-mail: hdsainfo@hdsa.org

International Joseph Disease Foundation, Inc.
P.O. Box 2550
Livermore, CA 94531-2550
Tel: 925-371-1288
Website: www.ijdf.net

International Polio Network/Gazette International
4207 Lindell Blvd., #110
St. Louis, MO 63108-2915
Tel: 314-534-0475
Fax: 314-534-5070
Website: www.post-polio.org
E-mail: gini_intl@msn.com

International Rett Syndrome Association
9121 Piscataway Rd.
Suite 2B
Clinton, MD 20735
Toll-Free: 800-818-7388
Tel: 301-856-3334
Fax: 301-856-3336
Website: www.rettsyndrome.org
E-mail: irsa@rettsyndrome.org

International Tremor Foundation
7046 West 105th Street
Overland Park, KS 66212-1803
Toll-Free: 888-387-3667
Tel: 913-341-3880
Fax: 913-341-1296
Website: www.essentialtremor.org
E-mail: staff@essentialtremor.org

Les Turner ALS Foundation
8142 North Lawndale Avenue
Skokie, IL 60076-3322
Toll-Free: 888-ALS-1107
Tel: 847-679-3311
Fax: 847-679-9109
Website: www.lesturnerals.org
E-mail: info@lesturnerals.org

Lipomyelomeningocele Family Support Net.
9217 Sayornis Court
Raleigh, NC 27615
Tel: 919-844-2043
Fax: 919-844-2044
Website: www.lfsn.org
E-mail: bborchert@mindspring.com

March of Dimes Birth Defects Foundation
1275 Mamaroneck Avenue
White Plains, NY 10605
Toll-Free: 888-MODIMES (663-4637)
Tel: 914-428-7100
Fax: 914-428-8203
Website: www.modimes.org
E-mail: resourcecenter@modimes.org

Moving Forward
2934 Glenmore Avenue
Kettering, OH 45409
Tel: 937-293-0409

Muscular Dystrophy Association
3300 East Sunrise Drive
Tucson, AZ 85718-3208
Toll-Free: 800-572-1717
Tel: 520-529-2000
Fax: 520-529-5300
Website: www.mdausa.org
E-mail: mda@mdausa.org

Muscular Dystrophy Family Foundation
2330 North Meridian Street
Indianapolis, IN 46208-5730
Toll-Free: 800-544-1213
Tel: 317-923-6333
Fax: 317-923-6334
Website: www.mdff.org
E-mail: mdff@mdff.org

Myoclonus Research Foundation, Inc.
200 Old Palisade Rd.
Fort Lee, NJ 07024
Tel: 201-585-0770
Website: www.myoclonus.com
E-mail: research@myoclonus.com

National Aphasia Association
29 John St., Suite 1103
New York, NY 10038
Toll-Free: 800-922-4NAA (4622)
Tel: 212-255-4329
Website: www.aphasia.org
E-mail: naa@aphasia.org

National Ataxia Foundation (NAF)
2600 Fernbrook Lane
Suite 119
Minneapolis, MN 55447-4752
Tel: 763-553-0020
Fax: 763-553-0167
Website: www.ataxia.org
E-mail: naf@ataxia.org

National Dysautonomia Research Foundation
421 West 4th Street
Red Wing, MN 55066-2555
Tel: 651-267-0525
Fax: 651-267-0524
Website: www.ndrf.org
E-mail: ndrf@ndrf.org

Easter Seals
230 West Monroe Street
Suite 1800
Chicago, IL 60606-4802
Toll-Free: 800-221-6827
Tel: 312-726-6200
Fax: 312-726-1494
TTY: 312-726-4258
Website: www.easter-seals.org
E-mail: info@easterseals.org

National Family Caregivers Association
10400 Connecticut Avenue
Suite 500
Kensington, MD 20895-3944
Toll-Free: 800-896-3650
Tel: 301-942-6430
Fax: 301-942-2302
Website: www.nfcacares.org
E-mail: info@nfccares.org

National Foundation for Jewish Genetic Diseases

250 Park Avenue
c/o Suite 1000
New York, NY 10177
Tel: 212-371-1030
Website: www.nfjgd.org

National Multiple Sclerosis Society

733 Third Avenue
6th Floor
New York, NY 10017-3288
Toll-Free: 800-344-4867
(FIGHTMS)
Tel: 212-986-3240
Fax: 212-986-7981
Website:
www.nationalmssociety.org
E-mail: nat@nmss.org

National Sleep Foundation

1522 K Street, N.W.
Suite 500
Washington, DC 20005
Tel: 202-347-3471
Fax: 202-347-3472
Website:
www.sleepfoundation.org
E-mail: nsf@sleepfoundation.org

National Society of Genetic Counselors, Inc.

233 Canterbury Drive
Wallingford, PA 19086-6617
Tel: 610-872-7608
Website: www.nsgc.org
E-mail: nsgc@nsgc.org

National Spasmodic Torticollis Association

9920 Talbert Avenue, Suite 233
Fountain Valley, CA 92708
Toll-Free: 800-HURTFUL (487-8385)
Tel: 714-378-7837
Fax: 714-378-7830
Website: www.torticollis.org
E-mail: NSTAmail@aol.com

NYU Center for the Study & Treatment of Movement Disorders

530 First Avenue
New York, NY 10016
Tel: 212-263-1483
Fax: 212-263-8031
E-mail:
anne@mcns10.med.nyu.edu

Opsoclonus Myoclonus Support Network, Inc.

c/o 420 Montezuma Way
West Covina, CA 91791
Tel: 626-339-7949
Website: www.geocities.com/
HotSprings/Spa2190

Parent Project for Muscular Dystrophy Research

1012 North University Blvd.
Middletown, OH 45042
Toll-Free: 800-714-KIDS (5437)
Tel: 513-424-0696
Fax: 513-425-9907
Website:
www.parentprojectmd.org
E-mail: ParentProject@aol.com

Polio Connection of America

P.O. Box 182
Howard Beach, NY 11414
Tel: 718-835-5536
Website: www.geocities.com/
w1066w
E-mail: w1066polio@hotmail.com

Project ALS

511 Avenue of the Americas
Suite 341
New York, NY 10011
Toll-Free: 800-603-0270
Tel: 212-969-0329
Fax: 212-337-9915
Website: www.projectals.org
E-mail: projectals@aol.com

Rett Syndrome Research Foundation

4600 Devitt Drive
Cincinnati, OH 45246
Tel: 513-874-3020
Fax: 513-874-2520
Website: www.rsrf.org

RLS (Restless Legs Syndrome) Foundation, Inc.

819 Second Street, S.W.
Rochester, MN 55902
Tel: 507-287-6465
Website: www.ris.org
E-mail: RLSFoundation@rls.org

Spina Bifida Association of America

4590 MacArthur Blvd. N.W.
Suite 250
Washington, DC 20007-4266
Toll-Free: 800-621-3141
Tel: 202-944-3285
Fax: 202-944-3295
Website: www.sbaa.org
E-mail: sbaa@sbaa.org

Shy-Drager/Multiple System Atrophy Support Group, Inc.

2004 Howard Lane
Austin, TX 78728
Toll-Free: 800-288-5582
Tel: 866-SDS-4999 (737-4999)
Fax: 512-251-3315
Website: www.shy-drager.com/
E-mail: Don.Summers@shy-drager.com

Society for Supranuclear Palsy

1838 Greene Tree Road
Suite 515
Baltimore, MD 21208
Toll-Free: 800-457-4777
Website: www.psp.org
E-mail: spsp@psp.org

Spastic Paraplegia Foundation (SPF)

P.O. Box 1208
Fortson, GA 31808
Tel: 978-256-2673
Website: www.sp-foundation.org

Tardive Dyskinesia/ Tardive Dystonia National Association
P.O. Box 45732
Seattle, WA 98145-0732
Tel: 206-522-3166
Fax: 206-528-2117
E-mail: skjaer@halcyon.com

United Cerebral Palsy Associations
1600 L Street, N.W., Suite 700
Washington, DC 20036
Toll-Free: 800-USA-5UCP (872-5827)
Tel: 202-776-0406
Fax: 202-776-0414
Website: www.ucp.org
E-mail: webmaster@ucp.org

Worldwide Education and Awareness for Movement Disorders (WE MOVE)
204 West 84th Street
New York, NY 10024
Toll-Free: 800-437-MOV2
Fax: 212-875-8389
Website: www.wemove.org
E-mail: wemove@wemove.org

Organizations for Families with Disabilities

Beach Center on Disability
The University of Kansas
Haworth Hall, Room 3136
1200 Sunnyside Ave.
Lawrence KS 66045-7534
Tel: 785-864-7600
Fax: 785-864-7605
Website: www.beachcenter.org
E-mail: beach@dole.lsi.ukans.edu

Through the Looking Glass
2198 Sixth Street
Suite 100
Berkeley, CA 94710-2204
Toll-Free: 800-644-2666
Tel: 510-848-1112
Fax: 510-848-4445
Website: www.lookingglass.org
E-mail: TLG@lookingglass.org

Parkinson's Disease

American Parkinson Disease Association
1250 Hylan Boulevard
Suite 4B
Staten Island, NY 10305-1946
Toll-Free: 800-223-APDA (2732)
Tel: 718-981-8001
Fax: 718-981-4399
Website: www.apdaparkinson.com
E-mail: apda@apdaparkinson.com

Michael J. Fox Foundation for Parkinson's Research
Grand Central Station
P.O. Box 4777
New York, NY 10163
Toll-Free: 800-708-7644
www.michaeljfox.com

National Parkinson Foundation, Inc.
1501 N.W. 9th Avenue
Bob Hope Research Center
Miami, FL 33136-1494
Toll-Free: 800-327-4545 (in Florida 800-433-7022)
Tel: 305-547-6666
Fax: 305-243-4402
Website: www.parkinson.org
E-mail: mailbox@Parkinson.org

Parkinson's Action Network
300 North Lee Street
Alexandria, VA 22314
Toll-Free: 800-850-4726
Fax: 703-518-0673
Website:
www.parkinsonaction.org
E-mail: info@parkinsonaction.org

Parkinson's Disease Foundation, Inc.
710 West 168th Street
New York, NY 10032-9982
Toll-Free: 800-457-6676
Tel: 212-923-4700
Fax: 212-923-4778
Website: www.parkinsons-foundation.org
E-mail: info@pdf.org

The Parkinson's Institute
1170 Morse Avenue
Sunnyvale, CA 94089-1605
Toll-Free: 800-786-2958
Tel: 408-734-2800
Fax: 408-734-8522
Website:
www.parkinsonsinstitute.org

Parkinson's Support Groups of America (PSGA)
11376 Cherry Hill Road, # 204
Beltsville, MD 20705
Tel: 301-937-1545

Worldwide Education and Awareness for Movement Disorders (WE MOVE)
204 W. 84th Street
New York, NY 10024
Toll-Free: 800-437-MOV2 (6682)
Fax: 212-875-8389
Website: www.wemove.org
E-mail: wemove@wemove.org

Spinal Cord Injury (SCI)

National Spinal Cord Injury Association
6701 Democracy Boulevard
Suite 300-9
Bethesda, MD 20817
Toll-Free: 800-962-9629
Tel: 301-588-6959
Fax: 301-588-9414
Website: www.spinalcord.org

American Spinal Injury Association
2020 Peachtree Road, N.W.
Atlanta, GA 30309-1402
Tel: 404-355-9772
Fax: 404-355-1826
Website: www.asia-spinalinjury.org

Paralyzed Veterans of America
801 18th St., N.W.
Washington, DC 20006
Toll-Free: 800-424-8200
E-mail: info@pva.org
Website: www.pva.org

RRTC on Aging with Spinal Cord Injury
Rancho Los Amigos Medical
Center
7601 E. Imperial Hwy.
800 West Annex
Downey, CA 90242-3456
Tel: 562-401-7402
Fax: 562-401-7011
Website: www.agingwithsci.org
E-mail: rrtcsci@aol.com

Medical RRTC on Secondary Conditions of SCI
UAB Spain Rehabilitation Center
1717 6th Ave. South
Birmingham, AL 35233-3334
Tel: 205-934-3334
TTD: 205-934-4642
Fax: 205-934-4642
Website: http://main.uab.edu/
show.asp?durki=8153#Contact
E-mail: rtc@sun.rehabm.uab.edu

Chapter 55

Directory of Resources for People with Movement Disorders

Assistive Technology Resources

Information in this section is adapted from ABLEDATA (online at www.abledata.com), a database project sponsored by the National Institute on Disability and Rehabilitation Research (NIDRR).

ABLEDATA
8630 Fenton Street, Suite 930
Silver Spring, MD 20910
Toll-Free: 800-227-0216
Tel: 301-608-8912 (TTY)
Fax: 301-608-8958
Website: www.abledata.com
E-mail: abledata@macroint.com

ABLEDATA is a federally funded project whose primary mission is to provide information on assistive technology and rehabilitation equipment available from domestic and international sources to consumers, organizations, professionals, and caregivers within the United States. It is sponsored by the National Institute on Disability and Rehabilitation Research (NIDRR), which is part of the Office of Special Education and Rehabilitative Services (OSERS) of the U.S. Department of Education. ABLEDATA is operated under Contract No. HN96015001.

Information in this chapter was compiled from the sources cited at the beginning of each section. All contact information was verified and updated in August 2002.

The ABLEDATA database contains information on more than 29,000 assistive technology products (over 19,000 of which are currently available), from white canes to voice output programs. The database contains detailed descriptions of each product including price and company information. The database also contains information on non-commercial prototypes, customized and one-of-a-kind products, and do-it-yourself designs. To select devices most appropriate to your needs, combine the ABLEDATA information with professional advice, product evaluations, and hands-on product trials. Note: ABLEDATA does not produce, distribute or sell any of the products listed on the database, but they will provide you with information on how to contact manufacturers or distributors of these products. They also do not produce any type of catalog.

This is a national assistive technology information exchange serving the nation's disability, rehabilitation, and senior communities. If you need information on assistive technology products and services, ABLEDATA can help.

The Assistive Technology Directory ($39) is a listing of companies with products listed in the database. This publication is available in print form from our information specialists.

ScootAround Inc.
584 Pembina Hwy.
Winnipeg, Canada R3M 3X7
Toll-Free: 888-441-7575
Tel: 204-982-0657
Fax: 204-478-1172
Website: www.scootaround.com
E-mail: info@scootaround.com

Provides scooter and wheelchair rentals for travelers to major cities throughout the United States.

Beneficial Designs
1617 Water Street, Suite 8
Minden, NV 89423-4310
Tel: 775-783-8822
Fax: 775-783-8823
Website: www.beneficialdesigns.com
E-mail: mail@beneficialdesigns.com

Designs assistive technologies to enable users of varying abilities to take part in recreational and leisure activities with *Tools for Play* and technologies for recreation in snow, on land, and in water.

Resources for Independent Living

The information in this section is from *Be Independent,* a booklet published by The American Parkinson Disease Association, 1250 Hylan Boulevard, Suite 4, Staten Island, NY 10305. © 1999 American Parkinson Disease Association. Reprinted with permission.

Adaptability
75 Mill Street
Colchester, CT 06415
Toll-Free: 800-937-3482
Website: www.adaptability.com

After Therapy Catalog
North Coast Medical
18305 Sutter Blvd.
Morgan Hill, CA 95037-2845
Toll-Free: 800-821-9319
Tel: 408-776-5000

Verizon Center for Customers with Disabilities
280 Locke Drive, 4th Floor
Marlboro, MA 01752
Toll-Free: 800-974-6006
Fax: 508-624-7645
Website: www22.verizon.com

Bruce Medical Supply
411 Waverly Oaks Rd., Suite 154
P.O. Box 9166
Waltham, MA 02452
Toll-Free: 800-225-8446
Fax: 781-894-9519
Website: www.brucemedical.com
E-mail: sales@brucemedical.com

Comfort House
189 Frelinghuysen Avenue
Newark, NJ 07114-1595
Toll-Free: 800-359-7701
Tel: 973-242-8080
Fax: 973-242-0131
Website: www.comforthouse.com
E-mail:
customerservice@comforthouse.com

Dr. Leonard's Health Care Catalog
P.O. Box 7821
Edison, NJ 08818
Toll-Free: 800-785-0880
Fax: 732-572-2118
Website: www.drleonards.com
E-mail:
custserv@drleonards.com

Dressing Tips and Clothing Res. for Making Life Easier
The Best 25 Catalogues Resources for Making Life Easier
9042 Aspen Grove Lane
Madison, WI 53717
Tel: 608-824-0402
Fax: 608-824-0403
Website:
www.meetinglifechallenges.com
E-mail:
help@meetinglifechallenges.com

Metro Medical Equipment
12985 Wayne Road
Livonia, MI 48150
Toll-Free: 800-877-7285
Fax: 734-522-9380

Durable Medical Equipment (over 3500) Plate Guards, Aids for Daily Living
Yes I Can
35-325 Date Palm Drive
Suite 131
Cathedral City, CA 92234
Toll-Free: 888-366-4226
Tel: 760-321-1717
Fax: 760-321-7780
Website: http://yesican.com
E-mail: info@yesican.com

Sammons Preston Rolyan
4 Sammons Court
Bolingbrook, IL 60440
Toll-Free: 800-323-5547
Fax: 800-547-4333
Website:
www.sammonspreston.com
E-mail:
ap@sammonspreston.com

Fashion Ease
1541 60th Street
Brooklyn, NY 11219
Toll-Free: 800-221-8929
Tel: 718-871-8188 (NY State)
Fax: 718-436-2067
Website: www.fashionease.com
E-mail: info@fashionease.com

Independent Living Aids Inc.
200 Robbins Lane
Jericho, NY 11753
Toll-Free: 800-537-2118
Tel: 516-937-1848
Fax: 516-937-3906
Website:
www.independentliving.com
E-mail: can-do@independentliving.com

Patients Transfer Systems
Beatrice M. Brantman, Inc.
207 E. Westminster
Lake Forest, IL 60045
Toll-Free: 800-232-7987
Fax: 847-615-8894
E-mail: beasyets@aol.com

Personal Pager
The Greatest of Ease Company
2443 Fillmore Street, #345
San Francisco, CA 94115
Tel: 415-441-6649
Fax: 415-441-4319
Website: http://
personalpagers.tripod.com/go
E-mail: greatestofease@aol.com

Sears Health Care Catalog
Sears Roebuck and Company
P.O. Box 804203
Chicago, IL 60680-4203
Toll-Free: 800-326-1750

The Speedo Aquatic Exercise System
7911 Haskell Avenue
Van Nuys, CA 91409
Toll-Free: 800-547-8770
Website: www.speedo.com

The Do Able Renewable Home
Consumer Affairs Program Dept.
American Association of Retired Persons (AARP)
P.O. Box 2240
Long Beach, CA 90801
Toll-Free: 800-424-3410

Voice Amplifiers

Rand Voice Amplifier
Park Surgical Company, Inc.
5001 New Utrecht Avenue
Brooklyn, NY 11219
Toll-Free: 800-633-7878
Tel: 718-436-9200
Fax: 718-854-2431
Website: www.parksurgical.com

Luminaud Inc.
8688 Tyler Blvd.
Mentor, OH 44060-4348
Toll-Free: 800-255-3408
Fax: 440-255-2250
Website: www.luminaud.com
E-mail: info@luminaud.com

Anchor Audio, Inc.
3415 Lomita Blvd.
Torrance, CA 90505
Toll-Free: 800-262-4671
Tel: 310-784-2300
Fax: 310-784-0066
Website: www.anchoraudio.com
E-mail: sales@anchoraudio.com

Walkers

Noble Motion Inc.
P.O. Box 5366
6741 Reynolds Street
Pittsburgh, PA 15206
Toll-Free: 800-234-9255
Fax: 412-363-7189
Website: www.wheels4walking.com
E-mail: info@noblemotion.com

Service Animals

The information in this section is excerpted from "A Wheeler's Best Friend," published in *New Mobility*, January 2002. © 2002 Bob Vogel; reprinted with permission.

Assistance Dogs International
980 Everett St.
Lakewood, CO 80215-5458
Tel: 303-238-5711
Website: www.assistance-dogs-intl.org.
E-mail: info@adionline.org

Canine Companions for Independence
P.O. Box 446
Santa Rosa, CA 95402
Tel: 707-577-1700
TDD: 707-577-1756
Website: www.caninecompanions.org
E-mail: info@caninecompanions.org

Discovery Dogs
P.O. Box 6050
San Rafael, CA 94903-0050
Tel: 415-479-9557
Fax: 415-472-4431
Website: www.discoverydogs.org.
E-mail: DiscoveryDogs@DiscoveryDogs.org

International Association of Assistance Dog Partners
38691 Filly Drive
Sterling Heights, MI 48310
Tel: 586-826-3938
Website: www.iaadp.org.
E-mail: info@iaadp.org

Assistive Technology Funding Resources

The information in this section is from "Assistive Technology Funding Resources." This document is reprinted with permission from "Finding the Money," by Candace Bennett, Managing Editor, Infinitec, Inc. Infinitec, a joint project of United Cerebral Palsy Association of Greater Chicago and United Cerebral Palsy Associations, Inc., is a non-profit corporation dedicated to helping individuals with disabilities and their families access life-enhancing technologies. Reprinted with permission of the author and UCP of Greater Chicago. © 1999. For additional information, visit www.infinitec.org.

The Alliance for Technology Access (ATA)
2173 E. Francisco Blvd., Suite L
San Rafael, CA 94901
Tel: 415-455-4575
TTY: 415-455-0491
Fax: 415-455-0654
Website: www.ataccess.org
E-mail: atainfo@ataccess.org

Information on parent support groups and on centers where equipment can be tried. Also offers information about evaluations for assistive technology related to computer use.

Center on Information Technology Accommodation (CITA)
1800 & F Street, N.W., Room 1234
Washington, DC 20405
Tel: 202-501-4906
Fax: 202-501-6269
TDD: 202-501-2010
Website: www.gsa.gov

Focuses on government legislation and policy concerning access to information. Also offers lists of equipment vendors, public and non-profit resources, and guidelines for technologies which enable access to information.

Direct Link for the Disabled, Inc.
P.O. Box 1036
Solvang, CA 93464
Tel: 805-688-1603

Provides personal responses to specific questions, information packets, and referrals.

Edlaw
1310 Minor Ave., #207
Seattle, WA 98101
Tel: 206-447-8050
Fax: 425-871-5266
Website: www.edlaw.net
E-mail: edlaw@edlaw.net

Provides information on the U.S. Individuals with Disabilities Education Act (IDEA) and Section 504 of the U.S. Rehabilitation Act. Includes links to disability law resources on the Internet.

Family Center on Technology and Disability
1660 L. Street, N.W.
Washington, DC 20036
Toll-Free: 800-USA-5UCP (voice)
TDD: 202-973-7197
Fax: 202-776-0414
Website: http://fctd.ucp.org

Assists organizations and programs that serve families of children with disabilities by providing information and support on accessing and using assistive technology. Many resources related to assistive technology and its funding.

Federation for Children with Special Health Care Needs
1135 Tremont Street, Suite 420
Boston, MA 02120
Toll-Free: 800-331-0688
Tel: 617-482-2915 (v/TDD)
Fax: 617-572-2094
Website: www.fcsn.org
E-mail: fcsninfo@fcsn.org

A parent training and information center, designed to help parents deal with schools. Call for the location of a center near you.

HEATH Resource Center / American Council on Education
2121 K Street, N.W., Suite 220
Washington, DC 20037
Toll-Free: 800-544-3284
Tel: 202-973-0904
Fax: 202-973-0908
Website: www.heath.gwu.edu
E-mail: askheath@heath.gwu.edu

National Early Childhood Technical Assistance System (NECTAS)
Campus Box 8040, UNC-CH
Chapel Hill, NC 27599
Tel: 919-962-2001
TDD: 919-843-3269
Fax: 919-966-7463
Website: www.nectas.unc.edu
E-mail: nectac@unc.edu

Provides information on Early Intervention Programs and who to contact in your state for more information.

National Information Center for Children and Youths with Disabilities (NICHCY)
P.O. Box 1492
Washington, DC 20013
Toll-Free: 800-695-0285 (v/TDD)
Fax: 202-884-8441
Website: www.nichcy.org
E-mail: nichcy@aed.org

Provides personal responses to specific questions, referrals to other sources of help, and technical assistance to parents and professionals.

National Rehabilitation Information Center (NARIC)
4200 Forbes Boulevard, Suite 202
Lanham, MD 20706
Toll-Free: 800-346-2742 (v)
Tel: 301-495-5900
Fax: 301-587-1967
Website: www.naric.com
E-mail: naricinfo@heitechservices.com

Provides information on disability and rehabilitation, including research, organizations, publications, journal articles, and Internet resources.

Neighborhood Legal Services
495 Ellicott Square Building
295 Main Street
Buffalo, NY 14203
Tel: 716-847-0650
TTY: 716-847-1322

Neighborhood Legal Services, continued
Fax: 716-847-1322
Website: www.nls.org
E-mail: feedback@nls.org

This organization trains attorneys to deal with assistive technology issues and also provides technical assistance.

Ready Access Program
State of Illinois
100 W. Randolph Street, Suite 4-100
Chicago, IL 60601
Tel: 312-814-1793
TDD: 312-814-6592
Website: www.state.il.us

The Illinois State Treasurer works with private lending institutions to help people with disabilities and their families who reside in Illinois obtain below-market interest rate loans for purchasing assistive technology. The maximum loan is $25,000; maximum pay-back, three years. Can be used only for purchasing assistive devices that demonstrably enhance a person's quality of life and enable increased independence.

RESNA
Technical Assistance Project
1700 N. Moore St., Suite 1540
Arlington, VA 22209-1903
Tel: 703-524-6686
TTY: 703-524-6639
Fax: 703-524-6630
Website: www.resna.org
E-mail: info@resna.org

Coordinates and provides information about the state Tech Act programs. Conducts annual conference and regional assistive technology conferences with exhibits. Funded by the U.S. Technology-Related Assistance for Individuals with Disabilities Act of 1988 and Amendments of 1994 [PL-103-28].

Almost all states in the U.S., the District of Columbia, Guam, the Northern Mariana Islands, and American Samoa, have a Tech Act program. Tech Act programs advise people with disabilities and their caregivers on all aspects of assistive technology including funding. Contact RESNA for a list of state Tech Act program locations, phone numbers, and general information.

TECH TOTS
United Cerebral Palsy Associations Inc.
3010 West Harvard Street
Santa Ana, CA 92704
Tel: 714-557-1291
Fax: 714-546-0943
Website: www.ucpa.org/techtots.htm

This program offers children with disabilities and their families hands-on experience with assistive technology; lends adapted toys and equipment for trial. There may be a Tech Tots center near you.

United Cerebral Palsy Associations, Inc.
1660 L Street, NW, Suite 700
Washington, DC 20036
Toll-Free: 800-872-5827
Tel: 202-776-0406
TTY: 202-973-7197
Fax: 202-776-0414
Website: www.ucpa.org

Index

Index

Page numbers followed by 'n' indicate a footnote. Page numbers in *italics* indicate a table or illustration.

A

ABLEDATA, contact information 366, 591–92
"About Wilson's Disease" (Sellner) 455n
acetophenazine 173, 499
acetylcholine 65, 239–42, 373–76, *376*
ACTH *see* adrenocorticotropic hormone
action myoclonus, described 27
action potentials, described 65–66
activities of daily living (ADL)
    bathroom safety 532–34
    bedroom safety 529–32
    dressing safety 534–37
    kitchen safety 538–40
    mealtime safety 540–41
    tremor 97
    walking safety 541–44
"Acute Cerebellar Ataxia" (Kleiner-Fisman) 185n
acute cerebellar ataxia, overview 185–86

A.D.A.M., Inc., publications
    creatinine test 59n
    muscle biopsy 53n
    preschooler test preparation 83n
Adaptability, contact information 593
adaptive devices, tremor 97
    see also assistive devices
adenine, described 328
ADHD *see* attention deficit hyperactivity disorder
ADL *see* activities of daily living
adolescents
    Angelman syndrome 198–99
    Huntington's disease 330–31
adrenocorticotropic hormone (ACTH) 362
After Therapy Catalog, contact information 593
age factor
    dystonia 126, 138
    essential tremor 92
    Friedreich's ataxia 317
    Huntington's disease 330–31
    Machado-Joseph disease 351
    multiple sclerosis 20, 357
    muscular dystrophy 12
    Parkinson's disease 105
    progressive supranuclear palsy 389
    restless legs syndrome 407

akathisia, described 8
akinesia
  defined 346, 571
  described 483
alcohol use
  restless legs syndrome 408
  tremor 98
The Alliance for Technology Access
  (ATA), contact information 597
Alliance of Genetic Support Groups,
  contact information 356, 581
alpha-synuclein protein 102
alprazolam 96
ALS *see* amyotrophic lateral sclerosis
ALSA *see* ALS Association of America
ALS Association of America (ALSA),
  contact information 305, 581
alternative therapies
  movement disorders 9
  multiple sclerosis 364
  tremor 97
amantadine 118–19, 364, 385, 397
Ambien (zolpidem) 397
American Association of Neurological
  Surgeons/Congress of Neurological
  Surgeons, neurological tests publication 45n
American Hippotherapy Association,
  contact information 523n
American Parkinson Disease Association, ADL publication 529n
American Parkinson Disease Foundation
  contact information 587
  independence publication 583
American Speech Language Hearing
  Association (ASHA), contact information 177, 355, 581
American Spinal Injury Association,
  contact information 588
aminoglycosides 64
amitriptyline 397
amoxapine 173, 499
"Amyotrophic Lateral Sclerosis"
  (NINDS) 297n
amyotrophic lateral sclerosis (ALS)
  causes 300–301
  cramps 16

amyotrophic lateral sclerosis (ALS),
  continued
  described 297–98
  diagnosis 299–300
  research 304–5
  statistics 298
  symptoms 298–99
  treatment 301–4
Anafranil (clomipramine) 287
Anchor Audio, Inc., contact information 595
anencephaly 263, 264
Angelman, Harry 187
Angelman syndrome
  genetic classes *191*
  overview 187–203
Angelman Syndrome Foundation,
  contact information 187n
angiography, described 45
animal studies
  Huntington's disease 340, 342, 343
  Parkinson's disease 101, 484
antagonistic muscle pairs, described 6
anteropulsion, described 107
anticholinergic medications
  cerebral palsy 226
  dystonia 143, 145–46, 175, 497, 498
  Parkinson's disease 118
anticipation, described 353
antidepressant medications
  amyotrophic lateral sclerosis 302
  progressive supranuclear palsy
    397
  Tourette syndrome 287
Apgar, Virginia 217
Apgar score
  cerebral palsy 217
  defined 233, 571
apraxia
  defined 233, 571
  Rett syndrome 251–52
"Areas of Research: Acquired Neurological Dysfunction" (Children's
  Neurobiological Solutions Foundation) 181n
"Areas of Research: Basic Cellular
  Developmental Neurobiology"
  (Children's Neurobiological Solutions Foundation) 181n

H

Hagberg, Bengt 251
Hain, Timothy C. 313n
Haldol (haloperidol) 130, 173, 287, 336, 499
Hallervorden-Spatz syndrome
  dystonia 146, 176–77
  overview 243–50
  Parkinson's disease 115
Hallervorden-Spatz Syndrome Association (HSSA), contact information 243n
haloperidol 130, 173, 287, 336, 499
hand preference, cerebral palsy 220
happiness, Angelman syndrome 193–94
Harati, Yadollah 55
Harvard Brain Tissue Resource Center, contact information 346
HDSA *see* Huntington's Disease Society of America
head injuries
  cerebral palsy 218
  spasticity 21
health care teams
  cerebral palsy 221–22
  described 35–41
  spasticity treatment 469
health insurance
  assistive technology 566–68
  genetic counseling 137
  plasmapheresis 522
heart disorders
  cardiologists 36
  Friedreich's ataxia 321, 323
  muscular dystrophy 12–13
HEATH Resource Center/American Council on Education, contact information 598
hemianopia
  defined 234, 574
  described 214
hemiballismus, described 8
hemi-dystonia, described 126
hemifacial spasm, described 160
hemiparesis 214
hemiparetic tremors, defined 234, 574

hemiplegia 214
hepatolenticular degeneration *see* Wilson's disease
hereditary ataxia, defined 10
hereditary Charcot disease *see* hereditary spastic paraplegia
hereditary chorea 327
Hereditary Disease Foundation, contact information 350, 582
hereditary motor and sensory neuropathies (HMSN) 308
hereditary spastic paraplegia (HSP) 415–30
heredity
  amyotrophic lateral sclerosis 298
  ataxia-telangiectasia 205
  cervical dystonia 165
  Charcot-Marie-Tooth disease 311, 312
  congenital myasthenic syndrome 241
  dystonia 132, 135–37, 149–58
  essential tremor 92
  Friedreich's ataxia 317–20
  hereditary spastic paraplegia 420–21
  Huntington's disease 328–29, 331
  Machado-Joseph disease 351, 352
  movement disorders 7
  oromandibular dystonia 162
  Parkinson's disease 100, 101, 102–4
  Rett syndrome 252
  spinal muscular atrophy 271–72
  Tourette syndrome 290
  Wilson's disease 456–58
  see also genetic defects
Herz, Ernst 125
hippotherapy 255, 523–25
histochemistry, described 54
histology tests, described 54
HMSN *see* hereditary motor and sensory neuropathies
horseback riding, neuromuscular function treatment 255, 523–25
HSP *see* hereditary spastic paraplegia
HSSA *see* Hallervorden-Spatz Syndrome Association
Human Genome Project Information, gene tests publication 79n

625

Health Reference Series
COMPLETE CATALOG

Adolescent Health Sourcebook

Basic Consumer Health Information about Common Medical, Mental, and Emotional Concerns in Adolescents, Including Facts about Acne, Body Piercing, Mononucleosis, Nutrition, Eating Disorders, Stress, Depression, Behavior Problems, Peer Pressure, Violence, Gangs, Drug Use, Puberty, Sexuality, Pregnancy, Learning Disabilities, and More

Along with a Glossary of Terms and Other Resources for Further Help and Information

Edited by Chad T. Kimball. 658 pages. 2002. 0-7808-0248-9. $78.

"A good starting point for information related to common medical, mental, and emotional concerns of adolescents." — *School Library Journal, Nov '02*

"This book provides accurate information in an easy to access format. It addresses topics that parents and caregivers might not be aware of and provides practical, useable information." — *Doody's Health Sciences Book Review Journal, Sep-Oct '02*

"Recommended reference source."
— *Booklist, American Library Association, Sep '02*

AIDS Sourcebook, 1st Edition

Basic Information about AIDS and HIV Infection, Featuring Historical and Statistical Data, Current Research, Prevention, and Other Special Topics of Interest for Persons Living with AIDS

Along with Source Listings for Further Assistance

Edited by Karen Bellenir and Peter D. Dresser. 831 pages. 1995. 0-7808-0031-1. $78.

"One strength of this book is its practical emphasis. The intended audience is the lay reader . . . useful as an educational tool for health care providers who work with AIDS patients. Recommended for public libraries as well as hospital or academic libraries that collect consumer materials."
— *Bulletin of the Medical Library Association, Jan '96*

"This is the most comprehensive volume of its kind on an important medical topic. Highly recommended for all libraries." — *Reference Book Review, '96*

"Very useful reference for all libraries."
— *Choice, Association of College and Research Libraries, Oct '95*

"There is a wealth of information here that can provide much educational assistance. It is a must book for all libraries and should be on the desk of each and every congressional leader. Highly recommended."
— *AIDS Book Review Journal, Aug '95*

"Recommended for most collections."
— *Library Journal, Jul '95*

AIDS Sourcebook, 2nd Edition

Basic Consumer Health Information about Acquired Immune Deficiency Syndrome (AIDS) and Human Immunodeficiency Virus (HIV) Infection, Featuring Updated Statistical Data, Reports on Recent Research and Prevention Initiatives, and Other Special Topics of Interest for Persons Living with AIDS, Including New Antiretroviral Treatment Options, Strategies for Combating Opportunistic Infections, Information about Clinical Trials, and More

Along with a Glossary of Important Terms and Resource Listings for Further Help and Information

Edited by Karen Bellenir. 751 pages. 1999. 0-7808-0225-X. $78.

"Highly recommended."
— *American Reference Books Annual, 2000*

"Excellent sourcebook. This continues to be a highly recommended book. There is no other book that provides as much information as this book provides."
— *AIDS Book Review Journal, Dec-Jan 2000*

"Recommended reference source."
— *Booklist, American Library Association, Dec '99*

"A solid text for college-level health libraries."
— *The Bookwatch, Aug '99*

Cited in *Reference Sources for Small and Medium-Sized Libraries*, American Library Association, 1999

Alcoholism Sourcebook

Basic Consumer Health Information about the Physical and Mental Consequences of Alcohol Abuse, Including Liver Disease, Pancreatitis, Wernicke-Korsakoff Syndrome (Alcoholic Dementia), Fetal Alcohol Syndrome, Heart Disease, Kidney Disorders, Gastrointestinal Problems, and Immune System Compromise and Featuring Facts about Addiction, Detoxification, Alcohol Withdrawal, Recovery, and the Maintenance of Sobriety

Along with a Glossary and Directories of Resources for Further Help and Information

Edited by Karen Bellenir. 613 pages. 2000. 0-7808-0325-6. $78.

"This title is one of the few reference works on alcoholism for general readers. For some readers this will be a welcome complement to the many self-help books on the market. Recommended for collections serving general readers and consumer health collections."
— *E-Streams, Mar '01*

"This book is an excellent choice for public and academic libraries."
— *American Reference Books Annual, 2001*

"Recommended reference source."
— *Booklist, American Library Association, Dec '00*

"Presents a wealth of information on alcohol use and abuse and its effects on the body and mind, treatment, and prevention." — *SciTech Book News, Dec '00*

"Important new health guide which packs in the latest consumer information about the problems of alcoholism." — *Reviewer's Bookwatch, Nov '00*

SEE ALSO *Drug Abuse Sourcebook, Substance Abuse Sourcebook*

■

Allergies Sourcebook, 1st Edition

Basic Information about Major Forms and Mechanisms of Common Allergic Reactions, Sensitivities, and Intolerances, Including Anaphylaxis, Asthma, Hives and Other Dermatologic Symptoms, Rhinitis, and Sinusitis

Along with Their Usual Triggers Like Animal Fur, Chemicals, Drugs, Dust, Foods, Insects, Latex, Pollen, and Poison Ivy, Oak, and Sumac; Plus Information on Prevention, Identification, and Treatment

Edited by Allan R. Cook. 611 pages. 1997. 0-7808-0036-2. $78.

■

Allergies Sourcebook, 2nd Edition

Basic Consumer Health Information about Allergic Disorders, Triggers, Reactions, and Related Symptoms, Including Anaphylaxis, Rhinitis, Sinusitis, Asthma, Dermatitis, Conjunctivitis, and Multiple Chemical Sensitivity

Along with Tips on Diagnosis, Prevention, and Treatment, Statistical Data, a Glossary, and a Directory of Sources for Further Help and Information

Edited by Annemarie S. Muth. 598 pages. 2002. 0-7808-0376-0. $78.

"This second edition would be useful to laypersons with little or advanced knowledge of the subject matter. This book would also serve as a resource for nursing and other health care professions students. It would be useful in public, academic, and hospital libraries with consumer health collections." — *E-Streams, Jul '02*

■

Alternative Medicine Sourcebook, 1st Edition

Basic Consumer Health Information about Alternatives to Conventional Medicine, Including Acupressure, Acupuncture, Aromatherapy, Ayurveda, Bioelectromagnetics, Environmental Medicine, Essence Therapy, Food and Nutrition Therapy, Herbal Therapy, Homeopathy, Imaging, Massage, Naturopathy, Reflexology, Relaxation and Meditation, Sound Therapy, Vitamin and Mineral Therapy, and Yoga, and More

Edited by Allan R. Cook. 737 pages. 1999. 0-7808-0200-4. $78.

"Recommended reference source."
—*Booklist, American Library Association, Feb '00*

"A great addition to the reference collection of every type of library." —*American Reference Books Annual, 2000*

Alternative Medicine Sourcebook, 2nd Edition

Basic Consumer Health Information about Alternative and Complementary Medical Practices, Including Acupuncture, Chiropractic, Herbal Medicine, Homeopathy, Naturopathic Medicine, Mind-Body Interventions, Ayurveda, and Other Non-Western Medical Traditions

Along with Facts about such Specific Therapies as Massage Therapy, Aromatherapy, Qigong, Hypnosis, Prayer, Dance, and Art Therapies, a Glossary, and Resources for Further Information

Edited by Dawn D. Matthews. 618 pages. 2002. 0-7808-0605-0. $78.

"An important alternate health reference."
—*MBR Bookwatch, Oct '02*

■

Alzheimer's, Stroke & 29 Other Neurological Disorders Sourcebook, 1st Edition

Basic Information for the Layperson on 31 Diseases or Disorders Affecting the Brain and Nervous System, First Describing the Illness, Then Listing Symptoms, Diagnostic Methods, and Treatment Options, and Including Statistics on Incidences and Causes

Edited by Frank E. Bair. 579 pages. 1993. 1-55888-748-2. $78.

"Nontechnical reference book that provides reader-friendly information."
—*Family Caregiver Alliance Update, Winter '96*

"Should be included in any library's patient education section." — *American Reference Books Annual, 1994*

"Written in an approachable and accessible style. Recommended for patient education and consumer health collections in health science center and public libraries." — *Academic Library Book Review, Dec '93*

"It is very handy to have information on more than thirty neurological disorders under one cover, and there is no recent source like it." — *Reference Quarterly, American Library Association, Fall '93*

SEE ALSO *Brain Disorders Sourcebook*

■

Alzheimer's Disease Sourcebook, 2nd Edition

Basic Consumer Health Information about Alzheimer's Disease, Related Disorders, and Other Dementias, Including Multi-Infarct Dementia, AIDS-Related Dementia, Alcoholic Dementia, Huntington's Disease, Delirium, and Confusional States

Along with Reports Detailing Current Research Efforts in Prevention and Treatment, Long-Term Care Issues, and Listings of Sources for Additional Help and Information

Edited by Karen Bellenir. 524 pages. 1999. 0-7808-0223-3. $78.

"Provides a wealth of useful information not otherwise available in one place. This resource is recommended for all types of libraries."
— American Reference Books Annual, 2000

"Recommended reference source."
— Booklist, American Library Association, Oct '99

Arthritis Sourcebook

Basic Consumer Health Information about Specific Forms of Arthritis and Related Disorders, Including Rheumatoid Arthritis, Osteoarthritis, Gout, Polymyalgia Rheumatica, Psoriatic Arthritis, Spondyloarthropathies, Juvenile Rheumatoid Arthritis, and Juvenile Ankylosing Spondylitis

Along with Information about Medical, Surgical, and Alternative Treatment Options, and Including Strategies for Coping with Pain, Fatigue, and Stress

Edited by Allan R. Cook. 550 pages. 1998. 0-7808-0201-2. $78.

". . . accessible to the layperson."
— Reference and Research Book News, Feb '99

Asthma Sourcebook

Basic Consumer Health Information about Asthma, Including Symptoms, Traditional and Nontraditional Remedies, Treatment Advances, Quality-of-Life Aids, Medical Research Updates, and the Role of Allergies, Exercise, Age, the Environment, and Genetics in the Development of Asthma

Along with Statistical Data, a Glossary, and Directories of Support Groups, and Other Resources for Further Information

Edited by Annemarie S. Muth. 628 pages. 2000. 0-7808-0381-7. $78.

"A worthwhile reference acquisition for public libraries and academic medical libraries whose readers desire a quick introduction to the wide range of asthma information." — Choice, Association of College & Research Libraries, Jun '01

"Recommended reference source."
— Booklist, American Library Association, Feb '01

"Highly recommended." — The Bookwatch, Jan '01

"There is much good information for patients and their families who deal with asthma daily."
— American Medical Writers Association Journal, Winter '01

"This informative text is recommended for consumer health collections in public, secondary school, and community college libraries and the libraries of universities with a large undergraduate population."
— American Reference Books Annual, 2001

Attention Deficit Disorder Sourcebook

Basic Consumer Health Information about Attention Deficit/Hyperactivity Disorder in Children and Adults, Including Facts about Causes, Symptoms, Diagnostic Criteria, and Treatment Options Such as Medications, Behavior Therapy, Coaching, and Homeopathy

Along with Reports on Current Research Initiatives, Legal Issues, and Government Regulations, and Featuring a Glossary of Related Terms, Internet Resources, and a List of Additional Reading Material

Edited by Dawn D. Matthews. 470 pages. 2002. 0-7808-0624-7. $78.

Back & Neck Disorders Sourcebook

Basic Information about Disorders and Injuries of the Spinal Cord and Vertebrae, Including Facts on Chiropractic Treatment, Surgical Interventions, Paralysis, and Rehabilitation

Along with Advice for Preventing Back Trouble

Edited by Karen Bellenir. 548 pages. 1997. 0-7808-0202-0. $78.

"The strength of this work is its basic, easy-to-read format. Recommended."
— Reference and User Services Quarterly, American Library Association, Winter '97

Blood & Circulatory Disorders Sourcebook

Basic Information about Blood and Its Components, Anemias, Leukemias, Bleeding Disorders, and Circulatory Disorders, Including Aplastic Anemia, Thalassemia, Sickle-Cell Disease, Hemochromatosis, Hemophilia, Von Willebrand Disease, and Vascular Diseases

Along with a Special Section on Blood Transfusions and Blood Supply Safety, a Glossary, and Source Listings for Further Help and Information

Edited by Karen Bellenir and Linda M. Shin. 554 pages. 1998. 0-7808-0203-9. $78.

"Recommended reference source."
— Booklist, American Library Association, Feb '99

"An important reference sourcebook written in simple language for everyday, non-technical users. "
— Reviewer's Bookwatch, Jan '99

Brain Disorders Sourcebook

Basic Consumer Health Information about Strokes, Epilepsy, Amyotrophic Lateral Sclerosis (ALS/Lou Gehrig's Disease), Parkinson's Disease, Brain Tumors, Cerebral Palsy, Headache, Tourette Syndrome, and More

Along with Statistical Data, Treatment and Rehabilitation Options, Coping Strategies, Reports on Current Research Initiatives, a Glossary, and Resource Listings for Additional Help and Information

Edited by Karen Bellenir. 481 pages. 1999. 0-7808-0229-2. $78.

"Belongs on the shelves of any library with a consumer health collection." —*E-Streams, Mar '00*

"Recommended reference source."
—*Booklist, American Library Association, Oct '99*

SEE ALSO *Alzheimer's Disease Sourcebook, 2nd Edition*

Breast Cancer Sourcebook

Basic Consumer Health Information about Breast Cancer, Including Diagnostic Methods, Treatment Options, Alternative Therapies, Self-Help Information, Related Health Concerns, Statistical and Demographic Data, and Facts for Men with Breast Cancer

Along with Reports on Current Research Initiatives, a Glossary of Related Medical Terms, and a Directory of Sources for Further Help and Information

Edited by Edward J. Prucha and Karen Bellenir. 580 pages. 2001. 0-7808-0244-6. $78.

"Recommended reference source."
—*Booklist, American Library Association, Jan '02*

"This reference source is highly recommended. It is quite informative, comprehensive and detailed in nature, and yet it offers practical advice in easy-to-read language. It could be thought of as the 'bible' of breast cancer for the consumer." —*E-Streams, Jan '02*

"The broad range of topics covered in lay language make the *Breast Cancer Sourcebook* an excellent addition to public and consumer health library collections."
—*American Reference Books Annual 2002*

"From the pros and cons of different screening methods and results to treatment options, *Breast Cancer Sourcebook* provides the latest information on the subject."
—*Library Bookwatch, Dec '01*

"This thoroughgoing, very readable reference covers all aspects of breast health and cancer. . . . Readers will find much to consider here. Recommended for all public and patient health collections."
—*Library Journal, Sep '01*

SEE ALSO *Cancer Sourcebook for Women, 1st and 2nd Editions, Women's Health Concerns Sourcebook*

Breastfeeding Sourcebook

Basic Consumer Health Information about the Benefits of Breastmilk, Preparing to Breastfeed, Breastfeeding as a Baby Grows, Nutrition, and More, Including Information on Special Situations and Concerns Such as Mastitis, Illness, Medications, Allergies, Multiple Births, Prematurity, Special Needs, and Adoption

Along with a Glossary and Resources for Additional Help and Information

Edited by Jenni Lynn Colson. 388 pages. 2002. 0-7808-0332-9. $78.

SEE ALSO *Pregnancy & Birth Sourcebook*

Burns Sourcebook

Basic Consumer Health Information about Various Types of Burns and Scalds, Including Flame, Heat, Cold, Electrical, Chemical, and Sun Burns

Along with Information on Short-Term and Long-Term Treatments, Tissue Reconstruction, Plastic Surgery, Prevention Suggestions, and First Aid

Edited by Allan R. Cook. 604 pages. 1999. 0-7808-0204-7. $78.

"This is an exceptional addition to the series and is highly recommended for all consumer health collections, hospital libraries, and academic medical centers."
—*E-Streams, Mar '00*

"This key reference guide is an invaluable addition to all health care and public libraries in confronting this ongoing health issue."
—*American Reference Books Annual, 2000*

"Recommended reference source."
—*Booklist, American Library Association, Dec '99*

SEE ALSO *Skin Disorders Sourcebook*

Cancer Sourcebook, 1st Edition

Basic Information on Cancer Types, Symptoms, Diagnostic Methods, and Treatments, Including Statistics on Cancer Occurrences Worldwide and the Risks Associated with Known Carcinogens and Activities

Edited by Frank E. Bair. 932 pages. 1990. 1-55888-888-8. $78.

Cited in *Reference Sources for Small and Medium-Sized Libraries, American Library Association, 1999*

"Written in nontechnical language. Useful for patients, their families, medical professionals, and librarians."
—*Guide to Reference Books, 1996*

"Designed with the non-medical professional in mind. Libraries and medical facilities interested in patient education should certainly consider adding the *Cancer Sourcebook* to their holdings. This compact collection of reliable information . . . is an invaluable tool for helping patients and patients' families and friends to take the first steps in coping with the many difficulties of cancer."
—*Medical Reference Services Quarterly, Winter '91*

"Specifically created for the nontechnical reader . . . an important resource for the general reader trying to understand the complexities of cancer."
—*American Reference Books Annual, 1991*

"This publication's nontechnical nature and very comprehensive format make it useful for both the general public and undergraduate students."
—*Choice, Association of College and Research Libraries, Oct '90*

New Cancer Sourcebook, 2nd Edition

Basic Information about Major Forms and Stages of Cancer, Featuring Facts about Primary and Secondary Tumors of the Respiratory, Nervous, Lymphatic, Circulatory, Skeletal, and Gastrointestinal Systems, and Specific Organs; Statistical and Demographic Data; Treatment Options; and Strategies for Coping

Edited by Allan R. Cook. 1,313 pages. 1996. 0-7808-0041-9. $78.

"An excellent resource for patients with newly diagnosed cancer and their families. The dialogue is simple, direct, and comprehensive. Highly recommended for patients and families to aid in their understanding of cancer and its treatment."

— *Booklist Health Sciences Supplement, American Library Association, Oct '97*

"The amount of factual and useful information is extensive. The writing is very clear, geared to general readers. Recommended for all levels." — *Choice, Association of College & Research Libraries, Jan '97*

■

Cancer Sourcebook, 3rd Edition

Basic Consumer Health Information about Major Forms and Stages of Cancer, Featuring Facts about Primary and Secondary Tumors of the Respiratory, Nervous, Lymphatic, Circulatory, Skeletal, and Gastrointestinal Systems, and Specific Organs

Along with Statistical and Demographic Data, Treatment Options, Strategies for Coping, a Glossary, and a Directory of Sources for Additional Help and Information

Edited by Edward J. Prucha. 1,069 pages. 2000. 0-7808-0227-6. $78.

"This title is recommended for health sciences and public libraries with consumer health collections."
— *E-Streams, Feb '01*

". . . can be effectively used by cancer patients and their families who are looking for answers in a language they can understand. Public and hospital libraries should have it on their shelves."
— *American Reference Books Annual, 2001*

"Recommended reference source."
— *Booklist, American Library Association, Dec '00*

■

Cancer Sourcebook for Women, 1st Edition

Basic Information about Specific Forms of Cancer That Affect Women, Featuring Facts about Breast Cancer, Cervical Cancer, Ovarian Cancer, Cancer of the Uterus and Uterine Sarcoma, Cancer of the Vagina, and Cancer of the Vulva; Statistical and Demographic Data; Treatments, Self-Help Management Suggestions, and Current Research Initiatives

Edited by Allan R. Cook and Peter D. Dresser. 524 pages. 1996. 0-7808-0076-1. $78.

". . . written in easily understandable, non-technical language. Recommended for public libraries or hospital and academic libraries that collect patient education or consumer health materials."
— *Medical Reference Services Quarterly, Spring '97*

"Would be of value in a consumer health library. . . . written with the health care consumer in mind. Medical jargon is at a minimum, and medical terms are explained in clear, understandable sentences."
— *Bulletin of the Medical Library Association, Oct '96*

"The availability under one cover of all these pertinent publications, grouped under cohesive headings, makes this certainly a most useful sourcebook." — *Choice, Association of College & Research Libraries, Jun '96*

"Presents a comprehensive knowledge base for general readers. Men and women both benefit from the gold mine of information nestled between the two covers of this book. Recommended."
— *Academic Library Book Review, Summer '96*

"This timely book is highly recommended for consumer health and patient education collections in all libraries." — *Library Journal, Apr '96*

■

Cancer Sourcebook for Women, 2nd Edition

Basic Consumer Health Information about Gynecologic Cancers and Related Concerns, Including Cervical Cancer, Endometrial Cancer, Gestational Trophoblastic Tumor, Ovarian Cancer, Uterine Cancer, Vaginal Cancer, Vulvar Cancer, Breast Cancer, and Common Non-Cancerous Uterine Conditions, with Facts about Cancer Risk Factors, Screening and Prevention, Treatment Options, and Reports on Current Research Initiatives

Along with a Glossary of Cancer Terms and a Directory of Resources for Additional Help and Information

Edited by Karen Bellenir. 604 pages. 2002. 0-7808-0226-8. $78.

"Highly recommended for academic and medical reference collections." — *Library Bookwatch, Sep '02*

"This is a highly recommended book for any public or consumer library, being reader friendly and containing accurate and helpful information."
— *E-Streams, Aug '02*

"Recommended reference source."
— *Booklist, American Library Association, Jul '02*

SEE ALSO *Breast Cancer Sourcebook, Women's Health Concerns Sourcebook*

Cardiovascular Diseases & Disorders Sourcebook, 1st Edition

Basic Information about Cardiovascular Diseases and Disorders, Featuring Facts about the Cardiovascular System, Demographic and Statistical Data, Descriptions of Pharmacological and Surgical Interventions, Lifestyle Modifications, and a Special Section Focusing on Heart Disorders in Children

Edited by Karen Bellenir and Peter D. Dresser. 683 pages. 1995. 0-7808-0032-X. $78.

". . . comprehensive format provides an extensive overview on this subject."
—*Choice, Association of College & Research Libraries, Jun '96*

". . . an easily understood, complete, up-to-date resource. This well executed public health tool will make valuable information available to those that need it most, patients and their families. The typeface, sturdy non-reflective paper, and library binding add a feel of quality found wanting in other publications. Highly recommended for academic and general libraries. "
—*Academic Library Book Review, Summer '96*

SEE ALSO *Healthy Heart Sourcebook for Women, Heart Diseases & Disorders Sourcebook, 2nd Edition*

Caregiving Sourcebook

Basic Consumer Health Information for Caregivers, Including a Profile of Caregivers, Caregiving Responsibilities and Concerns, Tips for Specific Conditions, Care Environments, and the Effects of Caregiving

Along with Facts about Legal Issues, Financial Information, and Future Planning, a Glossary, and a Listing of Additional Resources

Edited by Joyce Brennfleck Shannon. 600 pages. 2001. 0-7808-0331-0. $78.

"Essential for most collections."
—*Library Journal, Apr 1, 2002*

"An ideal addition to the reference collection of any public library. Health sciences information professionals may also want to acquire the *Caregiving Sourcebook* for their hospital or academic library for use as a ready reference tool by health care workers interested in aging and caregiving." —*E-Streams, Jan '02*

"Recommended reference source."
—*Booklist, American Library Association, Oct '01*

Colds, Flu & Other Common Ailments Sourcebook

Basic Consumer Health Information about Common Ailments and Injuries, Including Colds, Coughs, the Flu, Sinus Problems, Headaches, Fever, Nausea and Vomiting, Menstrual Cramps, Diarrhea, Constipation, Hemorrhoids, Back Pain, Dandruff, Dry and Itchy Skin, Cuts, Scrapes, Sprains, Bruises, and More

Along with Information about Prevention, Self-Care, Choosing a Doctor, Over-the-Counter Medications, Folk Remedies, and Alternative Therapies, and Including a Glossary of Important Terms and a Directory of Resources for Further Help and Information

Edited by Chad T. Kimball. 638 pages. 2001. 0-7808-0435-X. $78.

"A good starting point for research on common illnesses. It will be a useful addition to public and consumer health library collections."
—*American Reference Books Annual 2002*

"Will prove valuable to any library seeking to maintain a current, comprehensive reference collection of health resources. . . . Excellent reference."
—*The Bookwatch, Aug '01*

"Recommended reference source."
—*Booklist, American Library Association, July '01*

Communication Disorders Sourcebook

Basic Information about Deafness and Hearing Loss, Speech and Language Disorders, Voice Disorders, Balance and Vestibular Disorders, and Disorders of Smell, Taste, and Touch

Edited by Linda M. Ross. 533 pages. 1996. 0-7808-0077-X. $78.

"This is skillfully edited and is a welcome resource for the layperson. It should be found in every public and medical library." —*Booklist Health Sciences Supplement, American Library Association, Oct '97*

Congenital Disorders Sourcebook

Basic Information about Disorders Acquired during Gestation, Including Spina Bifida, Hydrocephalus, Cerebral Palsy, Heart Defects, Craniofacial Abnormalities, Fetal Alcohol Syndrome, and More

Along with Current Treatment Options and Statistical Data

Edited by Karen Bellenir. 607 pages. 1997. 0-7808-0205-5. $78.

"Recommended reference source."
—*Booklist, American Library Association, Oct '97*

SEE ALSO *Pregnancy & Birth Sourcebook*

Consumer Issues in Health Care Sourcebook

Basic Information about Health Care Fundamentals and Related Consumer Issues, Including Exams and Screening Tests, Physician Specialties, Choosing a Doctor, Using Prescription and Over-the-Counter Medications Safely, Avoiding Health Scams, Managing Common Health Risks in the Home, Care Options for Chronically or Terminally Ill Patients, and a List of Resources for Obtaining Help and Further Information

Edited by Karen Bellenir. 618 pages. 1998. 0-7808-0221-7. $78.

"Both public and academic libraries will want to have a copy in their collection for readers who are interested in self-education on health issues."
—*American Reference Books Annual, 2000*

"The editor has researched the literature from government agencies and others, saving readers the time and effort of having to do the research themselves. Recommended for public libraries."
— *Reference and User Services Quarterly, American Library Association, Spring '99*

"Recommended reference source."
—*Booklist, American Library Association, Dec '98*

■

Contagious & Non-Contagious Infectious Diseases Sourcebook

Basic Information about Contagious Diseases like Measles, Polio, Hepatitis B, and Infectious Mononucleosis, and Non-Contagious Infectious Diseases like Tetanus and Toxic Shock Syndrome, and Diseases Occurring as Secondary Infections Such as Shingles and Reye Syndrome

Along with Vaccination, Prevention, and Treatment Information, and a Section Describing Emerging Infectious Disease Threats

Edited by Karen Bellenir and Peter D. Dresser. 566 pages. 1996. 0-7808-0075-3. $78.

■

Death & Dying Sourcebook

Basic Consumer Health Information for the Layperson about End-of-Life Care and Related Ethical and Legal Issues, Including Chief Causes of Death, Autopsies, Pain Management for the Terminally Ill, Life Support Systems, Insurance, Euthanasia, Assisted Suicide, Hospice Programs, Living Wills, Funeral Planning, Counseling, Mourning, Organ Donation, and Physician Training

Along with Statistical Data, a Glossary, and Listings of Sources for Further Help and Information

Edited by Annemarie S. Muth. 641 pages. 1999. 0-7808-0230-6. $78.

"Public libraries, medical libraries, and academic libraries will all find this sourcebook a useful addition to their collections."
— *American Reference Books Annual, 2001*

"An extremely useful resource for those concerned with death and dying in the United States."
— *Respiratory Care, Nov '00*

"Recommended reference source."
—*Booklist, American Library Association, Aug '00*

"This book is a definite must for all those involved in end-of-life care." — *Doody's Review Service, 2000*

Depression Sourcebook

Basic Consumer Health Information about Unipolar Depression, Bipolar Disorder, Postpartum Depression, Seasonal Affective Disorder, and Other Types of Depression in Children, Adolescents, Women, Men, the Elderly, and Other Selected Populations

Along with Facts about Causes, Risk Factors, Diagnostic Criteria, Treatment Options, Coping Strategies, Suicide Prevention, a Glossary, and a Directory of Sources for Additional Help and Information

Edited by Karen Belleni. 602 pages. 2002. 0-7808-0611-5. $78.

■

Diabetes Sourcebook, 1st Edition

Basic Information about Insulin-Dependent and Non-insulin-Dependent Diabetes Mellitus, Gestational Diabetes, and Diabetic Complications, Symptoms, Treatment, and Research Results, Including Statistics on Prevalence, Morbidity, and Mortality

Along with Source Listings for Further Help and Information

Edited by Karen Bellenir and Peter D. Dresser. 827 pages. 1994. 1-55888-751-2. $78.

". . . very informative and understandable for the layperson without being simplistic. It provides a comprehensive overview for laypersons who want a general understanding of the disease or who want to focus on various aspects of the disease."
— *Bulletin of the Medical Library Association, Jan '96*

■

Diabetes Sourcebook, 2nd Edition

Basic Consumer Health Information about Type 1 Diabetes (Insulin-Dependent or Juvenile-Onset Diabetes), Type 2 (Noninsulin-Dependent or Adult-Onset Diabetes), Gestational Diabetes, and Related Disorders, Including Diabetes Prevalence Data, Management Issues, the Role of Diet and Exercise in Controlling Diabetes, Insulin and Other Diabetes Medicines, and Complications of Diabetes Such as Eye Diseases, Periodontal Disease, Amputation, and End-Stage Renal Disease

Along with Reports on Current Research Initiatives, a Glossary, and Resource Listings for Further Help and Information

Edited by Karen Bellenir. 688 pages. 1998. 0-7808-0224-1. $78.

"An invaluable reference." — *Library Journal, May '00*

Selected as one of the 250 "Best Health Sciences Books of 1999." — *Doody's Rating Service, Mar-Apr 2000*

"This comprehensive book is an excellent addition for high school, academic, medical, and public libraries. This volume is highly recommended."
—*American Reference Books Annual, 2000*

"Provides useful information for the general public."
— *Healthlines, University of Michigan Health Management Research Center, Sep/Oct '99*

Diabetes Sourcebook, 3rd Edition

Basic Consumer Health Information about Type 1 Diabetes (Insulin-Dependent or Juvenile-Onset Diabetes), Type 2 Diabetes (Noninsulin-Dependent or Adult-Onset Diabetes), Gestational Diabetes, Impaired Glucose Tolerance (IGT), and Related Complications, Such as Amputation, Eye Disease, Gum Disease, Nerve Damage, and End-Stage Renal Disease, Including Facts about Insulin, Oral Diabetes Medications, Blood Sugar Testing, and the Role of Exercise and Nutrition in the Control of Diabetes

Along with a Glossary and Resources for Further Help and Information

Edited by Dawn D. Matthews. 650 pages. 2003. 0-7808-0???-?. $78.

Diet & Nutrition Sourcebook, 1st Edition

Basic Information about Nutrition, Including the Dietary Guidelines for Americans, the Food Guide Pyramid, and Their Applications in Daily Diet, Nutritional Advice for Specific Age Groups, Current Nutritional Issues and Controversies, the New Food Label and How to Use It to Promote Healthy Eating, and Recent Developments in Nutritional Research

Edited by Dan R. Harris. 662 pages. 1996. 0-7808-0084-2. $78.

"Useful reference as a food and nutrition sourcebook for the general consumer." — *Booklist Health Sciences Supplement, American Library Association, Oct '97*

"Recommended for public libraries and medical libraries that receive general information requests on nutrition. It is readable and will appeal to those interested in learning more about healthy dietary practices."
— *Medical Reference Services Quarterly, Fall '97*

"An abundance of medical and social statistics is translated into readable information geared toward the general reader." — *Bookwatch, Mar '97*

"With dozens of questionable diet books on the market, it is so refreshing to find a reliable and factual reference book. Recommended to aspiring professionals, librarians, and others seeking and giving reliable dietary advice. An excellent compilation." — *Choice, Association of College and Research Libraries, Feb '97*

SEE ALSO *Digestive Diseases & Disorders Sourcebook, Gastrointestinal Diseases & Disorders Sourcebook*

Diet & Nutrition Sourcebook, 2nd Edition

Basic Consumer Health Information about Dietary Guidelines, Recommended Daily Intake Values, Vitamins, Minerals, Fiber, Fat, Weight Control, Dietary Supplements, and Food Additives

Along with Special Sections on Nutrition Needs throughout Life and Nutrition for People with Such Specific Medical Concerns as Allergies, High Blood Cholesterol, Hypertension, Diabetes, Celiac Disease, Seizure Disorders, Phenylketonuria (PKU), Cancer, and Eating Disorders, and Including Reports on Current Nutrition Research and Source Listings for Additional Help and Information

Edited by Karen Bellenir. 650 pages. 1999. 0-7808-0228-4. $78.

"This book is an excellent source of basic diet and nutrition information." — *Booklist Health Sciences Supplement, American Library Association, Dec '00*

"This reference document should be in any public library, but it would be a very good guide for beginning students in the health sciences. If the other books in this publisher's series are as good as this, they should all be in the health sciences collections."
— *American Reference Books Annual, 2000*

"This book is an excellent general nutrition reference for consumers who desire to take an active role in their health care for prevention. Consumers of all ages who select this book can feel confident they are receiving current and accurate information." — *Journal of Nutrition for the Elderly, Vol. 19, No. 4, '00*

"Recommended reference source."
— *Booklist, American Library Association, Dec '99*

SEE ALSO *Digestive Diseases & Disorders Sourcebook, Gastrointestinal Diseases & Disorders Sourcebook*

Digestive Diseases & Disorders Sourcebook

Basic Consumer Health Information about Diseases and Disorders that Impact the Upper and Lower Digestive System, Including Celiac Disease, Constipation, Crohn's Disease, Cyclic Vomiting Syndrome, Diarrhea, Diverticulosis and Diverticulitis, Gallstones, Heartburn, Hemorrhoids, Hernias, Indigestion (Dyspepsia), Irritable Bowel Syndrome, Lactose Intolerance, Ulcers, and More

Along with Information about Medications and Other Treatments, Tips for Maintaining a Healthy Digestive Tract, a Glossary, and Directory of Digestive Diseases Organizations

Edited by Karen Bellenir. 335 pages. 2000. 0-7808-0327-2. $78.

"This title would be an excellent addition to all public or patient-research libraries."
— *American Reference Books Annual, 2001*

"This title is recommended for public, hospital, and health sciences libraries with consumer health collections." — *E-Streams, Jul-Aug '00*

Disabilities Sourcebook

Basic Consumer Health Information about Physical and Psychiatric Disabilities, Including Descriptions of Major Causes of Disability, Assistive and Adaptive Aids, Workplace Issues, and Accessibility Concerns

Along with Information about the Americans with Disabilities Act, a Glossary, and Resources for Additional Help and Information

Edited by Dawn D. Matthews. 616 pages. 2000. 0-7808-0389-2. $78.

Domestic Violence & Child Abuse Sourcebook

Basic Consumer Health Information about Spousal/ Partner, Child, Sibling, Parent, and Elder Abuse, Covering Physical, Emotional, and Sexual Abuse, Teen Dating Violence, and Stalking; Includes Information about Hotlines, Safe Houses, Safety Plans, and Other Resources for Support and Assistance, Community Initiatives, and Reports on Current Directions in Research and Treatment

Along with a Glossary, Sources for Further Reading, and Governmental and Non-Governmental Organizations Contact Information

Edited by Helene Henderson. 1,064 pages. 2001. 0-7808-0235-7. $78.

Drug Abuse Sourcebook

Basic Consumer Health Information about Illicit Substances of Abuse and the Diversion of Prescription Medications, Including Depressants, Hallucinogens, Inhalants, Marijuana, Narcotics, Stimulants, and Anabolic Steroids

Along with Facts about Related Health Risks, Treatment Issues, and Substance Abuse Prevention Programs, a Glossary of Terms, Statistical Data, and Directories of Hotline Services, Self-Help Groups, and Organizations Able to Provide Further Information

Edited by Karen Bellenir. 629 pages. 2000. 0-7808-0242-X. $78.

Ear, Nose & Throat Disorders Sourcebook

Basic Information about Disorders of the Ears, Nose, Sinus Cavities, Pharynx, and Larynx, Including Ear Infections, Tinnitus, Vestibular Disorders, Allergic and Non-Allergic Rhinitis, Sore Throats, Tonsillitis, and Cancers That Affect the Ears, Nose, Sinuses, and Throat

Along with Reports on Current Research Initiatives, a Glossary of Related Medical Terms, and a Directory of Sources for Further Help and Information

Edited by Karen Bellenir and Linda M. Shin. 576 pages. 1998. 0-7808-0206-3. $78.

Eating Disorders Sourcebook

Basic Consumer Health Information about Eating Disorders, Including Information about Anorexia Nervosa, Bulimia Nervosa, Binge Eating, Body Dysmorphic Disorder, Pica, Laxative Abuse, and Night Eating Syndrome

Along with Information about Causes, Adverse Effects, and Treatment and Prevention Issues, and Featuring a Section on Concerns Specific to Children and Adolescents, a Glossary, and Resources for Further Help and Information

Edited by Dawn D. Matthews. 322 pages. 2001. 0-7808-0335-3. $78.

"Recommended for health science libraries that are open to the public, as well as hospital libraries. This book is a good resource for the consumer who is concerned about eating disorders." *— E-Streams, Mar '02*

"This volume is another convenient collection of excerpted articles. Recommended for school and public library patrons; lower-division undergraduates; and two-year technical program students." *— Choice, Association of College & Research Libraries, Jan '02*

"Recommended reference source." *— Booklist, American Library Association, Oct '01*

Emergency Medical Services Sourcebook

Basic Consumer Health Information about Preventing, Preparing for, and Managing Emergency Situations, When and Who to Call for Help, What to Expect in the Emergency Room, the Emergency Medical Team, Patient Issues, and Current Topics in Emergency Medicine

Along with Statistical Data, a Glossary, and Sources of Additional Help and Information

Edited by Jenni Lynn Colson. 494 pages. 2002. 0-7808-0420-1. $78.

Endocrine & Metabolic Disorders Sourcebook

Basic Information for the Layperson about Pancreatic and Insulin-Related Disorders Such as Pancreatitis, Diabetes, and Hypoglycemia; Adrenal Gland Disorders Such as Cushing's Syndrome, Addison's Disease, and Congenital Adrenal Hyperplasia; Pituitary Gland Disorders Such as Growth Hormone Deficiency, Acromegaly, and Pituitary Tumors; Thyroid Disorders Such as Hypothyroidism, Graves' Disease, Hashimoto's Disease, and Goiter; Hyperparathyroidism; and Other Diseases and Syndromes of Hormone Imbalance or Metabolic Dysfunction

Along with Reports on Current Research Initiatives

Edited by Linda M. Shin. 574 pages. 1998. 0-7808-0207-1. $78.

"Omnigraphics has produced another needed resource for health information consumers." *—American Reference Books Annual, 2000*

"Recommended reference source." *— Booklist, American Library Association, Dec '98*

Environmentally Induced Disorders Sourcebook

Basic Information about Diseases and Syndromes Linked to Exposure to Pollutants and Other Substances in Outdoor and Indoor Environments Such as Lead, Asbestos, Formaldehyde, Mercury, Emissions, Noise, and More

Edited by Allan R. Cook. 620 pages. 1997. 0-7808-0083-4. $78.

"Recommended reference source." *— Booklist, American Library Association, Sep '98*

"This book will be a useful addition to anyone's library." *— Choice Health Sciences Supplement, Association of College and Research Libraries, May '98*

". . . a good survey of numerous environmentally induced physical disorders . . . a useful addition to anyone's library." *— Doody's Health Sciences Book Reviews, Jan '98*

". . . provide[s] introductory information from the best authorities around. Since this volume covers topics that potentially affect everyone, it will surely be one of the most frequently consulted volumes in the Health Reference Series." *— Rettig on Reference, Nov '97*

Ethnic Diseases Sourcebook

Basic Consumer Health Information for Ethnic and Racial Minority Groups in the United States, Including General Health Indicators and Behaviors, Ethnic Diseases, Genetic Testing, the Impact of Chronic Diseases, Women's Health, Mental Health Issues, and Preventive Health Care Services

Along with a Glossary and a Listing of Additional Resources

Edited by Joyce Brennfleck Shannon. 664 pages. 2001. 0-7808-0336-1. $78.

"Recommended for health sciences libraries where public health programs are a priority." *—E-Streams, Jan '02*

"Not many books have been written on this topic to date, and the *Ethnic Diseases Sourcebook* is a strong addition to the list. It will be an important introductory resource for health consumers, students, health care personnel, and social scientists. It is recommended for public, academic, and large hospital libraries." *— American Reference Books Annual 2002*

"Recommended reference source." *— Booklist, American Library Association, Oct '01*

"Will prove valuable to any library seeking to maintain a current, comprehensive reference collection of health resources. . . . An excellent source of health information about genetic disorders which affect particular ethnic and racial minorities in the U.S." *— The Bookwatch, Aug '01*

Eye Care Sourcebook, 2nd Edition

Basic Consumer Health Information about Eye Care and Eye Disorders, Including Facts about the Diagnosis, Prevention, and Treatment of Common Refractive Problems Such as Myopia, Hyperopia, Astigmatism, and Presbyopia, and Eye Diseases, Including Glaucoma, Cataract, Age-Related Macular Degeneration, and Diabetic Retinopathy

Along with a Section on Vision Correction and Refractive Surgeries, Including LASIK and LASEK, a Glossary, and Directories of Resources for Additional Help and Information

Edited by Amy L. Sutton. 575 pages. 2003. 0-7808-0635-2. $78.

■

Family Planning Sourcebook

Basic Consumer Health Information about Planning for Pregnancy and Contraception, Including Traditional Methods, Barrier Methods, Hormonal Methods, Permanent Methods, Future Methods, Emergency Contraception, and Birth Control Choices for Women at Each Stage of Life

Along with Statistics, a Glossary, and Sources of Additional Information

Edited by Amy Marcaccio Keyzer. 520 pages. 2001. 0-7808-0379-5. $78.

"Recommended for public, health, and undergraduate libraries as part of the circulating collection."
— E-Streams, Mar '02

"Information is presented in an unbiased, readable manner, and the sourcebook will certainly be a necessary addition to those public and high school libraries where Internet access is restricted or otherwise problematic." — American Reference Books Annual 2002

"Recommended reference source."
— Booklist, American Library Association, Oct '01

"Will prove valuable to any library seeking to maintain a current, comprehensive reference collection of health resources. . . . Excellent reference."
— The Bookwatch, Aug '01

SEE ALSO Pregnancy & Birth Sourcebook

■

Fitness & Exercise Sourcebook, 1st Edition

Basic Information on Fitness and Exercise, Including Fitness Activities for Specific Age Groups, Exercise for People with Specific Medical Conditions, How to Begin a Fitness Program in Running, Walking, Swimming, Cycling, and Other Athletic Activities, and Recent Research in Fitness and Exercise

Edited by Dan R. Harris. 663 pages. 1996. 0-7808-0186-5. $78.

"A good resource for general readers." — Choice, Association of College and Research Libraries, Nov '97

"The perennial popularity of the topic . . . make this an appealing selection for public libraries."
— Rettig on Reference, Jun/Jul '97

Fitness & Exercise Sourcebook, 2nd Edition

Basic Consumer Health Information about the Fundamentals of Fitness and Exercise, Including How to Begin and Maintain a Fitness Program, Fitness as a Lifestyle, the Link between Fitness and Diet, Advice for Specific Groups of People, Exercise as It Relates to Specific Medical Conditions, and Recent Research in Fitness and Exercise

Along with a Glossary of Important Terms and Resources for Additional Help and Information

Edited by Kristen M. Gledhill. 646 pages. 2001. 0-7808-0334-5. $78.

"This work is recommended for all general reference collections."
— American Reference Books Annual 2002

"Highly recommended for public, consumer, and school grades fourth through college."
— E-Streams, Nov '01

"Recommended reference source." — Booklist, American Library Association, Oct '01

"The information appears quite comprehensive and is considered reliable. . . . This second edition is a welcomed addition to the series."
— Doody's Review Service, Sep '01

"This reference is a valuable choice for those who desire a broad source of information on exercise, fitness, and chronic-disease prevention through a healthy lifestyle." — American Medical Writers Association Journal, Fall '01

"Will prove valuable to any library seeking to maintain a current, comprehensive reference collection of health resources. . . . Excellent reference."
— The Bookwatch, Aug '01

■

Food & Animal Borne Diseases Sourcebook

Basic Information about Diseases That Can Be Spread to Humans through the Ingestion of Contaminated Food or Water or by Contact with Infected Animals and Insects, Such as Botulism, E. Coli, Hepatitis A, Trichinosis, Lyme Disease, and Rabies

Along with Information Regarding Prevention and Treatment Methods, and Including a Special Section for International Travelers Describing Diseases Such as Cholera, Malaria, Travelers' Diarrhea, and Yellow Fever, and Offering Recommendations for Avoiding Illness

Edited by Karen Bellenir and Peter D. Dresser. 535 pages. 1995. 0-7808-0033-8. $78.

"Targeting general readers and providing them with a single, comprehensive source of information on selected topics, this book continues, with the excellent caliber of its predecessors, to catalog topical information on health matters of general interest. Readable and thorough, this valuable resource is highly recommended for all libraries."
— Academic Library Book Review, Summer '96

"A comprehensive collection of authoritative information." — Emergency Medical Services, Oct '95

Food Safety Sourcebook

Basic Consumer Health Information about the Safe Handling of Meat, Poultry, Seafood, Eggs, Fruit Juices, and Other Food Items, and Facts about Pesticides, Drinking Water, Food Safety Overseas, and the Onset, Duration, and Symptoms of Foodborne Illnesses, Including Types of Pathogenic Bacteria, Parasitic Protozoa, Worms, Viruses, and Natural Toxins

Along with the Role of the Consumer, the Food Handler, and the Government in Food Safety; a Glossary, and Resources for Additional Help and Information

Edited by Dawn D. Matthews. 339 pages. 1999. 0-7808-0326-4. $78.

"**This book is recommended for public libraries and universities with home economic and food science programs.**" — *E-Streams, Nov '00*

"**Recommended reference source.**"
— *Booklist, American Library Association, May '00*

"**This book takes the complex issues of food safety and foodborne pathogens and presents them in an easily understood manner. [It does] an excellent job of covering a large and often confusing topic.**"
— *American Reference Books Annual, 2000*

∎

Forensic Medicine Sourcebook

Basic Consumer Information for the Layperson about Forensic Medicine, Including Crime Scene Investigation, Evidence Collection and Analysis, Expert Testimony, Computer-Aided Criminal Identification, Digital Imaging in the Courtroom, DNA Profiling, Accident Reconstruction, Autopsies, Ballistics, Drugs and Explosives Detection, Latent Fingerprints, Product Tampering, and Questioned Document Examination

Along with Statistical Data, a Glossary of Forensics Terminology, and Listings of Sources for Further Help and Information

Edited by Annemarie S. Muth. 574 pages. 1999. 0-7808-0232-2. $78.

"**Given the expected widespread interest in its content and its easy to read style, this book is recommended for most public and all college and university libraries.**"
— *E-Streams, Feb '01*

"**Recommended for public libraries.**"
— *Reference & User Services Quarterly, American Library Association, Spring 2000*

"**Recommended reference source.**"
— *Booklist, American Library Association, Feb '00*

"**A wealth of information, useful statistics, references are up-to-date and extremely complete. This wonderful collection of data will help students who are interested in a career in any type of forensic field. It is a great resource for attorneys who need information about types of expert witnesses needed in a particular case. It also offers useful information for fiction and nonfiction writers whose work involves a crime. A fascinating compilation. All levels.**" — *Choice, Association of College and Research Libraries, Jan 2000*

"**There are several items that make this book attractive to consumers who are seeking certain forensic data. . . . This is a useful current source for those seeking general forensic medical answers.**"
— *American Reference Books Annual, 2000*

∎

Gastrointestinal Diseases & Disorders Sourcebook

Basic Information about Gastroesophageal Reflux Disease (Heartburn), Ulcers, Diverticulosis, Irritable Bowel Syndrome, Crohn's Disease, Ulcerative Colitis, Diarrhea, Constipation, Lactose Intolerance, Hemorrhoids, Hepatitis, Cirrhosis, and Other Digestive Problems, Featuring Statistics, Descriptions of Symptoms, and Current Treatment Methods of Interest for Persons Living with Upper and Lower Gastrointestinal Maladies

Edited by Linda M. Ross. 413 pages. 1996. 0-7808-0078-8. $78.

"**. . . very readable form. The successful editorial work that brought this material together into a useful and understandable reference makes accessible to all readers information that can help them more effectively understand and obtain help for digestive tract problems.**"
— *Choice, Association of College & Research Libraries, Feb '97*

SEE ALSO *Diet & Nutrition Sourcebook, 1st and 2nd Editions, Digestive Diseases & Disorders*

∎

Genetic Disorders Sourcebook, 1st Edition

Basic Information about Heritable Diseases and Disorders Such as Down Syndrome, PKU, Hemophilia, Von Willebrand Disease, Gaucher Disease, Tay-Sachs Disease, and Sickle-Cell Disease, Along with Information about Genetic Screening, Gene Therapy, Home Care, and Including Source Listings for Further Help and Information on More Than 300 Disorders

Edited by Karen Bellenir. 642 pages. 1996. 0-7808-0034-6. $78.

"**Recommended for undergraduate libraries or libraries that serve the public.**"
— *Science & Technology Libraries, Vol. 18, No. 1, '99*

"**Provides essential medical information to both the general public and those diagnosed with a serious or fatal genetic disease or disorder.**" — *Choice, Association of College and Research Libraries, Jan '97*

"**Geared toward the lay public. It would be well placed in all public libraries and in those hospital and medical libraries in which access to genetic references is limited.**" — *Doody's Health Sciences Book Review, Oct '96*

Genetic Disorders Sourcebook, 2nd Edition

Basic Consumer Health Information about Hereditary Diseases and Disorders, Including Cystic Fibrosis, Down Syndrome, Hemophilia, Huntington's Disease, Sickle Cell Anemia, and More; Facts about Genes, Gene Research and Therapy, Genetic Screening, Ethics of Gene Testing, Genetic Counseling, and Advice on Coping and Caring

Along with a Glossary of Genetic Terminology and a Resource List for Help, Support, and Further Information

Edited by Kathy Massimini. 768 pages. 2001. 0-7808-0241-1. $78.

"Recommended for public libraries and medical and hospital libraries with consumer health collections."
— *E-Streams, May '01*

"Recommended reference source."
— *Booklist, American Library Association, Apr '01*

"Important pick for college-level health reference libraries." — *The Bookwatch, Mar '01*

Head Trauma Sourcebook

Basic Information for the Layperson about Open-Head and Closed-Head Injuries, Treatment Advances, Recovery, and Rehabilitation

Along with Reports on Current Research Initiatives

Edited by Karen Bellenir. 414 pages. 1997. 0-7808-0208-X. $78.

Headache Sourcebook

Basic Consumer Health Information about Migraine, Tension, Cluster, Rebound and Other Types of Headaches, with Facts about the Cause and Prevention of Headaches, the Effects of Stress and the Environment, Headaches during Pregnancy and Menopause, and Childhood Headaches

Along with a Glossary and Other Resources for Additional Help and Information

Edited by Dawn D. Matthews. 362 pages. 2002. 0-7808-0337-X. $78.

"Highly recommended for academic and medical reference collections." — *Library Bookwatch, Sep '02*

Health Insurance Sourcebook

Basic Information about Managed Care Organizations, Traditional Fee-for-Service Insurance, Insurance Portability and Pre-Existing Conditions Clauses, Medicare, Medicaid, Social Security, and Military Health Care

Along with Information about Insurance Fraud

Edited by Wendy Wilcox. 530 pages. 1997. 0-7808-0222-5. $78.

"Particularly useful because it brings much of this information together in one volume. This book will be a handy reference source in the health sciences library, hospital library, college and university library, and medium to large public library."
— *Medical Reference Services Quarterly, Fall '98*

Awarded "Books of the Year Award"
— *American Journal of Nursing, 1997*

"The layout of the book is particularly helpful as it provides easy access to reference material. A most useful addition to the vast amount of information about health insurance. The use of data from U.S. government agencies is most commendable. Useful in a library or learning center for healthcare professional students."
— *Doody's Health Sciences Book Reviews, Nov '97*

Health Reference Series Cumulative Index 1999

A Comprehensive Index to the Individual Volumes of the Health Reference Series, Including a Subject Index, Name Index, Organization Index, and Publication Index

Along with a Master List of Acronyms and Abbreviations

Edited by Edward J. Prucha, Anne Holmes, and Robert Rudnick. 990 pages. 2000. 0-7808-0382-5. $78.

"This volume will be most helpful in libraries that have a relatively complete collection of the Health Reference Series." — *American Reference Books Annual, 2001*

"Essential for collections that hold any of the numerous *Health Reference Series* titles."
— *Choice, Association of College and Research Libraries, Nov '00*

Healthy Aging Sourcebook

Basic Consumer Health Information about Maintaining Health through the Aging Process, Including Advice on Nutrition, Exercise, and Sleep, Help in Making Decisions about Midlife Issues and Retirement, and Guidance Concerning Practical and Informed Choices in Health Consumerism

Along with Data Concerning the Theories of Aging, Different Experiences in Aging by Minority Groups, and Facts about Aging Now and Aging in the Future; and Featuring a Glossary, a Guide to Consumer Help, Additional Suggested Reading, and Practical Resource Directory

Edited by Jenifer Swanson. 536 pages. 1999. 0-7808-0390-6. $78.

"Recommended reference source."
— *Booklist, American Library Association, Feb '00*

SEE ALSO Physical & Mental Issues in Aging Sourcebook

Healthy Heart Sourcebook for Women

Basic Consumer Health Information about Cardiac Issues Specific to Women, Including Facts about Major Risk Factors and Prevention, Treatment and Control Strategies, and Important Dietary Issues

Along with a Special Section Regarding the Pros and Cons of Hormone Replacement Therapy and Its Impact on Heart Health, and Additional Help, Including Recipes, a Glossary, and a Directory of Resources

Edited by Dawn D. Matthews. 336 pages. 2000. 0-7808-0329-9. $78.

"A good reference source and recommended for all public, academic, medical, and hospital libraries."
— *Medical Reference Services Quarterly, Summer '01*

"Because of the lack of information specific to women on this topic, this book is recommended for public libraries and consumer libraries."
—*American Reference Books Annual, 2001*

"Contains very important information about coronary artery disease that all women should know. The information is current and presented in an easy-to-read format. The book will make a good addition to any library." — *American Medical Writers Association Journal, Summer '00*

"Important, basic reference."
— *Reviewer's Bookwatch, Jul '00*

SEE ALSO Cardiovascular Diseases & Disorders Sourcebook, 1st Edition, Heart Diseases & Disorders Sourcebook, 2nd Edition, Women's Health Concerns Sourcebook

Heart Diseases & Disorders Sourcebook, 2nd Edition

Basic Consumer Health Information about Heart Attacks, Angina, Rhythm Disorders, Heart Failure, Valve Disease, Congenital Heart Disorders, and More, Including Descriptions of Surgical Procedures and Other Interventions, Medications, Cardiac Rehabilitation, Risk Identification, and Prevention Tips

Along with Statistical Data, Reports on Current Research Initiatives, a Glossary of Cardiovascular Terms, and Resource Directory

Edited by Karen Bellenir. 612 pages. 2000. 0-7808-0238-1. $78.

"This work stands out as an imminently accessible resource for the general public. It is recommended for the reference and circulating shelves of school, public, and academic libraries."
—*American Reference Books Annual, 2001*

"Recommended reference source."
—*Booklist, American Library Association, Dec '00*

"Provides comprehensive coverage of matters related to the heart. This title is recommended for health sciences and public libraries with consumer health collections."
— *E-Streams, Oct '00*

SEE ALSO Cardiovascular Diseases & Disorders Sourcebook, 1st Edition; Healthy Heart Sourcebook for Women

Household Safety Sourcebook

Basic Consumer Health Information about Household Safety, Including Information about Poisons, Chemicals, Fire, and Water Hazards in the Home

Along with Advice about the Safe Use of Home Maintenance Equipment, Choosing Toys and Nursery Furniture, Holiday and Recreation Safety, a Glossary, and Resources for Further Help and Information

Edited by Dawn D. Matthews. 606 pages. 2002. 0-7808-0338-8. $78.

"As a sourcebook on household safety this book meets its mark. It is encyclopedic in scope and covers a wide range of safety issues that are commonly seen in the home." — *E-Streams, Jul '02*

Immune System Disorders Sourcebook

Basic Information about Lupus, Multiple Sclerosis, Guillain-Barré Syndrome, Chronic Granulomatous Disease, and More

Along with Statistical and Demographic Data and Reports on Current Research Initiatives

Edited by Allan R. Cook. 608 pages. 1997. 0-7808-0209-8. $78.

Infant & Toddler Health Sourcebook

Basic Consumer Health Information about the Physical and Mental Development of Newborns, Infants, and Toddlers, Including Neonatal Concerns, Nutrition Recommendations, Immunization Schedules, Common Pediatric Disorders, Assessments and Milestones, Safety Tips, and Advice for Parents and Other Caregivers

Along with a Glossary of Terms and Resource Listings for Additional Help

Edited by Jenifer Swanson. 585 pages. 2000. 0-7808-0246-2. $78.

"As a reference for the general public, this would be useful in any library." — *E-Streams, May '01*

"Recommended reference source."
— *Booklist, American Library Association, Feb '01*

"This is a good source for general use."
—*American Reference Books Annual, 2001*

Injury & Trauma Sourcebook

Basic Consumer Health Information about the Impact of Injury, the Diagnosis and Treatment of Common and Traumatic Injuries, Emergency Care, and Specific Injuries Related to Home, Community, Workplace, Transportation, and Recreation

Along with Guidelines for Injury Prevention, a Glossary, and a Directory of Additional Resources

Edited by Joyce Brennfleck Shannon. 696 pages. 2002. 0-7808-0421-X. $78.

"Practitioners should be aware of guides such as this in order to facilitate their use by patients and their families."
— *Doody's Health Sciences Book Review Journal, Sep-Oct '02*

"Recommended reference source."
— *Booklist, American Library Association, Sep '02*

"Highly recommended for academic and medical reference collections."
— *Library Bookwatch, Sep '02*

■

Kidney & Urinary Tract Diseases & Disorders Sourcebook

Basic Information about Kidney Stones, Urinary Incontinence, Bladder Disease, End Stage Renal Disease, Dialysis, and More

Along with Statistical and Demographic Data and Reports on Current Research Initiatives

Edited by Linda M. Ross. 602 pages. 1997. 0-7808-0079-6. $78.

■

Learning Disabilities Sourcebook, 1st Edition

Basic Information about Disorders Such as Dyslexia, Visual and Auditory Processing Deficits, Attention Deficit/Hyperactivity Disorder, and Autism

Along with Statistical and Demographic Data, Reports on Current Research Initiatives, an Explanation of the Assessment Process, and a Special Section for Adults with Learning Disabilities

Edited by Linda M. Shin. 579 pages. 1998. 0-7808-0210-1. $78.

Named "Outstanding Reference Book of 1999."
— *New York Public Library, Feb 2000*

"An excellent candidate for inclusion in a public library reference section. It's a great source of information. Teachers will also find the book useful. Definitely worth reading."
— *Journal of Adolescent & Adult Literacy, Feb 2000*

"Readable . . . provides a solid base of information regarding successful techniques used with individuals who have learning disabilities, as well as practical suggestions for educators and family members. Clear language, concise descriptions, and pertinent information for contacting multiple resources add to the strength of this book as a useful tool."
— *Choice, Association of College and Research Libraries, Feb '99*

"Recommended reference source."
— *Booklist, American Library Association, Sep '98*

"A useful resource for libraries and for those who don't have the time to identify and locate the individual publications."
— *Disability Resources Monthly, Sep '98*

Learning Disabilities Sourcebook, 2nd Edition

Basic Consumer Health Information about Learning Disabilities, Including Dyslexia, Developmental Speech and Language Disabilities, Non-Verbal Learning Disorders, Developmental Arithmetic Disorder, Developmental Writing Disorder, and Other Conditions That Impede Learning Such as Attention Deficit/ Hyperactivity Disorder, Brain Injury, Hearing Impairment, Klinefelter Syndrome, Dyspraxia, and Tourette Syndrome

Along with Facts about Educational Issues and Assistive Technology, Coping Strategies, a Glossary of Related Terms, and Resources for Further Help and Information

Edited by Dawn D. Matthews. 621 pages. 2003. 0-7808-0626-3. $78.

■

Liver Disorders Sourcebook

Basic Consumer Health Information about the Liver and How It Works; Liver Diseases, Including Cancer, Cirrhosis, Hepatitis, and Toxic and Drug Related Diseases; Tips for Maintaining a Healthy Liver; Laboratory Tests, Radiology Tests, and Facts about Liver Transplantation

Along with a Section on Support Groups, a Glossary, and Resource Listings

Edited by Joyce Brennfleck Shannon. 591 pages. 2000. 0-7808-0383-3. $78.

"A valuable resource."
— *American Reference Books Annual, 2001*

"This title is recommended for health sciences and public libraries with consumer health collections."
— *E-Streams, Oct '00*

"Recommended reference source."
— *Booklist, American Library Association, Jun '00*

■

Lung Disorders Sourcebook

Basic Consumer Health Information about Emphysema, Pneumonia, Tuberculosis, Asthma, Cystic Fibrosis, and Other Lung Disorders, Including Facts about Diagnostic Procedures, Treatment Strategies, Disease Prevention Efforts, and Such Risk Factors as Smoking, Air Pollution, and Exposure to Asbestos, Radon, and Other Agents

Along with a Glossary and Resources for Additional Help and Information

Edited by Dawn D. Matthews. 678 pages. 2002. 0-7808-0339-6. $78.

"Highly recommended for academic and medical reference collections."
— *Library Bookwatch, Sep '02*
[Pain SB, 2nd ed.]

"A source of valuable information. . . . This book offers help to nonmedical people who need information about pain and pain management. It is also an excellent reference for those who participate in patient education."
— *Doody's Review Service, Sep '02*

■

Medical Tests Sourcebook

Basic Consumer Health Information about Medical Tests, Including Periodic Health Exams, General Screening Tests, Tests You Can Do at Home, Findings of the U.S. Preventive Services Task Force, X-ray and Radiology Tests, Electrical Tests, Tests of Blood and Other Body Fluids and Tissues, Scope Tests, Lung Tests, Genetic Tests, Pregnancy Tests, Newborn Screening Tests, Sexually Transmitted Disease Tests, and Computer Aided Diagnoses

Along with a Section on Paying for Medical Tests, a Glossary, and Resource Listings

Edited by Joyce Brennfleck Shannon. 691 pages. 1999. 0-7808-0243-8. $78.

■

Men's Health Concerns Sourcebook

Basic Information about Health Issues That Affect Men, Featuring Facts about the Top Causes of Death in Men, Including Heart Disease, Stroke, Cancers, Prostate Disorders, Chronic Obstructive Pulmonary Disease, Pneumonia and Influenza, Human Immunodeficiency Virus and Acquired Immune Deficiency Syndrome, Diabetes Mellitus, Stress, Suicide, Accidents and Homicides; and Facts about Common Concerns for Men, Including Impotence, Contraception, Circumcision, Sleep Disorders, Snoring, Hair Loss, Diet, Nutrition, Exercise, Kidney and Urological Disorders, and Backaches

Edited by Allan R. Cook. 738 pages. 1998. 0-7808-0212-8. $78.

■

Mental Health Disorders Sourcebook, 1st Edition

Basic Information about Schizophrenia, Depression, Bipolar Disorder, Panic Disorder, Obsessive-Compulsive Disorder, Phobias and Other Anxiety Disorders, Paranoia and Other Personality Disorders, Eating Disorders, and Sleep Disorders

Along with Information about Treatment and Therapies

Edited by Karen Bellenir. 548 pages. 1995. 0-7808-0040-0. $78.

■

Mental Health Disorders Sourcebook, 2nd Edition

Basic Consumer Health Information about Anxiety Disorders, Depression and Other Mood Disorders, Eating Disorders, Personality Disorders, Schizophrenia, and More, Including Disease Descriptions, Treatment Options, and Reports on Current Research Initiatives

Along with Statistical Data, Tips for Maintaining Mental Health, a Glossary, and Directory of Sources for Additional Help and Information

Edited by Karen Bellenir. 605 pages. 2000. 0-7808-0240-3. $78.

■

Mental Retardation Sourcebook

Basic Consumer Health Information about Mental Retardation and Its Causes, Including Down Syndrome, Fetal Alcohol Syndrome, Fragile X Syndrome, Genetic Conditions, Injury, and Environmental Sources

Along with Preventive Strategies, Parenting Issues, Educational Implications, Health Care Needs, Employment and Economic Matters, Legal Issues, a Glossary, and a Resource Listing for Additional Help and Information

Edited by Joyce Brennfleck Shannon. 642 pages. 2000. 0-7808-0377-9. $78.

"Public libraries will find the book useful for reference and as a beginning research point for students, parents, and caregivers."
—American Reference Books Annual, 2001

"The strength of this work is that it compiles many basic fact sheets and addresses for further information in one volume. It is intended and suitable for the general public. This sourcebook is relevant to any collection providing health information to the general public."
—E-Streams, Nov '00

"From preventing retardation to parenting and family challenges, this covers health, social and legal issues and will prove an invaluable overview."
—Reviewer's Bookwatch, Jul '00

Movement Disorders Sourcebook

Basic Consumer Health Information about Neurological Movement Disorders, Including Essential Tremor, Parkinson's Disease, Dystonia, Cerebral Palsy, Huntington's Disease, Myasthenia Gravis, Multiple Sclerosis, and Other Early-Onset and Adult-Onset Movement Disorders, Their Symptoms and Causes, Diagnostic Tests, and Treatments

Along with Mobility and Assistive Technology Information, a Glossary, and a Directory of Additional Resources

Edited by Joyce Brennfleck Shannon. 655 pages. 2003. 0-7808-0628-X. $78.

Obesity Sourcebook

Basic Consumer Health Information about Diseases and Other Problems Associated with Obesity, and Including Facts about Risk Factors, Prevention Issues, and Management Approaches

Along with Statistical and Demographic Data, Information about Special Populations, Research Updates, a Glossary, and Source Listings for Further Help and Information

Edited by Wilma Caldwell and Chad T. Kimball. 376 pages. 2001. 0-7808-0333-7. $78.

"The book synthesizes the reliable medical literature on obesity into one easy-to-read and useful resource for the general public."
—American Reference Books Annual 2002

"This is a very useful resource book for the lay public."
—Doody's Review Service, Nov '01

"Well suited for the health reference collection of a public library or an academic health science library that serves the general population." *—E-Streams, Sep '01*

"Recommended reference source."
—Booklist, American Library Association, Apr '01

" Recommended pick both for specialty health library collections and any general consumer health reference collection." *— The Bookwatch, Apr '01*

Ophthalmic Disorders Sourcebook

Basic Information about Glaucoma, Cataracts, Macular Degeneration, Strabismus, Refractive Disorders, and More

Along with Statistical and Demographic Data and Reports on Current Research Initiatives

Edited by Linda M. Ross. 631 pages. 1996. 0-7808-0081-8. $78.

SEE ALSO *Eye Care Sourcebook, 2nd Edition*

Oral Health Sourcebook

Basic Information about Diseases and Conditions Affecting Oral Health, Including Cavities, Gum Disease, Dry Mouth, Oral Cancers, Fever Blisters, Canker Sores, Oral Thrush, Bad Breath, Temporomandibular Disorders, and other Craniofacial Syndromes

Along with Statistical Data on the Oral Health of Americans, Oral Hygiene, Emergency First Aid, Information on Treatment Procedures and Methods of Replacing Lost Teeth

Edited by Allan R. Cook. 558 pages. 1997. 0-7808-0082-6. $78.

"Unique source which will fill a gap in dental sources for patients and the lay public. A valuable reference tool even in a library with thousands of books on dentistry. Comprehensive, clear, inexpensive, and easy to read and use. It fills an enormous gap in the health care literature." *— Reference and User Services Quarterly, American Library Association, Summer '98*

"Recommended reference source."
—Booklist, American Library Association, Dec '97

Osteoporosis Sourcebook

Basic Consumer Health Information about Primary and Secondary Osteoporosis and Juvenile Osteoporosis and Related Conditions, Including Fibrous Dysplasia, Gaucher Disease, Hyperthyroidism, Hypophosphatasia, Myeloma, Osteopetrosis, Osteogenesis Imperfecta, and Paget's Disease

Along with Information about Risk Factors, Treatments, Traditional and Non-Traditional Pain Management, a Glossary of Related Terms, and a Directory of Resources

Edited by Allan R. Cook. 584 pages. 2001. 0-7808-0239-X. $78.

"This would be a book to be kept in a staff or patient library. The targeted audience is the layperson, but the therapist who needs a quick bit of information on a particular topic will also find the book useful."
—Physical Therapy, Jan '02

"This resource is recommended as a great reference source for public, health, and academic libraries, and is another triumph for the editors of Omnigraphics."
—American Reference Books Annual 2002

"Recommended for all public libraries and general health collections, especially those supporting patient education or consumer health programs."
— *E-Streams, Nov '01*

"Will prove valuable to any library seeking to maintain a current, comprehensive reference collection of health resources. . . . From prevention to treatment and associated conditions, this provides an excellent survey."
— *The Bookwatch, Aug '01*

"Recommended reference source."
— *Booklist, American Library Association, July '01*

SEE ALSO Women's Health Concerns Sourcebook

Pain Sourcebook, 1st Edition

Basic Information about Specific Forms of Acute and Chronic Pain, Including Headaches, Back Pain, Muscular Pain, Neuralgia, Surgical Pain, and Cancer Pain

Along with Pain Relief Options Such as Analgesics, Narcotics, Nerve Blocks, Transcutaneous Nerve Stimulation, and Alternative Forms of Pain Control, Including Biofeedback, Imaging, Behavior Modification, and Relaxation Techniques

Edited by Allan R. Cook. 667 pages. 1997. 0-7808-0213-6. $78.

"The text is readable, easily understood, and well indexed. This excellent volume belongs in all patient education libraries, consumer health sections of public libraries, and many personal collections."
— *American Reference Books Annual, 1999*

"A beneficial reference." — *Booklist Health Sciences Supplement, American Library Association, Oct '98*

"The information is basic in terms of scholarship and is appropriate for general readers. Written in journalistic style . . . intended for non-professionals. Quite thorough in its coverage of different pain conditions and summarizes the latest clinical information regarding pain treatment." — *Choice, Association of College and Research Libraries, Jun '98*

"Recommended reference source."
— *Booklist, American Library Association, Mar '98*

Pain Sourcebook, 2nd Edition

Basic Consumer Health Information about Specific Forms of Acute and Chronic Pain, Including Muscle and Skeletal Pain, Nerve Pain, Cancer Pain, and Disorders Characterized by Pain, Such as Fibromyalgia, Shingles, Angina, Arthritis, and Headaches

Along with Information about Pain Medications and Management Techniques, Complementary and Alternative Pain Relief Options, Tips for People Living with Chronic Pain, a Glossary, and a Directory of Sources for Further Information

Edited by Karen Bellenir. 670 pages. 2002. 0-7808-0612-3. $78.

Pediatric Cancer Sourcebook

Basic Consumer Health Information about Leukemias, Brain Tumors, Sarcomas, Lymphomas, and Other Cancers in Infants, Children, and Adolescents, Including Descriptions of Cancers, Treatments, and Coping Strategies

Along with Suggestions for Parents, Caregivers, and Concerned Relatives, a Glossary of Cancer Terms, and Resource Listings

Edited by Edward J. Prucha. 587 pages. 1999. 0-7808-0245-4. $78.

"An excellent source of information. Recommended for public, hospital, and health science libraries with consumer health collections." — *E-Streams, Jun '00*

"Recommended reference source."
— *Booklist, American Library Association, Feb '00*

"A valuable addition to all libraries specializing in health services and many public libraries."
— *American Reference Books Annual, 2000*

Physical & Mental Issues in Aging Sourcebook

Basic Consumer Health Information on Physical and Mental Disorders Associated with the Aging Process, Including Concerns about Cardiovascular Disease, Pulmonary Disease, Oral Health, Digestive Disorders, Musculoskeletal and Skin Disorders, Metabolic Changes, Sexual and Reproductive Issues, and Changes in Vision, Hearing, and Other Senses

Along with Data about Longevity and Causes of Death, Information on Acute and Chronic Pain, Descriptions of Mental Concerns, a Glossary of Terms, and Resource Listings for Additional Help

Edited by Jenifer Swanson. 660 pages. 1999. 0-7808-0233-0. $78.

"This is a treasure of health information for the layperson." — *Choice Health Sciences Supplement, Association of College & Research Libraries, May 2000*

"Recommended for public libraries."
— *American Reference Books Annual, 2000*

"Recommended reference source."
— *Booklist, American Library Association, Oct '99*

SEE ALSO Healthy Aging Sourcebook

Podiatry Sourcebook

Basic Consumer Health Information about Foot Conditions, Diseases, and Injuries, Including Bunions, Corns, Calluses, Athlete's Foot, Plantar Warts, Hammertoes and Clawtoes, Clubfoot, Heel Pain, Gout, and More

Along with Facts about Foot Care, Disease Prevention, Foot Safety, Choosing a Foot Care Specialist, a Glossary of Terms, and Resource Listings for Additional Information

Edited by M. Lisa Weatherford. 380 pages. 2001. 0-7808-0215-2. $78.

"Recommended reference source."
— *Booklist, American Library Association, Feb '02*

"There is a lot of information presented here on a topic that is usually only covered sparingly in most larger comprehensive medical encyclopedias."
— *American Reference Books Annual 2002*

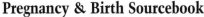

Pregnancy & Birth Sourcebook

Basic Information about Planning for Pregnancy, Maternal Health, Fetal Growth and Development, Labor and Delivery, Postpartum and Perinatal Care, Pregnancy in Mothers with Special Concerns, and Disorders of Pregnancy, Including Genetic Counseling, Nutrition and Exercise, Obstetrical Tests, Pregnancy Discomfort, Multiple Births, Cesarean Sections, Medical Testing of Newborns, Breastfeeding, Gestational Diabetes, and Ectopic Pregnancy

Edited by Heather E. Aldred. 737 pages. 1997. 0-7808-0216-0. $78.

"A well-organized handbook. Recommended."
— *Choice, Association of College and Research Libraries, Apr '98*

"Recommended reference source."
— *Booklist, American Library Association, Mar '98*

"Recommended for public libraries."
— *American Reference Books Annual, 1998*

SEE ALSO *Congenital Disorders Sourcebook, Family Planning Sourcebook*

Prostate Cancer Sourcebook

Basic Consumer Health Information about Prostate Cancer, Including Information about the Associated Risk Factors, Detection, Diagnosis, and Treatment of Prostate Cancer

Along with Information on Non-Malignant Prostate Conditions, and Featuring a Section Listing Support and Treatment Centers and a Glossary of Related Terms

Edited by Dawn D. Matthews. 358 pages. 2001. 0-7808-0324-8. $78.

"Recommended reference source."
— *Booklist, American Library Association, Jan '02*

"A valuable resource for health care consumers seeking information on the subject. . . .All text is written in a clear, easy-to-understand language that avoids technical jargon. Any library that collects consumer health resources would strengthen their collection with the addition of the *Prostate Cancer Sourcebook*."
— *American Reference Books Annual 2002*

Public Health Sourcebook

Basic Information about Government Health Agencies, Including National Health Statistics and Trends, Healthy People 2000 Program Goals and Objectives, the Centers for Disease Control and Prevention, the Food and Drug Administration, and the National Institutes of Health

Along with Full Contact Information for Each Agency

Edited by Wendy Wilcox. 698 pages. 1998. 0-7808-0220-9. $78.

"Recommended reference source."
— *Booklist, American Library Association, Sep '98*

"This consumer guide provides welcome assistance in navigating the maze of federal health agencies and their data on public health concerns."
— *SciTech Book News, Sep '98*

Reconstructive & Cosmetic Surgery Sourcebook

Basic Consumer Health Information on Cosmetic and Reconstructive Plastic Surgery, Including Statistical Information about Different Surgical Procedures, Things to Consider Prior to Surgery, Plastic Surgery Techniques and Tools, Emotional and Psychological Considerations, and Procedure-Specific Information

Along with a Glossary of Terms and a Listing of Resources for Additional Help and Information

Edited by M. Lisa Weatherford. 374 pages. 2001. 0-7808-0214-4. $78.

"An excellent reference that addresses cosmetic and medically necessary reconstructive surgeries. . . . The style of the prose is calm and reassuring, discussing the many positive outcomes now available due to advances in surgical techniques."
— *American Reference Books Annual 2002*

"Recommended for health science libraries that are open to the public, as well as hospital libraries that are open to the patients. This book is a good resource for the consumer interested in plastic surgery."
— *E-Streams, Dec '01*

"Recommended reference source."
— *Booklist, American Library Association, July '01*

Rehabilitation Sourcebook

Basic Consumer Health Information about Rehabilitation for People Recovering from Heart Surgery, Spinal Cord Injury, Stroke, Orthopedic Impairments, Amputation, Pulmonary Impairments, Traumatic Injury, and More, Including Physical Therapy, Occupational Therapy, Speech/ Language Therapy, Massage Therapy, Dance Therapy, Art Therapy, and Recreational Therapy

Along with Information on Assistive and Adaptive Devices, a Glossary, and Resources for Additional Help and Information

Edited by Dawn D. Matthews. 531 pages. 1999. 0-7808-0236-5. $78.

"This is an excellent resource for public library reference and health collections."
— *American Reference Books Annual, 2001*

"Recommended reference source."
— *Booklist, American Library Association, May '00*

Respiratory Diseases & Disorders Sourcebook

Basic Information about Respiratory Diseases and Disorders, Including Asthma, Cystic Fibrosis, Pneumonia, the Common Cold, Influenza, and Others, Featuring Facts about the Respiratory System, Statistical and Demographic Data, Treatments, Self-Help Management Suggestions, and Current Research Initiatives

Edited by Allan R. Cook and Peter D. Dresser. 771 pages. 1995. 0-7808-0037-0. $78.

"Designed for the layperson and for patients and their families coping with respiratory illness. . . . an extensive array of information on diagnosis, treatment, management, and prevention of respiratory illnesses for the general reader." — *Choice, Association of College and Research Libraries, Jun '96*

"A highly recommended text for all collections. It is a comforting reminder of the power of knowledge that good books carry between their covers." — *Academic Library Book Review, Spring '96*

"A comprehensive collection of authoritative information presented in a nontechnical, humanitarian style for patients, families, and caregivers." — *Association of Operating Room Nurses, Sep/Oct '95*

■

Sexually Transmitted Diseases Sourcebook, 1st Edition

Basic Information about Herpes, Chlamydia, Gonorrhea, Hepatitis, Nongonoccocal Urethritis, Pelvic Inflammatory Disease, Syphilis, AIDS, and More

Along with Current Data on Treatments and Preventions

Edited by Linda M. Ross. 550 pages. 1997. 0-7808-0217-9. $78.

■

Sexually Transmitted Diseases Sourcebook, 2nd Edition

Basic Consumer Health Information about Sexually Transmitted Diseases, Including Information on the Diagnosis and Treatment of Chlamydia, Gonorrhea, Hepatitis, Herpes, HIV, Mononucleosis, Syphilis, and Others

Along with Information on Prevention, Such as Condom Use, Vaccines, and STD Education; And Featuring a Section on Issues Related to Youth and Adolescents, a Glossary, and Resources for Additional Help and Information

Edited by Dawn D. Matthews. 538 pages. 2001. 0-7808-0249-7. $78.

"Recommended for consumer health collections in public libraries, and secondary school and community college libraries." — *American Reference Books Annual 2002*

"Every school and public library should have a copy of this comprehensive and user-friendly reference book." — *Choice, Association of College & Research Libraries, Sep '01*

"This is a highly recommended book. This is an especially important book for all school and public libraries." — *AIDS Book Review Journal, Jul-Aug '01*

"Recommended reference source." — *Booklist, American Library Association, Apr '01*

"Recommended pick both for specialty health library collections and any general consumer health reference collection." — *The Bookwatch, Apr '01*

■

Skin Disorders Sourcebook

Basic Information about Common Skin and Scalp Conditions Caused by Aging, Allergies, Immune Reactions, Sun Exposure, Infectious Organisms, Parasites, Cosmetics, and Skin Traumas, Including Abrasions, Cuts, and Pressure Sores

Along with Information on Prevention and Treatment

Edited by Allan R. Cook. 647 pages. 1997. 0-7808-0080-X. $78.

". . . comprehensive, easily read reference book." — *Doody's Health Sciences Book Reviews, Oct '97*

SEE ALSO Burns Sourcebook

■

Sleep Disorders Sourcebook

Basic Consumer Health Information about Sleep and Its Disorders, Including Insomnia, Sleepwalking, Sleep Apnea, Restless Leg Syndrome, and Narcolepsy

Along with Data about Shiftwork and Its Effects, Information on the Societal Costs of Sleep Deprivation, Descriptions of Treatment Options, a Glossary of Terms, and Resource Listings for Additional Help

Edited by Jenifer Swanson. 439 pages. 1998. 0-7808-0234-9. $78.

"This text will complement any home or medical library. It is user-friendly and ideal for the adult reader." — *American Reference Books Annual, 2000*

"A useful resource that provides accurate, relevant, and accessible information on sleep to the general public. Health care providers who deal with sleep disorders patients may also find it helpful in being prepared to answer some of the questions patients ask." — *Respiratory Care, Jul '99*

"Recommended reference source." — *Booklist, American Library Association, Feb '99*

■

Sports Injuries Sourcebook, 1st Edition

Basic Consumer Health Information about Common Sports Injuries, Prevention of Injury in Specific Sports, Tips for Training, and Rehabilitation from Injury

Along with Information about Special Concerns for Children, Young Girls in Athletic Training Programs, Senior Athletes, and Women Athletes, and a Directory of Resources for Further Help and Information

Edited by Heather E. Aldred. 624 pages. 1999. 0-7808-0218-7. $78.

"While this easy-to-read book is recommended for all libraries, it should prove to be especially useful for public, high school, and academic libraries; certainly it should be on the bookshelf of every school gymnasium." —E-Streams, Mar '00

"Public libraries and undergraduate academic libraries will find this book useful for its nontechnical language." —American Reference Books Annual, 2000

■

Sports Injuries Sourcebook, 2nd Edition

Basic Consumer Health Information about the Diagnosis, Treatment, and Rehabilitation of Common Sports-Related Injuries in Children and Adults

Along with Suggestions for Conditioning and Training, Information and Prevention Tips for Injuries Frequently Associated with Specific Sports and Special Populations, a Glossary, and a Directory of Additional Resources

Edited by Joyce Brennfleck Shannon. 614 pages. 2002. 0-7808-0604-2. $78.

■

Stress-Related Disorders Sourcebook

Basic Consumer Health Information about Stress and Stress-Related Disorders, Including Stress Origins and Signals, Environmental Stress at Work and Home, Mental and Emotional Stress Associated with Depression, Post-Traumatic Stress Disorder, Panic Disorder, Suicide, and the Physical Effects of Stress on the Cardiovascular, Immune, and Nervous Systems

Along with Stress Management Techniques, a Glossary, and a Listing of Additional Resources

Edited by Joyce Brennfleck Shannon. 610 pages. 2002. 0-7808-0560-7. $78.

"I am impressed by the amount of information. It offers a thorough overview of the causes and consequences of stress for the layperson. . . . A well-done and thorough reference guide for professionals and nonprofessionals alike." —Doody's Review Service, Dec '02

■

Substance Abuse Sourcebook

Basic Health-Related Information about the Abuse of Legal and Illegal Substances Such as Alcohol, Tobacco, Prescription Drugs, Marijuana, Cocaine, and Heroin; and Including Facts about Substance Abuse Prevention Strategies, Intervention Methods, Treatment and Recovery Programs, and a Section Addressing the Special Problems Related to Substance Abuse during Pregnancy

Edited by Karen Bellenir. 573 pages. 1996. 0-7808-0038-9. $78.

"A valuable addition to any health reference section. Highly recommended." —The Book Report, Mar/Apr '97

". . . a comprehensive collection of substance abuse information that's both highly readable and compact. Families and caregivers of substance abusers will find the information enlightening and helpful, while teachers, social workers and journalists should benefit from the concise format. Recommended." —Drug Abuse Update, Winter '96/'97

SEE ALSO *Alcoholism Sourcebook, Drug Abuse Sourcebook*

■

Surgery Sourcebook

Basic Consumer Health Information about Inpatient and Outpatient Surgeries, Including Cardiac, Vascular, Orthopedic, Ocular, Reconstructive, Cosmetic, Gynecologic, and Ear, Nose, and Throat Procedures and More

Along with Information about Operating Room Policies and Instruments, Laser Surgery Techniques, Hospital Errors, Statistical Data, a Glossary, and Listings of Sources for Further Help and Information

Edited by Annemarie S. Muth and Karen Bellenir. 596 pages. 2002. 0-7808-0380-9. $78.

■

Transplantation Sourcebook

Basic Consumer Health Information about Organ and Tissue Transplantation, Including Physical and Financial Preparations, Procedures and Issues Relating to Specific Solid Organ and Tissue Transplants, Rehabilitation, Pediatric Transplant Information, the Future of Transplantation, and Organ and Tissue Donation

Along with a Glossary and Listings of Additional Resources

Edited by Joyce Brennfleck Shannon. 628 pages. 2002. 0-7808-0322-1. $78.

"Recommended for libraries with an interest in offering consumer health information." —E-Streams, Jul '02

"This is a unique and valuable resource for patients facing transplantation and their families." —Doody's Review Service, Jun '02

■

Traveler's Health Sourcebook

Basic Consumer Health Information for Travelers, Including Physical and Medical Preparations, Transportation Health and Safety, Essential Information about Food and Water, Sun Exposure, Insect and Snake Bites, Camping and Wilderness Medicine, and Travel with Physical or Medical Disabilities

Along with International Travel Tips, Vaccination Recommendations, Geographical Health Issues, Disease Risks, a Glossary, and a Listing of Additional Resources

Edited by Joyce Brennfleck Shannon. 613 pages. 2000. 0-7808-0384-1. $78.

Vegetarian Sourcebook

Basic Consumer Health Information about Vegetarian Diets, Lifestyle, and Philosophy, Including Definitions of Vegetarianism and Veganism, Tips about Adopting Vegetarianism, Creating a Vegetarian Pantry, and Meeting Nutritional Needs of Vegetarians, with Facts Regarding Vegetarianism's Effect on Pregnant and Lactating Women, Children, Athletes, and Senior Citizens

Along with a Glossary of Commonly Used Vegetarian Terms and Resources for Additional Help and Information

Edited by Chad T. Kimball. 360 pages. 2002. 0-7808-0439-2. $78.

Women's Health Concerns Sourcebook

Basic Information about Health Issues That Affect Women, Featuring Facts about Menstruation and Other Gynecological Concerns, Including Endometriosis, Fibroids, Menopause, and Vaginitis; Reproductive Concerns, Including Birth Control, Infertility, and Abortion; and Facts about Additional Physical, Emotional, and Mental Health Concerns Prevalent among Women Such as Osteoporosis, Urinary Tract Disorders, Eating Disorders, and Depression

Along with Tips for Maintaining a Healthy Lifestyle

Edited by Heather E. Aldred. 567 pages. 1997. 0-7808-0219-5. $78.

SEE ALSO Breast Cancer Sourcebook, Cancer Sourcebook for Women, 1st and 2nd Editions, Healthy Heart Sourcebook for Women, Osteoporosis Sourcebook

Workplace Health & Safety Sourcebook

Basic Consumer Health Information about Workplace Health and Safety, Including the Effect of Workplace Hazards on the Lungs, Skin, Heart, Ears, Eyes, Brain, Reproductive Organs, Musculoskeletal System, and Other Organs and Body Parts

Along with Information about Occupational Cancer, Personal Protective Equipment, Toxic and Hazardous Chemicals, Child Labor, Stress, and Workplace Violence

Edited by Chad T. Kimball. 626 pages. 2000. 0-7808-0231-4. $78.

Worldwide Health Sourcebook

Basic Information about Global Health Issues, Including Malnutrition, Reproductive Health, Disease Dispersion and Prevention, Emerging Diseases, Risky Health Behaviors, and the Leading Causes of Death

Along with Global Health Concerns for Children, Women, and the Elderly, Mental Health Issues, Research and Technology Advancements, and Economic, Environmental, and Political Health Implications, a Glossary, and a Resource Listing for Additional Help and Information

Edited by Joyce Brennfleck Shannon. 614 pages. 2001. 0-7808-0330-2. $78.

Teen Health Series

Helping Young Adults Understand, Manage, and Avoid Serious Illness

Diet Information for Teens
Health Tips about Diet and Nutrition

Including Facts about Nutrients, Dietary Guidelines, Breakfasts, School Lunches, Snacks, Party Food, Weight Control, Eating Disorders, and More

Edited by Karen Bellenir. 399 pages. 2001. 0-7808-0441-4. $58.

"Full of helpful insights and facts throughout the book. ... An excellent resource to be placed in public libraries or even in personal collections."
— *American Reference Books Annual 2002*

"Recommended for middle and high school libraries and media centers as well as academic libraries that educate future teachers of teenagers. It is also a suitable addition to health science libraries that serve patrons who are interested in teen health promotion and education." — *E-Streams, Oct '01*

"This comprehensive book would be beneficial to collections that need information about nutrition, dietary guidelines, meal planning, and weight control. ... This reference is so easy to use that its purchase is recommended." — *The Book Report, Sep-Oct '01*

"This book is written in an easy to understand format describing issues that many teens face every day, and then provides thoughtful explanations so that teens can make informed decisions. This is an interesting book that provides important facts and information for today's teens." — *Doody's Health Sciences Book Review Journal, Jul-Aug '01*

"A comprehensive compendium of diet and nutrition. The information is presented in a straightforward, plain-spoken manner. This title will be useful to those working on reports on a variety of topics, as well as to general readers concerned about their dietary health."
— *School Library Journal, Jun '01*

Drug Information for Teens
Health Tips about the Physical and Mental Effects of Substance Abuse

Including Facts about Alcohol, Anabolic Steroids, Club Drugs, Cocaine, Depressants, Hallucinogens, Herbal Products, Inhalants, Marijuana, Narcotics, Stimulants, Tobacco, and More

Edited by Karen Bellenir. 452 pages. 2002. 0-7808-0444-9. $58.

Mental Health Information for Teens
Health Tips about Mental Health and Mental Illness

Including Facts about Anxiety, Depression, Suicide, Eating Disorders, Obsessive-Compulsive Disorders, Panic Attacks, Phobias, Schizophrenia, and More

Edited by Karen Bellenir. 406 pages. 2001. 0-7808-0442-2. $58.

"In both language and approach, this user-friendly entry in the *Teen Health Series* is on target for teens needing information on mental health concerns." — *Booklist, American Library Association, Jan '02*

"Readers will find the material accessible and informative, with the shaded notes, facts, and embedded glossary insets adding appropriately to the already interesting and succinct presentation."
— *School Library Journal, Jan '02*

"This title is highly recommended for any library that serves adolescents and parents/caregivers of adolescents." — *E-Streams, Jan '02*

"Recommended for high school libraries and young adult collections in public libraries. Both health professionals and teenagers will find this book useful."
— *American Reference Books Annual 2002*

"This is a nice book written to enlighten the society, primarily teenagers, about common teen mental health issues. It is highly recommended to teachers and parents as well as adolescents."
— *Doody's Review Service, Dec '01*

Sexual Health Information for Teens
Health Tips about Sexual Development, Human Reproduction, and Sexually Transmitted Diseases

Including Facts about Puberty, Reproductive Health, Chlamydia, Human Papillomavirus, Pelvic Inflammatory Disease, Herpes, AIDS, Contraception, Pregnancy, and More

Edited by Deborah A. Stanley. 400 pages. 2003. 0-7808-0445-7. $58.

Health Reference Series

Adolescent Health Sourcebook

AIDS Sourcebook, 1st Edition

AIDS Sourcebook, 2nd Edition

Alcoholism Sourcebook

Allergies Sourcebook, 1st Edition

Allergies Sourcebook, 2nd Edition

Alternative Medicine Sourcebook, 1st Edition

Alternative Medicine Sourcebook, 2nd Edition

Alzheimer's, Stroke & 29 Other Neurological Disorders Sourcebook, 1st Edition

Alzheimer's Disease Sourcebook, 2nd Edition

Arthritis Sourcebook

Asthma Sourcebook

Attention Deficit Disorder Sourcebook

Back & Neck Disorders Sourcebook

Blood & Circulatory Disorders Sourcebook

Brain Disorders Sourcebook

Breast Cancer Sourcebook

Breastfeeding Sourcebook

Burns Sourcebook

Cancer Sourcebook, 1st Edition

Cancer Sourcebook (New), 2nd Edition

Cancer Sourcebook, 3rd Edition

Cancer Sourcebook for Women, 1st Edition

Cancer Sourcebook for Women, 2nd Edition

Cardiovascular Diseases & Disorders Sourcebook, 1st Edition

Caregiving Sourcebook

Childhood Diseases & Disorders Sourcebook

Colds, Flu & Other Common Ailments Sourcebook

Communication Disorders Sourcebook

Congenital Disorders Sourcebook

Consumer Issues in Health Care Sourcebook

Contagious & Non-Contagious Infectious Diseases Sourcebook

Death & Dying Sourcebook

Depression Sourcebook

Diabetes Sourcebook, 1st Edition

Diabetes Sourcebook, 2nd Edition

Diet & Nutrition Sourcebook, 1st Edition

Diet & Nutrition Sourcebook, 2nd Edition

Digestive Diseases & Disorder Sourcebook

Disabilities Sourcebook

Domestic Violence & Child Abuse Sourcebook

Drug Abuse Sourcebook

Ear, Nose & Throat Disorders Sourcebook

Eating Disorders Sourcebook

Emergency Medical Services Sourcebook

Endocrine & Metabolic Disorders Sourcebook

Environmentally Induced Disorders Sourcebook

Ethnic Diseases Sourcebook

Eye Care Sourcebook, 2nd Edition

Family Planning Sourcebook

Fitness & Exercise Sourcebook, 1st Edition

Fitness & Exercise Sourcebook, 2nd Edition

Food & Animal Borne Diseases Sourcebook

Food Safety Sourcebook

Forensic Medicine Sourcebook